Richard J. Simonsen

Dentistry in the 21st Century
A Global Perspective

Dentistry in the 21st Century
A Global Perspective

Proceedings of the International Symposium
on Dentistry in the 21st Century, Berlin, September 10, 1989

Edited by

Richard J. Simonsen, DDS, MS

Global Professional Services Manager
Dental Products Division
3M Health Care
St. Paul, Minnesota
and
Professor, College of Dentistry
University of Minnesota
Minneapolis, Minnesota

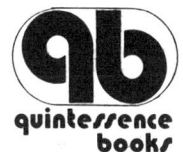

Quintessence Publishing Co, Inc
Chicago, London, Berlin, São Paulo, Hong Kong, and Tokyo

Library of Congress Cataloging-in-Publication Data

International Symposium on Dentistry in the 21st Century (1989 :
  Berlin, Germany)
    Dentistry in the 21st century : a global perspective : proceedings
  of the International Symposium on Dentistry in the 21st Century,
  Berlin, Federal Republic of Germany, September 10, 1989 / edited by
  Richard J. Simonsen.
       p. cm.
    Symposium held in conjunction with the 6th International
  Quintessence Symposium.
    Includes bibliographical references.
    ISBN 0-86715-228-1
    1. Dentistry–Congresses.   2. Dentistry–Cross-cultural studies–
  Congresses.   I. Simonsen, Richard J.   II. International
  Quintessence Symposium (6th : 1989 : Berlin, Germany)   III. Title.
  IV. Title: Dentistry in the twenty-first century.
    [DNLM: 1. Cross-Cultural Comparison–congresses.   2. Dentistry–
  trends–congresses.   WU 100 I61d 1989]
  RK21.I65 1989
  617.6–dc20
  DNLM/DLC   90-9233
  for Library of Congress   CIP

© 1991 by Quintessence Publishing Co, Inc, Chicago, Illinois.
All rights reserved.

This book or any part thereof must not be reproduced by any means or in any form without the written permission of the publisher.

Lithography: JUP, Industrie- und Presseklischee GmbH, Berlin
Composition, printing, and binding: Franz W. Wesel, Druckerei und Verlag GmbH & Co. KG, Baden-Baden

Printed in Germany

Contents

Participants				7
Preface			R. J. Simonsen	9
Chapter 1	World — Research		H. Löe	13
Chapter 2	German Democratic Republic		C. Thierfelder	25
Chapter 3	South America		P. A. M. Bastos	29
Chapter 4	Spain		J. A. Gil	39
Chapter 5	USA — Education/Practice		A. A. Dugoni	43
Chapter 6	Japan		S. Hobo	59
Chapter 7	USSR		V. K. Leontiev	71
Chapter 8	People's Republic of China		Z.-K. Zhang	85
Chapter 9	Austria		R. Slavicek	91
Chapter 10	Africa		J. Reddy	103
Chapter 11	Denmark		B. Melsen	115
Chapter 12	Canada		G. A. Zarb	121
Chapter 13	Singapore		K.-M. Yii	135
Chapter 14	United Kingdom		J. W. McLean	141
Chapter 15	Hong Kong		T. C. Wong	149
Chapter 16	Yugoslavia		M. Rode	157
Chapter 17	Switzerland		P. Schärer	165
Chapter 18	USA — Education		R. P. White	173
Chapter 19	Federal Republic of Germany — Research		H. Weber	191
Chapter 20	Scandinavia		I. A. Mjör	199
Chapter 21	Italy		M. Martignoni	207
Chapter 22	Poland		W. Józefowicz	213
Chapter 23	Federal Republic of Germany – Practice		F. Braun	221
Chapter 24	Fédération Dentaire Internationale		R. Gonzales-Giralda	235
Discussion				239

Participants

Dr Pedro Américo Machado Bastos
Av. 9 de Julho
5483 São Paulo
Brazil

Dr Frank Braun
Immermannstr. 35
D-4000 Düsseldorf 1
Federal Republic of Germany

Professor Arthur A. Dugoni
Dean, University of the Pacific
2155 Webster Street
San Francisco, CA 94115, USA

Dr Jaime A. Gil
Edificio Albia T-13
S. Vincente 8
48001 Bilbao, Spain

Dr Sumiya Hobo
Shibuya-ku
150 Tokyo
Japan

Professor Dr Wlodzimierz Józefowicz
90-202 Iodé
PL-21 Nawotki
Poland

Dr Yii Kie-Mung
P.O. Box 1140
Raffles City 9117
Singapore

Professor Valery K. Leontiev
Timur Frunze Str. 16
Moscow 119840
USSR

Dr Harald Löe
Director, NIDR
NIH Building 31, Room 2C39
Bethesda, MD 20892, USA

Professor Dr Mario Martignoni
Via Maria Adelaide, 6
I-00196 Rome
Italy

Dr John W. McLean
38 Devonshire Street
London W1N 1LD
England

Professor Dr Birte Melsen
Vennelyst Boulevard
DK-8000 Århus
Denmark

Dr Ivar A. Mjör
NIOM, Postboks 70
N-1344 Haslum
Norway

Professor Jairam Reddy
University of Durban Westville
Private Bag X54001
Durban 4000, South Africa

Dr sc Matjaz Rode
Bratov Ucakar 16
YU-61000 Ljubljana
Yugoslavia

Professor Dr Peter Schärer
Plattenstr. 11
CH-8028 Zürich
Switzerland

Participants

Dr Rudolf Slavicek
Wahrunger Str. 56
A-1090 Vienna
Austria

Professor Christian Thierfelder
Schumannstrasse 20–21
DDR-1040 Berlin
German Democratic Republic

Dr Wong Tin Chun
15 Hennessy Road, 8th Floor
Hong Kong

Professor Dr Heiner Weber
Osianderstr. 2–8
D-7400 Tübingen 1
Federal Republic of Germany

Dr Raymond P. White, Jr
University of North Carolina
CB 7570, Brauer Hall
Chapel Hill, NC 27599, USA

Dr George A. Zarb
124 Edward Street
Toronto, M5G 1G6
Ontario, Canada

Dr Zhang Zehn-kang
Wei Gon Cun
Beijing
People's Republic of China

Chairman

Professor Richard J. Simonsen
University of Minnesota
School of Dentistry
515 Delaware Street SE
Minneapolis, MN 55455, USA

Guests

Professor Nikolay Bazhanov
Pogodinskaja Str. 5
Moscow 119435
USSR

Dr Roberto Gonzalez-Giralda
Suarez Guerra 42
Santa Cruz de Tenerife 38002
Canary Islands, Spain

Dr Larisa Panova
47 Ostozhenka
Moscow 119034
USSR

Host

Horst-Wolfgang Haase
Quintessence Publishing Co
Ifenpfad 2–4
D-1000 Berlin 42
Federal Republic of Germany

Preface

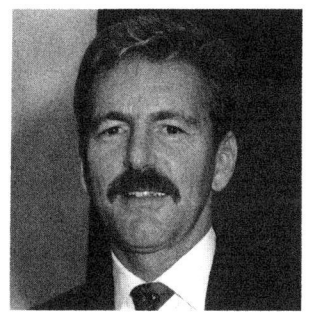

Richard J. Simonsen
Minneapolis, Minnesota

The year 1989 was an historic year. The reason for this book pales in comparison to the political events of late 1989 and early 1990. The great city of Berlin, where this World Symposium was held on September 10, 1989, was, at that time, divided by a concrete wall. In a matter of weeks the wall was down. But who, at our symposium in September, could have predicted the events of November 9, 1989? Likewise, who are we to predict the future of dentistry into the next century? – but we try here to define the present state of dentistry in our countries, and at the same time predict the future of the profession into the 21st century.

This gathering of experts discussing the state of the dental profession at the end of the 1980s, and attempting to project into the future the prospects for the profession into the 21st century, was a significant event for the profession. Rarely do 26 participants, from nearly as many different countries, gather together in one room with a group of invited guests from additional parts of the world.

The particular time for the symposium was chosen by the publisher, Mr H. W. Haase, to celebrate the 40th anniversary of the International Quintessence Publishing Group and the 20th anniversary of *Quintessence International.* The World Symposium was held in conjunction with the 6th International Quintessence Symposium.

It is intended that this publication will be distributed as a gift to the libraries of all dental universities in the world, and that it be donated to the national dental associations of all countries in the world. This is done as a commemoration of the anniversaries and to celebrate the progress in our chosen profession.

Each speaker invited to this symposium was asked to prepare some words on the state of dentistry in their respective area of the world, and to attempt to predict the future of dentistry in their country, or continent, based on its own unique problems. Each participant presented his or her opinions and data. Then an open discussion was held to further clarify some issues of mutual interest.

Preface

It was clear from our discussions that scientific research must be the basis of all progress in dental health care. Furthermore, aggressive preventive efforts are particularly necessary in developing countries to cut off the predictable increase in dental diseases that industrialized nations have already experienced. It was also clear from the large number of countries represented that a health system for one country may not be the ideal system for another.

It is hoped that this major undertaking by the International Quintessence Publishing Group to foster goodwill, and to cast some light on international understanding and cooperation in our profession, will be put to good use. Certainly, the camaraderie felt by all who participated, from many diverse cultures and backgrounds, will live on in our memories.

In the spirit of the unexpected and historic events that followed this symposium by just a few weeks, it is hoped that we can continue our cooperative international efforts to promote optimal dental health care for all, irrespective of national origin, race, religion, or socioeconomic background.

I am sure that all the participants join me in thanking Mr H. W. Haase for making this opportunity possible and for his dedication to the betterment of dental health on a global basis.

Richard J. Simonsen
Editor and Symposium Chairman

The participants at the Quintessence International World Symposium of 1989 gather around Mr H. W. Haase to congratulate him on the 40th anniversary of the International Quintessence Publishing Group and the 20th anniversary of *Quintessence International*.

1. Professor Richard J. Simonsen
2. Professor Jairam Reddy
3. Professor Valery K. Leontiev
4. Professor Arthur A. Dugoni
5. Dr Larisa Panova
6. Dr Roberto Gonzalez-Giralda
7. Professor Dr Wlodzimierz Jósefowicz
8. Professor Nikolay Bazhanov
9. Dr Harald Löe
10. Dr Rudolf Slavicek
11. Dr Zhang Zehn-kang
12. Mr H. W. Haase
13. Dr Wong Tin Chun
14. Dr sc Matjaz Rode
15. Dr Ivar A. Mjör
16. Professor Dr Heiner Weber
17. Dr Sumiya Hobo
18. Professor Dr Birte Melsen
19. Dr Raymond P. White, Jr
20. Professor Dr Mario Martignoni
21. Dr Yii Kie-Mung
22. Dr Jaime A. Gil
23. Dr George A. Zarb
24. Professor Dr Peter Schärer
25. Dr Frank Braun
26. Dr Pedro Américo Machado Bastos

Preface

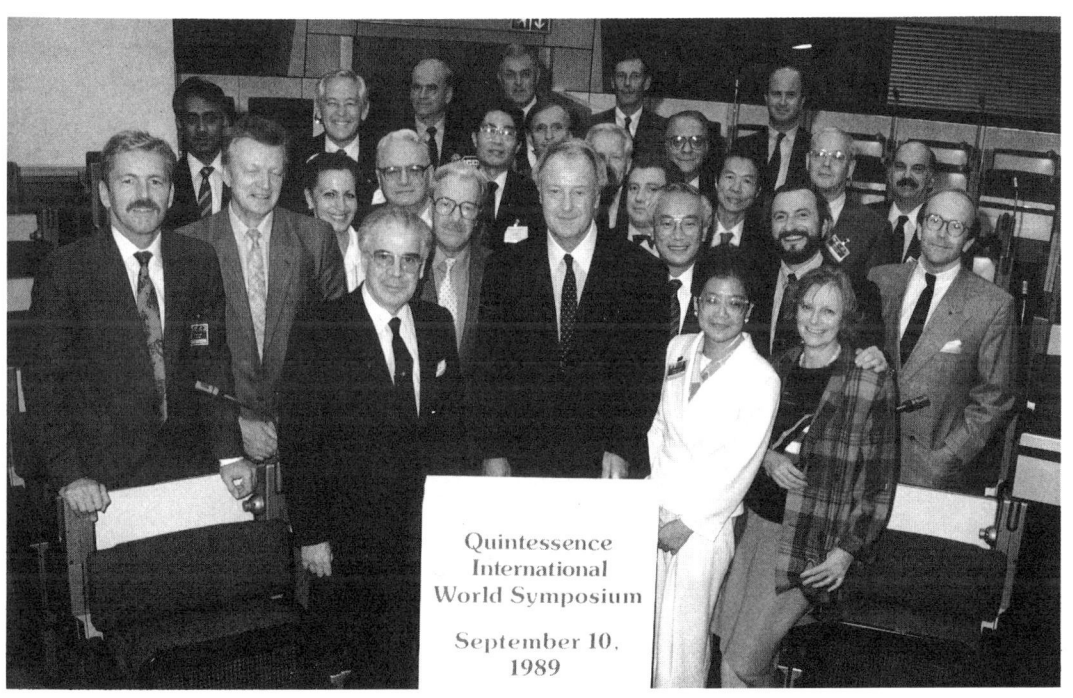

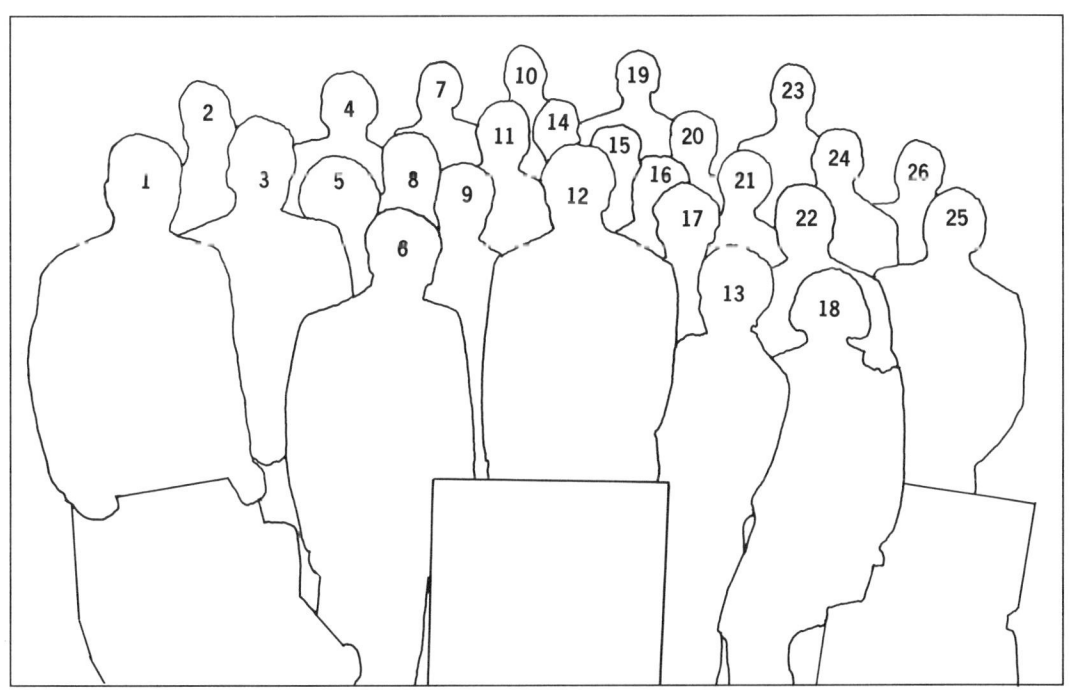

Chapter 1

Dentistry in the 21st Century

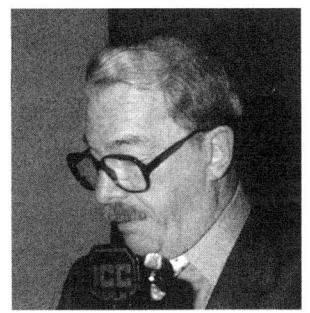

Harald Löe
Bethesda, Maryland

Abstract

Recent surveys indicate major improvements in the oral health of Americans, reflecting 40 years of advances in dental research. Many older Americans, some children, and people who are medically compromised or handicapped remain at high risk for disease, however. Cell and molecular biology techniques are being applied to identify those at risk and are leading to improved methods of diagnosis, treatment, and prevention for a wide range of oral health problems. The education of future dentists must prepare them for an expanded role as practitioners able to diagnose and treat all the diseases and disorders that affect the oral tissues.

We are living in times of extraordinary change. New knowledge, new discoveries and inventions are transforming the way we live now and the way our children will live tomorrow. New means of communication are enabling the peoples of the world to see and hear and read about these changes as they happen. The result is a world drawn closer than ever, a global village united by common dreams and aspirations for the good life, the healthy life.

It is our privilege — and responsibility — as health science professionals to promote the good and healthy life by exchanging information and ideas based on the experience of our native countries. At the same time we acknowledge the universal nature of science: we speak a common language and celebrate a common heritage of techniques and accomplishments that have revolutionized health science in our time.

From the perspective of the United States, progress in dental science has been nothing short of spectacular. Dra-

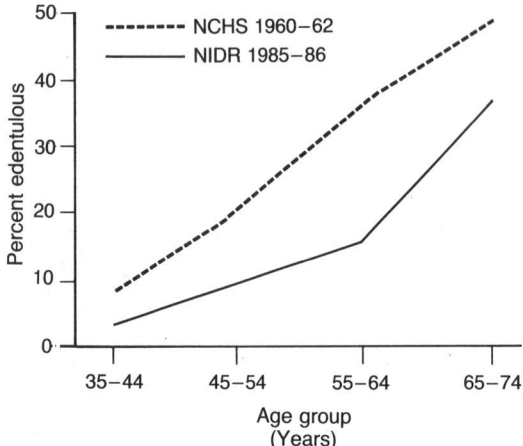

Fig 1 Percent of edentulous persons among adult US population.

Fig 2 Loss of attachment in dentate working adults in the United States, 1985–1986, expressed in percent of sample.

matic shifts in the patterns of dental disease are evident from the latest national surveys conducted by the National Institute of Dental Research (NIDR): A study of employed adults and older Americans in 1985–1986[1] and a study of schoolchildren in 1986–1987.[2] Both surveys show impressive gains in the oral health of the American people — even when compared to studies conducted as recently as 1980.

The adult survey was based on oral examinations of more than 15,000 employed adults, aged 18 to 64 years, seen at 800 worksites, and more than 5,000 older Americans, aged 65 to 103 years, seen at 200 senior citizen centers. Collectively, the sample represents 104 million Americans.

The most striking finding in the survey was that only 4% of working adults have lost all their teeth (Fig 1). Moreover, half the workers have lost at most a single tooth.

As a whole, the employed group averaged 23 decayed or restored tooth surfaces, of which 95% were already restored. The prevalence of root caries was about 20%. The mean number of decayed or restored root surfaces per person was less than 1, and close to half the root lesions were already restored.

The periodontal health of the workers has also significantly improved. Although gingivitis was common, and most individuals showed some loss of attachment (Fig 2), less than 2% of the periodontal pocket had a depth greater than 5 mm (Table 1).

The children's survey looked at nearly 40,000 schoolchildren between 5 and 17 years old, a sample representing 43 million elementary and secondary school students in America. The significant finding here was that half the children were caries free, never having had a carious lesion and never having had a restoration (Table 2). This is an increase over the

Table 1 Percent and cumulative percent of persons by most severe pocket, employed dentate population, US 1985–1986

Pocket depth (mm)	Male Pct	Male Cum Pct	Female Pct	Female Cum Pct	Both Pct	Both Cum Pct
2	50.52	96.36	56.51	93.69	53.18	95.18
3	28.76	45.85	25.47	37.18	27.74	42.00
4	11.86	17.09	7.58	10.71	9.96	14.26
5	3.05	5.23	2.05	3.14	2.61	4.30
6	1.39	2.18	0.72	1.08	1.09	1.70
7	0.53	0.80	0.30	0.37	0.43	0.61
8	0.11	0.27	0.05	0.06	0.08	0.18
9	0.06	0.16	0.01	0.01	0.04	0.09
10	0.07	0.10	0.01	0.01	0.04	0.06
11	0.00	0.03	0.00	0.00	0.00	0.01
12+	0.02	0.02	0.00	0.00	0.01	0.01

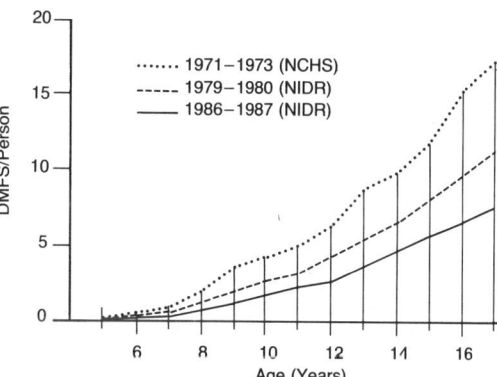

Oral health of US schoolchildren, NIDR 1987

Fig 3 Age-specific prevalence of dental caries (DMFS) in the three US national surveys.

Table 2 Percent of children caries free in two national surveys

Age	1979–1980	1986–1987
5	95.4	97.3
6	89.7	94.4
7	76.5	84.2
8	58.6	75.0
9	50.6	65.5
10	37.9	55.7
11	33.7	45.0
12	26.9	41.7
13	21.1	34.0
14	19.6	27.7
15	14.9	21.8
16	11.8	20.0
17	10.7	15.6
All Ages	**36.6**	**49.9**

Table 3 Age-specific prevalence of caries in permanent teeth, 1979–1980 and 1986–1987

	Mean DMFS	
Age	1979–1980	1986–1987
5	0.11	0.07
6	0.20	0.13
7	0.58	0.41
8	1.25	0.71
9	1.90	1.14
10	2.60	1.69
11	3.00	2.33
12	4.18	2.66
13	5.41	3.76
14	6.53	4.68
15	8.07	5.71
16	9.58	6.68
17	11.04	8.04
Total	**4.77**	**3.07**

37% who were found to be caries free in a similar survey completed only 7 years earlier in 1980 (Fig 3). Furthermore, the children who still have decay have significantly fewer and smaller carious lesions than children in the earlier survey. The overall caries prevalence rate dropped from a mean DMFS of 4.8 to a mean of 3.1 in 1987 (Table 3).

Taken together, the surveys indicate

that dental caries and periodontal diseases — the two most prevalent, painful, and costly dental diseases in the world and the major causes of tooth loss — are rapidly declining in the United States among children and younger adults. No question about it, we are witnessing dramatic proof that 40 years' improvement in dental research in America is paying off. Indeed, the savings to Americans in terms of reductions in caries treatment expenditure alone are estimated to be between $2 and $3 billion a year.

It was a little over 40 years ago, in 1948, that the US Congress established the National Institute of Dental Research to address the serious oral health problems of the American people. World War II had revealed that 10% of Army recruits could not meet the minimal dental requirements. Indeed, the standards had to be relaxed and dentists recruited into the Army so that they could fit dentures to young men to enable them to serve.

The 1940s and 1950s marked a turning point. Charged with a mission to improve the oral health of Americans, the NIDR invested its energies into research on fluorine, conducting the classic controlled clinical trials that established the value of water fluoridation in preventing caries. These advances were followed by the revolutionary discoveries by researchers in America and abroad that caries and periodontal diseases were bacterial infections associated with dental plaque. All at once was born a rationale for treatment — and, even more important — an understanding that these diseases could be prevented.

Research is not the whole explanation for the improvements in oral health that are now literally changing the faces of Americans, however. It took the combined efforts of dental researchers working with dental practitioners and community leaders to establish water fluoridation in the nation's cities. It took the ingenuity of private industry to develop fluoride dentifrices, mouthrinses, gels, and other fluoride vehicles now everywhere in use. And it took improvements in the standard of living and in education to produce today's generation of health-conscious Americans, each owning and using a toothbrush. So what research had discovered about the cause and prevention of disease was translated into better oral hygiene practices, improved knowledge and understanding by the general public, and, of course, rapid adoption of the results of research by the dental practitioners themselves.

If society is to reap the benefits of continued advances in dental research, it will take the same kind of concerted action, the same collaborative effort of researchers with dental practitioners and educators, with industry and the general public, to work toward a better, healthier life.

In that regard, the recent surveys are very instructive. For example, the children's survey showed that two thirds of the carious lesions that remain are on the pits and fissures of the occlusal surfaces of the teeth. These are the areas least affected by fluoride, but they can be protected from decay by dental sealants. Yet the survey indicates that only 8% to 10% of the children receive this caries-preventive measure, so sealants — products of restorative materials research that have been available for over a decade — are not in wide use. The lesson is clear: a scientific advance is not truly an advance if no one uses it.

The adult survey has been instructive for what it says about older Americans. In sharp contrast to the employed group, 42% of adults 65 years and older have lost all their teeth. Those who still have teeth continue to experience coronal caries at about the same rate as the younger adults, but they have three times the rate of root caries and suffer the most severe and extensive periodontal diseases. Moreover, these data were obtained from older Americans well enough to attend senior citizens centers.

We have very little information on the oral health of the homebound, frail, or institutionalized. The lesson here is that dental research must enlarge its horizons; it must go beyond the oral health needs of children and younger adults to address the whole spectrum of oral diseases and conditions that affect adults and the elderly. This need is especially great given the dramatic increase in numbers of older individuals not only in the United States but in many nations of the world. Indeed, the need to look at individuals or groups of any age who are at risk for oral health problems is essential. These categories include the poor, the handicapped, and the many different special patient populations with medical conditions and/or treatments that adversely affect the oral tissues.

The new biology

Fortunately, these epidemiologic imperatives find dental research ready, willing, and able to take full advantage of the new cell and molecular approaches that have revolutionized biomedical research in the last decade. Not only have these "new biology" techniques transformed basic research studies, they are also dramatically expanding our options for the identification of risk patients in diagnosis, treatment, and prevention.

Diagnostic molecules

Already there are diagnostic kits available or under development that employ genetic probes or monoclonal antibodies to detect disease-causing bacteria or the by-products of disease in oral tissues and fluids. These tests are not time- and labor-intensive procedures, but tests that can be performed in the dental office or clinic to identify and treat individuals at high risk for dental caries. Some test kits are available for detecting periodontal disease pathogens,[3] including bacteria associated with severe forms of disease such as prepubertal or juvenile periodontitis. Because these severe forms appear to run in families, investigators can also make use of new genetic techniques to search for markers to identify relatives at risk. Eventually such genetic analyses could lead to ways of correcting the defective gene or genes.

Anti-attachment approaches

At the molecular level we now are beginning to understand the processes by which the normal oral flora become established in the mouth. Specific proteins on the surface of bacteria have been identified that are responsible for bacterial adherence to oral tissues and co-aggregations with other species.[4] Genetic and immunologic studies are now being applied to develop mutant forms of bacteria that are unable to attach or adhere.[5] Other studies are discovering which surface receptors may be common to different species of bacteria. Here there is a potential for developing a kind of broad-spectrum anti-attachment agent or rinse that could be used in home care.

Replacement therapy

In other approaches employing genetic manipulations, researchers are developing harmless forms of oral pathogens to replace pathogens in the mouth. This "replacement therapy" relies on the ability of the mutant forms to compete successfully with their virulent relatives and colonize the oral tissues.[6]

New vaccines

An understanding of the genetics of oral bacteria is also leading to new approaches to the development of oral vaccines. Caries researchers have identified several virulence factors of the surface of *Streptococcus mutans* bacteria. The genes coding for these proteins have been cloned and introduced into a harmless strain of bacteria that normally inhabits the intestine. The idea is to use these genetically engineered bacteria as an oral vaccine. Once swallowed, the bacteria would settle in the intestine, express the *S mutans* proteins, and stimulate lymphoid tissue lining the intestine. The activated lymph cells would generate anticaries antibodies that then are released in the mouth via salivary secretion.[7]

With regard to periodontal diseases, one of the problems that has confronted research has been the difficulty of isolating and cultivating the many species of bacteria recovered from diseased sites. The newer molecular approaches are proving far more efficient in this respect. Should this line of research establish that a few pathogens play roles in the transition from periodontal health to disease, it might pave the way for new, genetically engineered periodontal disease vaccines.

New antibodies

Molecular technology should also help to resolve the issue of periodontal disease activity/inactivity by allowing the probing of a local site for the existence of bacteria or host cells and their metabolic products. In turn, these findings could permit a more selective approach to treatment — perhaps the use of "narrow spectrum" antibiotics, agents specifically directed against the bacterial species identified.

In the meantime, new therapeutic agents are appearing that are themselves the product of molecular engineering, such as chemically modified tetracycline (CMT). This is tetracycline with its antibiotic property removed through a manipulation of its molecular structure.[8] The new drug appears to be nontoxic and has the useful properties of inhibiting tissue production of collagenase and bone resorption. Because it lacks antibiotic properties, it might be used for long periods of time without inducing bacterial resistance.

Repair and regeneration

One of the most exciting results of recent research has been to change traditional ways of thinking about disease and its consequences. Genetic disease is no longer thought to be incurable. The regeneration of nerve tissue is no longer an idle dream. In terms of oral disease, advanced periodontitis is no longer thought to be irreversible. New insights into the cellular biology of the attachment apparatus have led to the concept of guided tissue regeneration.[9,10] This concept is based on the hypothesis that a subpopulation of periodontal ligament cells has the potential for developing new connective tissue attachment and bone at sites affected by advanced disease.[11]

A major reason for the new optimism with regard to the healing and regeneration of tissue has been the discovery of whole new populations of cells and extracellular molecules involved in the critical processes of growth and repair. Dental investigators have now isolated many of these molecules — growth factors, chemoattractants, immune cell activators — in the extracellular matrices of bones, teeth, and soft tissues. They are isolating and cloning the associated genes and purifying the protein products to enhance wound healing and bony repairs.

Some of this research involves studies of basement membrane, the thin layer of extracellular material that surrounds nerves and blood vessels and also separates organs of the body. Dental investigators have discovered a molecule in basement membrane — laminin — which plays a role in the process of cancer metastasis. Detailed structural and chemical analyses of the molecules have now led to the synthesis of drugs designed to block metastasias.[12]

Saliva studies

Salivary secretions have also been the source of great interest as investigators continue to discover components of saliva involved in the defense, maintenance, and repair of the oral tissue. One goal of this research is to develop synthetic solutions, "designer salivas," that would combine calcium and phosphates or other minerals with fluoride and other components, to aid in remineralizing carious lesions, especially for use in individuals at high risk for disease.[13]

Teeth for life

An emphasis on individuals at high risk makes sense in industrialized countries where substantial gains in oral and general health have been made. It is the approach the NIDR is advocating in a new initiative we are calling the Research and Action Program for Improving the Oral Health of All Americans — more briefly, "Teeth for Life." The goals are to eliminate toothlessness in the next generation; to prevent further deterioration of the oral health of those with already compromised dentition; and to ensure that adults already in good oral health maintain the state as they advance to the retirement years.

We have every reason to believe that these goals coincide with the hopes and expectations of Americans today. Our surveys indicate that more people than ever before are seeing their dentists on a regular basis. The drugstores and supermarkets are stocked with enormous quantities of oral health care products ranging from toothbrushes and toothpastes of every shape and style to fancy toothpicks, flosses, and oral rinses. Clearly, behind these consumer products are cultural and esthetic demands that teeth can be clean, white, and disease free. The growth in adult orthodontics would indicate as well that more and more Americans want their teeth to be straight and properly aligned. There is no doubt that these younger adults differ substantially from their parents and grandparents; they fully expect to keep their natural teeth; they do not accept the very idea of toothlessness and dentures.

And we in dental research intend to help them. All the advances that the new biology is making possible in diagnostics, in prevention, in treatment, are geared to furthering the goal of teeth for life. Complementing those approaches are the more traditional lines of dental research, which have also been making rapid progress. Investigators are perfecting techniques for digital subtraction x-rays and three-dimensional radiography — CT scans of the mouth.[14] Development in nuclear medicine techniques and magnetic resonance imagery will permit earlier and better diagnoses of orofacial hard and soft tissue.

Biomaterials research has enjoyed its own explosive growth. In addition to ever-improving, more durable composite resins, techniques for bonding to dentin are being perfected.[15] The newer chapter alloys will eventually replace silver and gold, and implants will be the treatment of choice for individuals who need even single-tooth replacements. The emphasis in restorative dentistry will be on conservative concepts and approaches to produce the least trauma and loss of healthy tooth substance. Restorative materials and sealants may incorporate systems for the controlled release of fluoride or other therapeutic agents.

But what about today's generation of older Americans? What about the individuals and groups at any stage or age of life who are in poor oral or general health, or who are unwilling or unable to maintain good oral health?

The NIDR intends to focus on these individuals as well, to find out who they are and where they are and why they are at risk. We will analyze past surveys and conduct new epidemiological studies, looking at selected groups that include minorities, the poor, the unemployed, and those who are frail, homebound, or in institutions or nursing homes. These studies will take into consideration systemic diseases and treatments, personal and cultural attitudes and behaviors, and other non–disease-related factors such as the cost of oral health care, access to and utilization of services, and previous dental history.

The NIDR will also conduct and support basic research on normal changes in the oral tissue associated with aging. These include changes in the oral microecology, in the immune system, in the capacity for tissue repair, as well as research on the various oral conditions and how they affect and are affected by systemic disease and treatments.

These activities are designed to expand the knowledge base, guiding and coordinating the research component of the Research and Action Program. The action side will solicit the participation of the practitioner, community, and individuals who can help move the research into public and professional knowledge and application — exactly the kind of concerted action and commitment that has worked so successfully in the past to advance the oral health of the American people.

Dental practice in the new millennium

The action side clearly will have an impact on the nature of dental practice and the education of future practitioners. The restoration of carious lesions will cease to be the mainstay of general dentists and pedodontists. However, caries in all its forms—coronal, secondary, and root surface caries—will continue to be seen in adults and the elderly, and treatments emphasizing conservative and prophylactic approaches will be expected. Periodontal diseases have already ceased to be a major cause of tooth loss in American adults. Gingivitis and milder forms of periodontitis will probably remain prevalent, however, and will be amenable to treatment by primary care practitioners. The need for endodontic care should dissipate. The need for removable prosthodontics will decline or disappear as a result of more teeth being saved. In their place will be fixed prosthodontics and implants to replace single teeth.

The role of the general dentist will expand to include the diagnosis and treatment of *all* oral diseases and disorders. Besides caries and periodontal diseases, dental practitioners will be concerned with detecting and treating oral cancer and precancerous lesions, herpes virus and other soft tissue infections, acute and chronic orofacial pain, temporomandibular joint problems, salivary gland dysfunctions, and disorders of taste and smell and swallowing. Here the profession is well served by significant growth and progress of oral health research in the fields of oral biology, wound healing, and repair. Examples of recent advances include the development of experimental vaccines against herpes virus infections, the use of novel drugs in combination with low-dose analgesics to provide long-lasting pain relief, and the demonstration of the effectiveness of the drug pilocarpine in relieving dry mouth in patients with residually functioning salivary gland tissue.

Dentists of the future will routinely record data on the general health of their patients, medications used, dietary and tobacco habits, and other relevant information. They will advise patients on how systemic diseases or treatments can affect the oral cavity, and, conversely, how oral problems and treatments may affect general health. This more comprehensive view on the part of the dentist will be especially important as the population shifts toward older-aged groups where prevalences of diabetes, cancer, heart diseases, arthritis, and other chronic conditions are higher.

As a result of these changes in their role, dental practitioners themselves will be perceived differently. They will be recognized as specialists among other biomedical specialists contributing to an integrated approach to patient care.

There is already dramatic evidence that this is happening with regard to AIDS patients. Clinical dental investigators were quick to recognize unusual oral signs and symptoms in patients later diagnosed as having AIDS. Dental scientists continue to conduct basic research on the AIDS virus and the immune system, while their clinical investigator colleagues clarify the natural history and prognosis of the disease in relation to oral manifestations. Recognition and treatment of the oral signs and symptoms of infection with the human immunodeficiency virus (HIV) can only be expected to increase if present forecasts are borne out, and will demand great sensitivity in diagnosing, counseling, and referring patients for testing if the HIV status is not known.

agnose and manage the many categories of special patients who are at risk for oral health problems for whatever reason. This more expanded scope of dental practice will also demand new levels of sophistication in communication skills and in clinical decision making aimed at designing treatment options tailored to the needs and abilities of the individual patient.

These new demands are already having an impact on dental education: They are mobilizing forces for changes in curricula that recognize that dentists in the new millenium will no longer be focused on one disease, one technique, or one mode of treatment. The new practitioners will be generalists depending as much on analytical abilities as on manual skills, rich in knowledge as well as in technique. These "physicians of the mouth" will be the men and women who oversee the next stage in the evolution of our profession — the passage from restorative dentistry and repairs to a practice dominated by prevention of the two main oral diseases and the management of a multitude of "orphan" diseases. However, the all-important achievement will be: preservation of the natural teeth for life!

Implications for dental education

All this necessitates an increase in the depth and breadth of predoctoral preparation of future dentists. More internal medicine and clinical pharmacology, more immunology, more genetics and molecular biology will be necessary to di-

References

1. National Institute of Dental Research: *Oral Health of United States Adults: The National Survey of Oral Health in U. S. Employed Adults and Seniors: 1985–1986.* NIH Pub. No. 87-2868, 1987.
2. National Institute of Dental Research: *Oral Health of United States Children: The National Survey of Dental Caries in U. S. School Children 1986–1987, National and Regional Findings.* NIH Pub. No. 89-2247, in press.
3. French CK, Savitt ED, Simon SL, Eklund SM, Chen MC, Klotz LC, Vaccaro KK: DNA Probe detection of periodontal pathogens. *Oral Microbiol Immunol* 1986; 1:58–62.
4. Kolenbrander PE: Intergeneric coaggregation among human oral bacteria and ecology of dental plaque. *Ann Rev Microbiol* 1988; 42:627–656.
5. Cisar JO, Vatter AE, Clark WB, Curl SH, Hurst-Calderone S, Sandberg AL: Mutants of *Actinomyces viscosus* TI4V lacking type 1, type 2, or both types of fimbriae. *Infect Immun* 1988; 56:2984–2989.
6. Hillman JD, Socransky SS: Replacement therapy for the prevention of dental disease. *Adv Dent Res* 1987; 1(1):119–125.
7. Curtiss R III: Genetic analysis of *Streptococcus mutans* virulence and prospects for an anticaries vaccine. *J Dent Res* 1986; 65(8):1034–1045.
8. Golub LM, McNamara TF, D'Angelo G, Greenwald RA, Ramamurthy NS: A non-antibacterial chemically-modified tetracycline inhibits mammalian collagenase activity. *J Dent Res* 1987; 66(8):1310–1314.
9. Karring T, Nyman S, Lindhe J: Healing following implantation of periodontitis affected roots into bone tissue. *J Clin Periodontol* 1980; 7:96–105.
10. Nyman S, Karring T, Lindhe J, Planten S: Healing following implantation of periodontitis affected roots into gingival connective tissue. *J Clin Periodontol* 1980; 7:394–401.
11. Gottlow J, Nyman S, Lindhe J, Karring T, Wennström J: New attachment formation in the human periodontium by guided tissue regeneration. *J Clin Periodontol* 1986; 13:597–603.
12. Iwamoto Y, Robey FA, Graf J, Sasaki M, Kleinman HK, Yamada Y, Martin GR: YIGSR, a synthetic laminin pentapeptide, inhibits experimental metastasis formation. *Science* 1987; 238:1132–1134.
13. Levine MJ, Aguirre, Hatton MN, Tabak LA: Artificial salivas: present and future. *J Dent Res* 1987; 66(Spec Iss):693–698.
14. Ruttiman UE: Computer-based reconstruction and temporal subtraction of radiographs. *Adv Dent Res* 1987; 1(1):72–79.
15. Bowen RL, Eichmiller FC, Marjenhoff WA, Rupp NW: Adhesive bonding of composites. *J Am Col Dentists* 1989; 56(2):10–13.

Chapter 2

Stomatology in the German Democratic Republic: Historic Record and Prospects

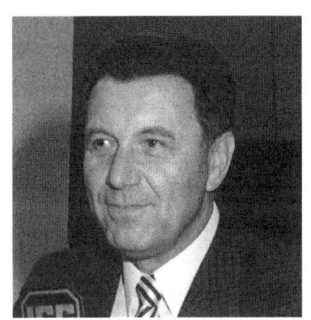

Christian Thierfelder
Berlin, German
Democratic Republic

Abstract

Dental education has a very long tradition at Berlin University. The educational concept has undergone continual change and has been systematically raised to a higher level. A comprehensive presentation is given on the third stage of reforms in higher education, with details on the respective contents.

The study of stomatology is followed by further compulsory education to the level of dental specialist. The corresponding provisions are discussed. An outlook is also given on the further scheduled changes in this field of study.

A characterization is given on developments that have taken place since 1949 in the personnel situation with regard to dentists and auxiliary dental staff.

The discussions are based on the situation from September 1989 onwards; the changes that have been taking place since then will certainly also have consequences on dentistry in the eastern part of Germany.

The first institute for academic training of dentists in what was then the German Reich was opened in Berlin in October 1884. At about the same time, similar institutions were established in Halle and Leipzig. Nevertheless, the Berlin institute was the first center founded and run by a university. Affiliated with it were numerous outstanding dentists and scholars who made substantial contributions to the erection of a building for science-based and medically oriented stomatology.

However, the real birth of the German dental profession had occurred even earlier, in Prussia in 1826, when in a ministerial edict dentistry was officially recognized as an independent profession in its own right.

Stomatological education used to be quite irregular, especially in the 19th century, and it took some time for it to assume, in a stepwise manner, a college-type profile linking research and practice.

Substantially new patterns were introduced to the German Democratic Republic after World War II by three higher education reforms (1945/46, 1951/52, 1967/68).

Stomatological education, according to the new university curriculum of 1953, was extended from 4 to 5 years. The major purpose of this curriculum was to produce stomatological practitioners for public health. Three compulsory in-service training periods were inserted to the 1st, 3rd, and 5th academic years to meet the demand for unity between theory and practice.

Yet it was only in the wake of the third higher education reform that conditions could be created to elevate stomatology to the status of a fully independent branch of university study. Science-related and theoretical-experimental principles began to be taught in separate lectures and seminars with specific reference to stomatology. In the clinical-medical disciplines specific teaching programs clearly defined for stomatology were introduced. New subjects were added, such as military and emergency medicine. Clinical-stomatological programs were set up on an interdisciplinary basis, that is, in conjunction with all stomatological subdisciplines. More emphasis began to be placed on prophylactic stomatology, and pediatric stomatology as well as periodontology were expanded.

Also, new rules and regulations were issued for taking academic degrees. All undergraduates are expected to become capable of independent scientific performance. On successful completion of the 5-year course, they earn the lowest academic degree, stomatologist. The diploma is awarded upon presentation of a graduation paper that has to satisfy minimal scientific standards. Only then, in accordance with the National Doctorate Conferment Rules, can the second academic degree, Dr med, be bestowed on a graduate.

The regular 5-year course is followed by compulsory 4-year postgraduate specialization in general stomatology (74% of all graduates), pediatric stomatology (20%), orthodontics (4%), or dental surgery (2%). Those programs are offered at separate postgraduate specialization centers that boast highly skilled personnel and first-rate equipment. Stomatological specialization is based on one clearly defined nationwide program providing for working visits at hospitals, practice exercises, theoretical instruction, and formal examinations supervised by a panel of professors.

Postgraduate stomatological specialization in medicotheoretical disciplines was introduced in 1978. There are about 50 stomatological specialists at present in anatomy, biochemistry, physiology, pathology, microbiology, and pharmacology. These specialists are expected to contribute to the theoretical expansion and consolidation of stomatology and ultimately to teach in their fields.

Stomatological education in the GDR is distributed among six universities (Berlin, Leipzig, Halle, Rostock, Greifswald, and Jena) and two medical academies (Dresden and Erfurt). Education at the two latter institutions is confined to clinical training, beginning in the third academic year, while preclinical training is available for undergraduates in Berlin, Leipzig, and Halle.

The emergence of stomatology as an independent branch of university study was accompanied by organizational modifications to the centers of medical education. Departments of stomatology began to be established.

Our department of stomatology is made up of outpatient clinics for restorative, prosthetic, surgical, and orthodontic stomatology, subsections in these outpatient clinics for pediatric stomatology and periodontology, a hospital and outpatient clinic for dentofacial surgery, as well as separate sections for dental technology, stomatological radiology, patient registration, and documentation. Departments at other GDR universities have sections for prophylactic stomatology and for stomatological research as well. Affiliated with our department of stomatology at Humboldt-Universität zu Berlin is a division for experimental stomatology and biomaterials research.

We are now working on restructuring stomatological education. The new system is to come into effect in 1990. This has become necessary because the dentists we are educating now will have to meet the challenge of the next millenium. This will require the following qualitative alterations:

1. Intensified replacement of curative by preventive action in general stomatological practice
2. More emphasis on professional ethics in undergraduate education
3. Increased active scientific commitment of undergraduates, with a view to making positive contributions to technological scientific progress
4. More effective orientation of clinical training to the epidemiological situation in the general public, with particular consideration of high-risk patients and selected social groups

We shall teach the fundamentals of medicine under the aspect of unity between regular and postgraduate education, with equal emphasis being placed on knowledge, skills, and motivation. The issues and subjects of teaching will have to be more strongly oriented toward real long-term demands on practice. Some future-oriented reserves will have to be created in education for easier understanding and adoption of new ideas and methods.

No general decline of caries has so far been noted in the population of the GDR, notwithstanding fluoridation of drinking water and other complex programs for the prevention of caries. A noticeable decline in this disease will not be achievable unless more is done on an individual basis with regard to oral hygiene.

We also expect an increase in the incidence of diseases unrelated to plaque, such as pain dysfunction syndrome. Efforts are being made for early diagnosis of, and thus early therapy for, reversible pathological alterations. Orthodontic treatment is increasingly in demand for both adolescents and adults. In prosthodontic therapy there will be more fixed dentures and implants.

A decline in morbidity is not obtainable solely from undifferentiated collective measures. Clear-cut progress, with preservation and improvement of oral health, will be achievable only by individual action, with due consideration of individual disposition.

The number of dentists in the GDR between 1949 and 1970 was about 7,000

Table 1 Dentists in the GDR, according to Statistical Yearbook 1988

Year/region (1987)	No. dentists	Ratio to 10,000 citizens	No. citizens to one dentist
1949	7,100	3.8	2,661
1955	7,259	4.1	2,457
1960	6,361	3.7	2,702
1965	6,207	3.6	2,743
1970	7,349	4.3	2,321
1975	7,968	4.7	2,115
1980	9,709	5.8	1,724
1985	11,757	7.1	1,416
1986	12,185	7.3	1,364
1987	12,527	7.5	1,328
Berlin	1,150	9.2	1,084
Cottbus	611	6.9	1,446
Dresden	1,377	7.8	1,283
Erfurt	979	7.9	1,263
Frankfurt	507	7.1	1,403
Gera	631	8.5	1,172
Halle	1,191	6.7	1,495
Karl-Marx-Stadt	1,290	6.9	1,444
Leipzig	1,065	7.8	1,285
Magdeburg	901	7.2	1,386
Neubrandenburg	420	6.8	1,477
Potsdam	794	7.1	1,413
Rostock	764	8.4	1,193
Schwerin	434	7.3	1,367
Suhl	413	7.5	1,330

(Table 1). It has gradually increased to approximately 13,000, after enrollment figures doubled and later quadrupled. This has brought the dentist-citizen ratio to 1:1,300. Within the next years we intend to reach 1:1,200, the ratio recommended by the World Health Organization. Nevertheless, enrollment figures will be reduced because it will be necessary only to make up for mortality and to level out regional differences. The annual enrollment figure at Berlin University, for example, will be cut from 100 to 60.

We have not yet managed to ensure adequate availability of personnel in the fields of dental mechanics and stomatological assistance. The ratio of dentists to dental technicians is at the unsatisfactory level of 1:0.6 despite many efforts already taken. Similarly, the ratio of dentists to stomatological nurses is insufficient, being 1:0.9. These two paramedical professions are based on 3-year technical school courses, and great efforts are being taken to recruit more candidates for training. For additional motivation and because of need, postgraduate education is generally available to paramedical personnel. Roughly 50% of all dental technologists go in for specialization in ceramics, prosthodontic cast fabrication, orthodontics, and special fields in prosthetics. Stomatological nurses can take courses for specialization in dental and oral hygiene.

We estimate that in spite of the international caries decline, demands on dental care will not quantitatively decrease as the forthcoming millenium approaches. The substance of stomatological care, however, will undergo qualitative change. We should raise our sights to these forthcoming developments in formulating efficient strategies for more effective education and practice. This will prove crucial if stomatology is to meet the challenge of the future.

Chapter 3

Dentistry in Latin America: The 21st Century

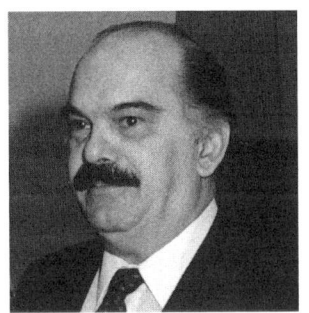

Pedro Américo
Machado Bastos
São Paulo, Brazil

Abstract

Latin American health care problems cannot be dissociated from their socioeconomic context, and projections on the future can only be analyzed in light of the economic particularities, social conditions, and political realities of Latin America. In Latin American countries, poverty increases at a fast rate; economic growth is losing speed; the real value of salaries has slid backward; the employment level has dropped, prices for basic goods and agricultural products for export have collapsed and public investments have been drastically reduced. The outlook for the future is no better.

All things considered, we believe that prevention and technology will exert a considerable influence over every area of the profession: research, teaching, and professional practice. South American dentistry will probably follow the development of worldwide dentistry, although at a slower pace.

South America, with about 18 million square kilometers and a population of about 300 million inhabitants, is a region of many facets and high contrasts. Within the continent and even within each country, we find underdeveloped deserts and oases of prosperity. This situation is closely related to the economic, social, and cultural characteristics of our colonization. The European conquerors were much more interested in exploring our natural riches and establishing trading posts aimed exclusively at commercial objectives rather than developing the countries. This policy was not completely reversed with the political independence of the South American nations and in fact persists today through the economic power exercised by the oligarchy that still rules the area and is effectively backed by international economic powers.

However, during the last decades, South America has experienced a certain degree of progress in terms of industrialization. This is mainly the case of Brazil, which stands out and today is ranked as the seventh nation of the industrialized

Table 1 Brazilian income distribution, 1985

Population	Share of total income (%)
Poorest 10%	1.05
Poorest 50%	12.99
Wealthiest 50%	87.00
Wealthiest 10%	47.16

Source: Pinto, VG, 1988.[8]

nations in the capitalist world. With a gross national product of $350 billion and a trade balance of $20 billion in 1988, the Brazilian economy, however, follows a badly managed path, with an external debt of $120 billion, a high inflation rate (175% in 1989), and an unfair income distribution (Table 1). As can be seen from the table, the wealthiest 10% of the population receives nearly half the total personal income in Brazil.

External debt has been impairing South American development. In Brazil, from 9% growth in 1980 we experienced a reversal to 0.4% negative growth in 1988. The increase in the interest rates in the world market, in past years mainly in the United States, has increased this debt to levels that make payment impossible. In 1976, the Brazilian external debt was $70 billion; by 1988, $70 billion was paid in interest rates and services, nevertheless the debt went up to $120 billion. At the same time, a very small amount of money for investment entered the country. The situation in the other South American countries is quite similar but they have even less possibility of overcoming their crises.

Health conditions

Because the available data are insufficient for South American countries, I will analyze the Brazilian picture and whenever possible extend my discussion to other countries. Brazil occupies half of the continental area and its population represents 50% of the total South American population. It should adequately represent the average South American situation.

Considering the facts, it is not a surprise if we find a precarious oral health condition in the region. The financial resources are small and insufficient for the area, and most of the areas are susceptible to general diseases, which, because of their more serious consequences, are considered priorities. As we all know, the World Health Organization and the Fédération Dentaire Internationale have established as a target for the year 2000, in children, a maximum of three caries-affected teeth at age 12. The DMFT values for Brazil are shown in Table 2, while the situation in several other South American countries for children within the 12-year age group is indicated in Table 3.

The Brazilian situation gets more serious when one considers the DMFT index at the age of 12 (Table 4).

Further, when we include the adult population, the situation becomes alarming: the continuous growth of the DMFT average occurs at the expense of the teeth lost through extractions. These, in the beginning, represent only 8% in the group from 6 to 14 years of age but soon stand for 46% between 20 and 29 years, and 68% and 90% among the older groups (Fig 1).

Health conditions

Table 2 Brazilian DMFT index

Age (yr)	Rate
6	1.25
9	3.61
12	6.65

Table 3 DMFT indices for 12-year-olds in selected South American countries

Country	Rate
Argentina	3.36
Chile	4.84
Uruguay	7.00
Paraguay	5.99
Colombia	5.99

Table 4 DMFT index for 12-year-old children in Brazil

Index	No. teeth affected (%)
Decayed	60%
Extraction indicated	6%
Missing	5%
Filled	29%

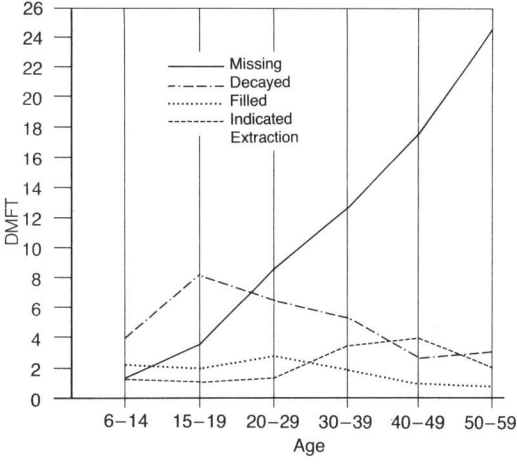

Fig 1 *(right)* Evolution of caries index according to its components from 6 to 59 years — Brazil 1983.

An epidemiological survey carried out by the Brazilian Ministry of Health subdivided the population into four groups, and the results are summarized in Table 5–8.

In the whole epidemiological survey, the worst results were always found within the lower-income groups, as one might well expect.

Besides caries and periodontal diseases, it is estimated that in Brazil 45% of the children show malocclusion; 1 out of 800 children has a cleft lip, with or without cleft palate; and 8.5% of the malignant tumors in males and 2.3% in females occur in the mouth.

Table 5 DMFT rates of the Brazilian population

DMFT rate		% population
DMFT 0.0 to 3	(ideal)	19.5%
DMFT 3.1 to 5	(average)	27.5%
DMFT 5.1 to 7	(high)	18.0%
DMFT over 7	(very high)	35.0%

Table 6 Percentage of Brazilian children unaffected by caries

Age (yr)	% unaffected
6	48.0%
12	3.7%
6 to 12	13.8%

Table 7 Periodontal status of Brazilians

Condition	% population affected		
	15–19 yr	35–44 yr	50–59 yr
Healthy	51.7	16.6	5.5
Bleeding	19.9	11.3	4.9
Calculi	23.1	23.6	12.0
Pockets	2.3	8.5	6.9
Nulls	2.9	40.1	70.4

Table 8 Prosthodontic status of Brazilians (urban population) aged 50–59 yr

Status	% population
All teeth extracted in at least one dental arch	72%
Prosthesis used	45%
No prosthesis used	14%
Only maxillary prosthesis used	11%

Treatment of oral diseases

As we can see, the oral health conditions in Brazil are worrying. The same is true for other South American countries. The demand for treatment is high but its fulfillment is impaired by the lack of financial resources, both public and private. To give an overall view, in 1986 the resources allocated to health care, general and oral, in Brazil, were as shown in Fig 2. As one can see, the health care area received only 4.7% of the gross national product. Of this 4.7%, the medical areas received 96.5% and the dental area 3.5%. In short, dentistry used only 0.16% of the GNP ($434 million).

The demand for dental treatment and the necessary resources to meet it can be seen in Table 9.

Dental services

Currently, Brazil has about 100,000 dentists, or 1 per 1,500 inhabitants, which may seem reasonable. However, considering the irregular distribution of professionals, with concentration in the richest urban areas, the small amount of public resources, and the low purchasing power of the population, there is today an excessive supply of services.

In Brazil, the liberal exercise of the profession is predominant. However, the access to a private office is a privilege of 10% of the Brazilian population. Today, the vast majority use the services provided by agreements between corporations and health care enterprises, or by the health insurance. A radical change that puts emphasis on preventive measures in the oral health care policy has become inevitable.

In South America, a joint effort by the Brazilian, Argentinian, Chilean, Uruguayan, and Paraguayan governments, with the help of the World Health Organization, is trying to change this unfavorable picture through a policy of effective action toward the more significant problems and the more destitute groups.

Education

As absurd as it may seem, Brazil currently has about 80 dental schools. The lobby of the private teaching community has defeated every attempt aimed at closing the deficient schools and preventing the opening of new ones. No doubt the

Education

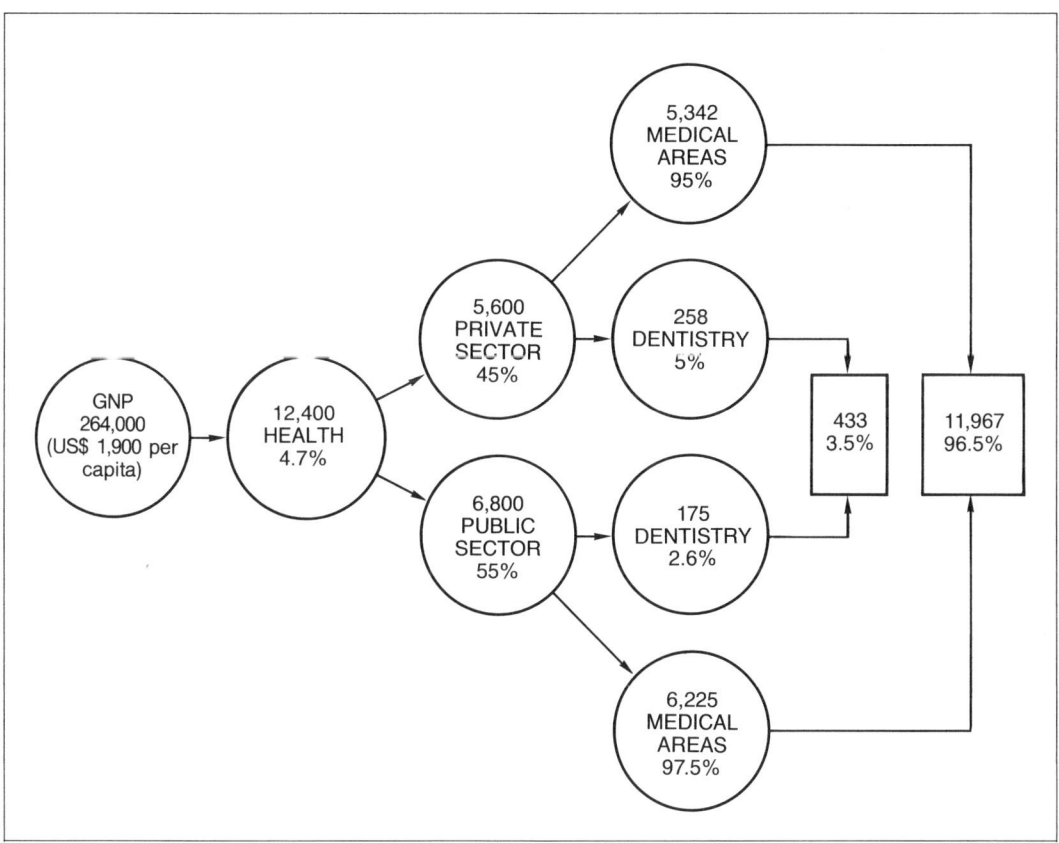

Fig 2 Health financial allocation — Brazil 1986 (US$ million).

Table 9 Demand for dental treatment Brazil 1988; estimate based on 1980 data (Viegas, AR)

Problem	Age group	Population (millions)	Needs	Dentists needed (thousands)	Problem	Age group	Population (millions)	Needs	Dentists needed (thousands)
Restorations and extractions of primary teeth	0–12	51.0	171	85.0	Prostheses (crowns; fixed, removable, and complete dentures)	15–70	77.5	160	130.0
Restorations and extractions of permanent teeth	7–14	26.0	152	75.0	Periodontal treatment (conservative)	15–70	77.5	146	150.0
Extractions	15–70	77.5	152	17.5					
Restorations	15–70	77.5	256	128.0	Periodontal treatment (surgical)	15–70	77.5	24	41.0

Source: Ministry of Social Welfare and Assistance, 1983.

teaching quality is not good for most schools. It is worth adding that many schools do show a high level of teaching and research, thanks to both the efforts of teachers with high pedagogical and scientific standards, and to the continuous interchange with the best odontologic centers in the world.

Prevention

Prevention of oral diseases should be seen from a wide-ranging approach, as it embodies the public health programs of fluoridation and the people's education provided by both public communication and by the private dental offices. The ideal solution is the fluoridation of the public water supplied by the cities' governments. We have enjoyed in Brazil considerable progress: in 1984, 28 million people were covered by fluoridation, and in 1988 this benefit reached 60 million. The forecast for the year 2000 is that 70% of the Brazilian population, approximately 105 million people, will be protected by fluoride. In the public school network, 3.5 million children already use weekly mouthwashes with sodium fluoride.

Sugar consumption in South America is a highly negative factor affecting caries control. Brazil is the third major sugar producer in the world, and its consumption is 137 g/day per capita (the maximum acceptable intake is 50 g/day per capita). Argentina consumes 92 g/day per capita, Chile 92 g/day per capita, Paraguay 68 g/day per capita, and Uruguay 88 g/day per capita. It is worth mentioning that our effort to discipline the population as to sugar consumption has been an inglorious task. We are always fighting the immense power of advertising promotions and the big candy, juice, and refreshment producers.

As paradoxical as it may seem, nutrition is a serious problem in terms of South American health care. Countries like Brazil and Argentina enjoy a privileged position in the world market of food production. Unfortunately, most of this production is exported. Most South American people do not eat proper diets, and there is a disquieting lack of basic nutritional factors in the diet of the poor population.

The 21st century

As stated previously, dentistry cannot be dissociated from the economic, social, and political contexts in which it exists. Thus, its future will depend on how the current structures of the region will evolve. In the beginning, the structural changes will probably be slow, but as the midpoint of the century approaches, great changes will influence dentistry and its practice, teaching, and social organization. Such changes, generated by advanced technological development, will dramatically affect such areas as prevention and treatment.

All things considered, South American dentistry will probably follow the development of worldwide dentistry, thanks to the increasing exchange of knowledge facilitated by mass communication and transportation means, which will transform the progress achieved universally. More and more, the world is becoming the global village anticipated by McLuhan. Prevention and technology will exert a considerable influence over every area of the profession: research, teaching, and professional practice.

Prevention

The more relevant and more foreseeable fact is unquestionably the impact of preventive measures. The use of fluoride and/or other preventive measures (which certainly will be developed) will have a more intense and universal application, thus reducing caries to negligible levels. A more comprehensive knowledge of the mouth, saliva, and oral microflora will allow the control of the harmful effects of dental plaque, thus dramatically decreasing caries and periodontal disease. The diet should be modified by mass education and public control of consumer goods, becoming healthier, with a lower consumption of carbohydrates.

Without caries and without periodontal disease, at least in the current levels, what will dentistry be? Certainly, professional activity will be very limited and directed to areas such as oral surgery, traumatology, orthodontics, preventive dentistry, oral medicine, and so forth. Work in restorative dentistry, prosthodontics, and endodontics, which are now the mainstream of dental practice, will be placed in the background and restricted to the treatment of traumatic injuries, surgical deformations, and esthetic repairs.

Another prevailing factor in the foreseeable changes in dentistry for the next century will be the technical-scientific development already on its way, in all areas of human activity, as we will see later.

Research

The volume of new knowledge, already considerable, will grow to vast proportions, thanks to the opportunities offered by technology. This large amount of information, notwithstanding its beneficial effects, will bring many difficulties to the process of incorporating them to scientific knowledge. Universities will require specialized teams to capture, analyze, and select new information so that it can be used in teaching and research. The information will be essential to this process because it provides more speed and flexibility for gathering, analyzing, and comparing data. It will also allow us to orient our research toward the most important areas, avoiding unnecessary repetition.

Research, which in the last decades has provided great help to the improvement of the quality of our profession, will certainly be the major drive for a progress never before dreamed of in prevention, diagnosis, and treatment of oral diseases.

Teaching

With the foreseeable results of caries and periodontal disease prevention, dentistry will lose many of its mechanical-surgical characteristics and will become prominently biological. Adhesive dentistry, already on its way, will dramatically reduce the need for cavity preparation in the treatment of caries. As a result, we will have great changes in teaching: the dental professional will be, necessarily, a specialist physician. Would the cost be justified, then, for the professional education of a dentist in a school specially designed for such purposes? Probably not. The technical training, which today occupies a considerable part of the curriculum, will be so reduced and restricted that it will not justify the time spent today with dental teaching. Perhaps we will be able to see the integration of dentistry to its natural place: medicine. Even medicine will probably undergo some modification once the volume of new knowledge makes unrealistic the education of a general physician in a 6-year course. The most feasible course may be to educate a general physician in a 4-year course and then offer specialization in specific areas (major surgery, psychiatry, etc) in which dentistry would be included.

The modus operandi of teaching will also be involved in the process of transformation, still by the influence of technology and communication breakthroughs. The main innovation should be, in my view, the possibility of remote teaching. Students and teachers would only need to come together for practical instruction and evaluations. Television and computers would bring to the students, in their homes, classes, seminars, and other conventional theoretical activities. Schools would broadcast their courses through the country or all over the world, and the students would have the chance to select the best ones in each specific curriculum area and "attend" them at home. In the same way, extracurricular activities such as congresses and other scientific events would be watched around the world in the same way we watch a live football game today. Complete courses could be recorded in video and made available to universities in every continent.

Organizing dental practices

The liberal practice of dentistry, predominant nowadays in Brazil and some South American countries, will not be the most common way of assisting patients. Also in this area, prevention and technology will be the determining factors of change.

The increasing specialization trend, generated by the high cost of technology and the results of prevention, will lead professionals to work in teams in private institutions under health care agreements, where the continuous exchange of information, ease in assisting patients, and reducing operational costs are possible. The technology that provides better treatment conditions through the use of instruments, equipment, and sophisticated materials also generates a considerable increase in costs. It will be difficult for the dentist to subsist individually, having to cope with the expenses derived from the acquisition of expensive equipment and instruments, on periodic continuing education and the management of a private clinic.

The predominant liberal practice system should be replaced in one of two ways: by team-working in private institutions under health care agreements, or by assistance financed by public resources, as is found today not only in South America but all around the world.

The predominance of one type of service or the other will depend on the economic conditions and sociopolitical systems existing in each country. In Brazil, and other South American countries, the tendency is for dentistry, like medicine, to be almost completely socialized.

Technology

The changes generated by technology will be much wider and numerous during the transition into the 21st century than they were from the past century to the present one. They will be much more evident in the field of biology and will lead to a greater knowledge of the human body, its function, and, most of all, the organism's reaction and defense processes. Immunology and genetic engineering will substantially alter the current concepts and practices of the dental treatment. New techniques and medicines will be available for prevention and treatment of infections, neoplasias, and other affections that occur in the mouth. We can already foresee the tremendous progress in the fields of diagnosis and planning with the recent introductions of new techniques, some of which are already available (television minicamera for intraoral use, digital x-ray equipment, magnetic resonance imaging, etc).

As to treatment itself, we expect as clinicians — and as patients too — that our forecast can become, as soon as possible, reality. First, we must look for an anesthetic system that eliminates pain without loss of consciousness and without the side effects provoked by the general anesthesia currently used. Perhaps the puncture might be one of the ways for developing a new anesthetic method. We still want a more effective and more rapid cavity preparation, without vibration, that is silent and less traumatic than the current system.

As to indirect restorations, we expect the development of new techniques and materials for impression and fabrication. More accurate impression and computerized fabrication can be already seen with the recent introduction of CAD/CAM systems. The current techniques for manufacture of metallic, ceramic, and polymer prostheses still present great difficulties and high cost, which makes them a benefit for the elite only. One can anticipate, before long, the advent of a polymer material with hardness, longevity, and biological compatibility — properties of porcelain — allied with the resilience, ease of handling, and lower cost of the current resins.

As to direct restorations, the great step should be the development of materials with the same characteristics of manipulation and marginal sealing as amalgam, the strength and corrosion resistance of the gold alloys, the adhesiveness and fluoride release of glass ionomers, and the esthetics of composite resins. In fact, what we want is an esthetic material that can substitute not for amalgam or gold, but for dental enamel and dentin.

In the field of pulp vitality protection, we will certainly have techniques and materials that will permit the biological sealing of dental tubules through a mineralization process generated by the pulp. In endodontics, we dream about the possibility of a noninvasive treatment, with sterilization and natural obliteration of the canals that nature does without our knowing today.

We hope that the new century brings agreement among the several schools of occlusion, and that the enlightened people of that fundamental area of dentistry find the ideal occlusion and feasible methods for its attainment.

Esthetics will become a greater concern of our patients, and to satisfy them we will need an effective and lasting process to bleach the dental structures as well as a truly adhesive esthetic material, durable and stable in color.

Also in the field of dental treatment, we entrust our hopes in the improvement of laser beams. The soft laser, which has been successfully used in the treatment of neuralgias and joint pains, could have, in the future, a larger application in the treatment of several injuries in the soft tissue of the mouth. The hard lasers, which have been widely applied in medical surgery, probably will be incorporated in the armamentarium of the dental surgeon for surgical intervention without bleeding and with local sterilization by the beam. Other applications of the hard lasers, some in advanced stages of research, are sealing of pits and fissures on the tooth enamel surface; treatment of white enamel lesions; cavity preparation; soldering of extracted teeth to the remaining ones for the building of immediate natural fixed partial dentures; attaching brackets in orthodontics; direct cementation of etched fixed partial dentures; splinting mobile teeth; building of space maintainers; soldering of metals inside the mouth; sterilization and sealing of root canals, etc. The use of lasers is still in an experimental stage, but technology has been evolving at a fast rate and harmful side effects such as heat release should be under control in the very near future.

A great need with a promising future is the attainment of oral implant systems. We believe that an implant system can be developed without the current clinical restrictions and at a cost within the reach of the majority of the population.

These are my forecasts and my hopes. However, as fantastic and fascinating the technological advances may be, none of them will be more important and more desirable than the eradication of oral diseases. I hope that, when the ideal products and techniques are developed, prevention will have already made them useless.

Further reading

Chesnais, J-C: La Revanche du Tiers-Monde, Portuguese translation, Editora Espaço e Tempo, Rio de Janeiro, 1989.

Coopers and Lyland: Relatório Anual da Economia Mundial, in *O Estado de São Paulo*, Brasil, 1989.

Instituto Nacional de Assistência Médica da Previdência Social: Programa de Orientação da Assistência Odontológica, MPAS/CCS, Rio de Janeiro, 1983.

International Bank for Reconstruction and Development/World Bank: World Development Report 1988, Washington, DC, 1988.

Ministério da Saúde do Brasil: Levantamento Epidemiológico em Saúde Bucal; Brasil Zona Urbana, 1986, CDMS, Brasília, 1988.

Ministério da Saúde do Brasil: Política Nacional de Saúde Bucal, Brasília, October 1988.

Pinto, VG: Perfil da Odontologia Brasileira, Documento Técnico 01/88, Divisão Nacional de Saúde Bucal, Brasil, 1988.

Pinto, VG: Informe Consolidado sobre el Sistema de Salud Bucal en Argentina, Brasil, Chile, Paraguay y Uruguay, OPS/OMS, July 1984.

Souza, PR: Quem Paga a Conta? Editora Brasiliense, São Paulo, Brasil, 1989.

Chapter 4

21st-Century Dentistry in Spain

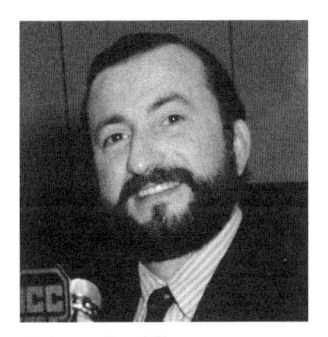

Jaime A. Gil
Bilbao, Spain

Abstract

Dentistry in Spain will experience very important changes in the next century.

Since Spain became a member of the European Community, a new 5-year dental curricula has been established through which students graduate with a dental degree.

The major concern of Spanish dentistry is the enormous competition that may develop between the new national graduates, the European dentists that will be coming to practice in Spain after 1992, and the great number of Latin American dentists already practicing in our country.

This can develop into a situation where they all might be trying to fight unemployment working on a salary for the Spanish National Health Service, on a percentage for an insurance company, or on a special partnership with the Spanish government—the so-called capitation system.

For the first half of this century, dental students were able to graduate in Spain with a DDS degree; it was not until 1948 that dentistry was considered to be a medical specialty and students were obliged to undertake 6 years of medical studies before they could begin dental training.

At that time there were only two dental schools in the whole country and that situation remained until 1987. The increasing demand for dental treatment by the Spanish population compelled the government to open several new dental schools that accepted only medical graduates.

When Spain became a member of the European Community it was requested that a dental curriculum be developed that would offer a dental degree similar to those available in the other European countries. Now the dental schools in Spain are gradually switching to the new curriculum that consists of a 5-year program specifically devoted to dentistry.

The increasing number of applicants to these new dental studies has obliged

39

the government to limit the number of students accepted in each school, because almost 1,000 dentists will be graduating each year among the nine schools. Furthermore, cultural agreements between Spain and some Latin American countries enable dentists from those countries to practice in Spain. For political and financial reasons, there are currently more than 2,000 Latin American dentists who have elected to emigrate from their native countries and practice in Spain; many more are considering moving into our country. Moreover, Spain will open its doors to all European dentists in 1992. Thus, although the awareness for dental treatment is increasing in the Spanish population, the Spanish General Dental Council is indeed very worried because many of our new dental graduates of the new curricula may be unemployed from the day they graduate.

In the past, all dentistry in Spain has been under private enterprise, and the patient had to pay the total amount of his or her dental treatment. Insurance companies have become aware of this situation and are proliferating tremendously as many dentists that are already suffering a shortage of patients become interested in this type of partnership with an insurance company. Unemployment among dentists will make insurance companies more and more attractive because dentists will find in them a good source of patients.

This may create a situation where the insurance companies will make the investment and the dentists will end up being salaried. The same kind of situation could result if the Spanish National Health Service develops its future project toward dental public health. Only a few years ago, no dentist working in Spain would have even considered working on a salary for the National Health Service.

The biggest problem the state will have in developing this project to provide a more comprehensive dental treatment is cost. The amount of the investment for public dental health centers is so great that the government could consider establishing a capitation system in the near future.

One may expect, then, that the overriding concern of Spanish dentistry will be the competition among national, Latin American, and European dentists trying to fight unemployment by working on a salary for the Spanish National Health Service, on a percentage for an insurance company, or in a special partnership with the Spanish social government — the so-called capitation system.

Trying to fight unemployment, dentists will go back to school to become specialists by pursuing postdoctoral studies. However, specialists need referrals, and no general dentists will be ready to refer patients when they will actually be lacking patients themselves.

Competition will oblige the general dentists to increase their knowledge and improve their techniques in the different fields of dentistry, and will create a higher demand for clinical courses in continuing education.

As the number of unemployed dentists increases, the demand for applications to study dentistry will decrease, and dental schools will have to lower the requirements for the entering students; most will probably even have to start marketing their own programs, to make them attractive for prospective students, by offering courses in the newest topics — cosmetic dentistry and implants. As a result, the general dentist will be trained in a broad spectrum of treatment modalities but probably with no great depth in any of them. This would certainly affect the quality of available dental treatment, and eventually pressure would be put on dental schools to turn out better qualified dentists. This situation, together with the decrease in the number of applications, will inevitably result in the closure of several dental schools.

Nevertheless, the question that will always remain is: How do we improve the quality of applicants entering dental schools? It would not be the least surprising if the answer would be to accept applicants with a medical degree. This, of course, will take generations to occur, because the average age of the Spanish dentist in the year 2000 will be in the middle 30s. History would prove to repeat itself if dentistry would again be considered a medical specialty in the second half of the next century.

Further reading

Alijarde J: Demografia Profesional en la 1° Región. *Profesión Dental* 1986; XV (3):9–22.

Bascones Martinez A: El odontólogo y estomatòlogo ante la Comunidad Económica Europea. *Profesión Dental* 1986; XIV (1):9–12.

Bracco P: La Odontología en los Paises de la Comunidad Económica Europea: Italia. *Profesión Dental* 1986;XIV(2):9–16.

Monlleo Pons J: Informe de la Colegiación de Odontólogos y Estomatólogos en España: Madrid. *Consejo General de Colegios de Odontólogos y Estomatólogos de España* 1987:32.

Moreno Gonzalez JP: Reflexiones sobre el número de Odonto-Estomatólogos y su formación. *Boletín de Información Dental* 1982; XLII (318):43–52.

Chapter 5

Dentistry in the 21st Century: The Future Will Be Different — But Better!

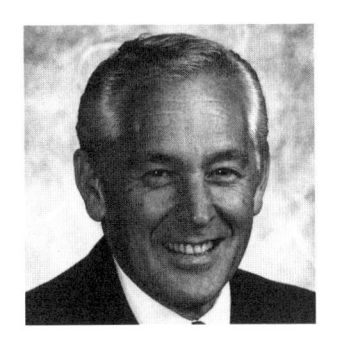

Arthur A. Dugoni*
San Francisco, California

Abstract

As the 21st century approaches, the dental profession faces serious challenges to its future. Dentistry's environment has changed. Society's emphasis over the next 20 years will shift from the needs of the young to the concerns and demands of Americans in their middle years and to the elderly.

The future for dentistry will lie in more noninvasive options: less mechanical/surgical repair; more care dependent on an indepth knowledge of chemistry and biology; more sophisticated diagnosis and treatment planning alternatives; and more systemic and topical use of antibiotics and other chemicals to prevent and treat.

Senator Robert Kennedy said the following: "Some men see things as they are and say why. I dream of things that never were and say why not?" It is obvious to me that this outstanding international meeting continues to ask that question, "Why not?" Why not an outstanding educational meeting? Why not one of the best meetings in the world? Why not provide an opportunity for the communication of knowledge? The American Dental Association is proud to share with you several commitments:

- To prevent dental disease and improve the health of the citizens of the world.
- To educate those citizens to the new technological and scientific advances that will improve the quality of their lives.
- To improve the skill and knowledge of dentists all over the world.

This meeting is a major commitment and contribution to that effort.

As the 21st century approaches, the dental profession faces serious chal-

* At the time of this symposium, Dr Dugoni was President of the American Dental Association.

lenges to its future. Whether it be a biological species or a profession, survival depends on successful adaptation to change. Dentistry's environment has changed — we cannot wish the changes away — and they are a part of our social and economic milieu. We will need to utilize our best talent to help us successfully adapt to a different future.

Recent history

To better understand some of the issues related to practice, education, and licensure, it is important to review some of the recent history and concerns of the dental profession in the United States. In 1926, Dr William Gies published his classic evaluation of dental education. The results described dentistry as a technical trade rather than a profession. Dr Gies indicated that most students were enrolled in proprietary schools and no attention was paid to the basic or clinical sciences. The professional community responded to the challenge he set forth. Currently, dental education takes place only in accredited universities, and students are given a strong foundation in the basic and clinical sciences. Over the last 60 years, dentistry has developed from a trade to a respected and learned profession; from ignorance to understanding because of the standards and quality of education and the standards and quality of practice; and our clinical and scientific research efforts, which are the hallmark of a profession.

The 1960s were characterized by expansion and growth. The federal government provided approximately $250 million for the rebuilding and development of new dental schools, and dental enrollments were markedly increased in anticipation of increased demand for dental care. The 1970s revealed that the demands for care were being met by the profession but that dental schools were continuing to produce dentists at an ever increasing rate. This factor, coupled with other events, led to a period of deep concern, characterized by pessimism, which permeated the profession during the late 1970s and early 1980s. The national economy was in a period of recession, the profession was over-producing dentists, and the results of our preventive techniques were beginning to be most evident.

Future demand for care

Dentistry is a young profession and its research efforts are younger yet. Most of the progress in dental research has been accomplished over the past 50 years. In 1950 only $300,000 was spent for dental research in contrast to over $140 million in 1989. What we have accomplished in prevention, diagnosis and treatment, and new technological advances has rarely been equalled by any learned profession. Billions of dollars have been saved annually in dental treatment because of our outstanding research efforts, especially those related to prevention and treatment of caries and periodontal disease.

It is generally assumed that the decline

in tooth decay will lead to a reduction in the demand for dental services. As dental caries declines, so will the demand for basic restorative dentistry, but this does not mean there will be an overall reduction in the demand for dental services. Many factors other than the incidence of caries will continue to influence demand; factors such as education, insurance coverage, affluence, age, and the employment of our citizens are equally important.

Although fluoride, fluoridation, and emphasis on community and personal preventive practices have resulted in a marked decrease in caries in children in the United States and in many other developed countries, major dental diseases are not disappearing, but their patterns in the population are changing and other services are expanding. From 1971 to 1980, approximal caries decreased about 50% in the 5- to 7-year-old age group. In 1980, 37% of these children were free of caries, and in 1987 almost 50% were caries free. The major beneficiaries of multiple fluorides and other preventive practices have been the younger age groups, but 25% of children still have very high dental decay rates. In addition, some significant changes are occurring in the adult population. The adult population is increasing in number, and a greater proportion will retain their teeth for a longer period of time. As these older adults increase in number, their dental health becomes increasingly important. The number of middle-aged and older adults who will retain their teeth over the next 20 to 30 years becomes a major factor in looking at future demands for dental care.

It has been estimated that in the next 10 to 40 years, even assuming a continued decline in caries prevalence, the hours of operative dentistry treatment needs for adults aged 35 to 44 years will increase dramatically. Using 1972 as a base year, the number of hours needed was 21.6 million hours; in 1990 the need will be 32.8 million hours; and in 2030 the need will be 34.9 million hours. This represents a 62% increase from 1972 to 2030. This trend is largely due to the increasing number of dentulous adults who will be present in the older age groups by the year 2000. This estimate does not take into account the increased demand that has developed for the treatment of periodontal disease, cosmetic dentistry, orthodontics, orthognathic surgery, sealants, and dental implants. Reinhardt and Douglass reported on a regional survey in the Northeast that found that dentists were generating 10% of their gross income from esthetic treatment of noncarious teeth. What we will see over the next several decades is not an elimination of the need for restorative dentistry but a change in target populations and changes in procedures with new materials and techniques, hence an increased scope of services. With fewer extractions (as a result of the reduction in dental decay), the demand for fixed partial dentures and complicated restorative dentistry should actually increase, because traditionally, the edentulous patient has had a very low rate of utilization. With more teeth at dental risk, adults will have more dental needs.

NIDR study (21,000 working adults)

Preliminary data from a 1986 National Institute of Dental Research study of 21,000 working adults aged 18 to 64 years and seniors aged 65 years and above has added to our data base.

- Only 4% of persons aged 18 to 64 years are edentulous (average 24 to 25 teeth per person); 50% have lost at most one permanent tooth. This represents a significant drop in tooth loss from what was seen in a 1971 to 1974 survey.
- A total of 42% of persons over age 65 were missing all of their teeth; only 2% had all 28 permanent teeth.

Data to date

Coronal caries

- The incidence of coronal caries has declined in persons aged 18 to 35 years.
- In persons above age 35 years, little change in coronal caries incidence has been noted.
- In persons aged 18 to 64 years, 95% of coronal caries have been restored. An extraordinarily high level of dental care is seen.
- We are eliminating edentulism.
- Caries improvement has been shown in younger adults.

Root caries

- There is a fair amount of root caries secondary to recession.
- A total of 21% of employed adults have root caries.
- A total of 63% of persons over age 65 have root caries.
- Only 50% of caries (in both groups) have been restored.

Periodontal disease in working adults (aged 18 to 64 years)

- A total of 43% had one or more gingival sites with gingivitis.
- Some 77% had at least one site with periodontal attachment losses.
- A total of 2% had pockets measuring 6 mm or more.
- Fully 24% had 4 mm or more of attachment loss.

Periodontal disease in seniors (over age 65 years)

- Of these, 47% had gingivitis.
- Fully 95% had at least one site with periodontal attachment loss.
- A total of 4% had pockets measuring 6 mm or deeper.
- Some 68% had 4 mm or more of attachment loss.

Summary

- Up to age 40 to 45 years dental health is surprisingly good.
- After age 50 years dental health declines.
- As for persons over age 65 years, Dr Harald Löe, NIDR director, states:

"Clearly, the worst problems are in the older segments of the population. This group has high rates of caries, periodontal disease, and tooth loss with all the attendant pain and suffering, plus the need for dental services."

Periodontal disease

The new concepts of the periodontal disease process and the trend toward simpler treatment methods should produce significant changes in periodontal education and practice. Surveys indicate that periodontal disease accounts for only 4% to 5% of practice time. However, the severe form of the disease — periodontitis — is seen predominantly in lower socioeconomic patients, and these patients have comparatively low rates of utilization of dental care. Although the need is clearly there, the demand for periodontal care is not predictable. Periodontal disease receives very little attention by today's practitioners because of dental education's past emphasis on restorative techniques. With an aging population and a growing appreciation of the desirability of retaining teeth, we can anticipate an increased need for periodontal care.

Science and technology

The relevance of basic science and clinical research is expanding into clinical practice. We are all aware of innovations in dental treatment, such as the new restorative materials that allow dentists to produce more services per unit of practice time. Other changes include more sophisticated diagnosis and treatment planning alternatives; more systemic and topical use of antibiotics and other chemicals; and the effects of new developments in medicine, genetic engineering, and immunology as they impact the dental profession.

The future of dentistry holds more non-invasive options; less mechanical/surgical repair, and more treatment that depends on an in-depth knowledge of chemistry and biology. In addition, enamel remineralization, microbiological testing for caries and periodontal disease, enamel and dentin bonding, sealants, and dental implants will become vital components of dental education and practice for the 1990s.

Demand for orthodontics

The orthodontist of the next decade will be challenged and stimulated by more innovation and change than in the previous history of orthodontics. The next decade will demand an orthodontist who is more occlusally sophisticated and who has an increasing awareness of the periodontal implications of adult therapy. Orthodontics will be heavily involved in joint clinical treatment plans with oral surgeons, fixed prosthodontists, and restorative dentists. Orthodontists will find themselves involved more in surgical orthodontic correction, in functional appliances, in primary and mixed dentition treatment, in a greater appreciation of the effects of the airways on growth, development, and treatment, and thus more consultation with otolaryngologists. The orthodontic practice, both management and diagnosis, will become more heavily involved with computer technology. Rigid endosseous implants will provide exciting abutments for the correction of malocclusions and craniofacial anomalies.

Orthodontics may be a unique field in dentistry because malocclusion is largely determined by genetic factors and the need for care does not fluctuate widely, as may be the case for caries or periodontal diseases. Yet orthodontic care has experienced tremendous growth, particularly for adults. In the past 20 years the number of adults being treated in specialty orthodontic practices has increased from 5% to 35%. The prospect that this was caused by a fivefold increase in disease prevalence is unrealistic.

It is estimated that approximately two thirds of preadolescent American children would benefit from orthodontic treatment, roughly half of these having definite to severe malocclusions. The percentages of adolescents aged 12 to 17 years who could benefit or that might require care are slightly higher. No accurate estimate for the adult population is available.

Sociodemographics

The sociodemographic trends indicate an increase in the demand for dental care. The nation is growing middle aged and more solitary. Men and women are delaying marriage, postponing childbirth, having few or no children at all. The data show that our environment has changed. It is imperative for the dental profession and dental education to adapt if the profession as we know it is to prosper. Most of the changes have been triggered by the baby boom generation — individuals born between 1946 and 1964 and numbering 75 million strong (one out of every three Americans, the largest generation in United States history). The oldest members of this generation have turned 40 years old. The generation that could hum television jingles before they could hum the national anthem, that made rock and roll and protest as "rites of passage," and that swore never to trust anyone over 30 is becoming middle aged. This group, with the highest buying power, has the greatest number of restored teeth. As this group continues to mature in the 1990s it will constitute the largest market for replacement restorations, fixed partial dentures, endodontics, periodontics, cosmetic dentistry, implants, and orthodontics.

In 1986 the median age of the population reached 31.4 years; this is the oldest median ever, and it is expected to exceed 36 years by the year 2000. By the early 1990s one half of our households will be headed by baby boomers, one fourth of our population will be elderly, and these two groups will define our society for a very long time. There are more Americans over age 65 than there are teenagers. Single persons now account for 23% of all United States households. As many as 8% of today's adults will never marry. Families with single heads of households grew by 69% from 1970 to 1983. One out of every five children, and more than half of all black children, live in a one-parent household. Fifteen years ago 45% of all households consisted of a husband, wife, and children; today that figure is less than 28%. The stereotypical nuclear family of mom, dad, and two kids now accounts for less than 11% of all households.

The number of female-headed households with one or more children under 18 more than doubled from 1970 to 1982, from 2.9 million to 5.9 million. In 1960 only 19% of women with children under 16 years of age were in the workforce; today half of them are.

In spite of decreasing birth rates, immigration will keep the population in the United States from shrinking. If the projected rates of immigration and fertility are realized, 100 years from now the United States will have a population of about 300 million, of whom 16% will be black, 16% Hispanic, 10% Asian, and a diminishing majority of 58% non-Hispanic whites.

Demographers predict that population shifts in the South and West will continue over the next two decades; however, they are likely to occur at a slower rate as the population ages, the natural resources of these areas (notably energy sources and water supplies) are depleted, and their tax rates rise. Population shifts are also occurring within each region of the country. Although three quarters of the population currently live in metropolitan areas and only one quarter live in rural areas, data from the 1980 census indicate that more people moved away from metropolitan areas than moved to them during the 1970s, reversing a long established trend. The growth of small towns and rural areas not adjacent to a metropolitan area was particularly impressive because it does not reflect metropolitan sprawl or spillover.

In 1980, for the first time, the majority of Americans lived in the South and West. During the 1970s, California, Florida, and Texas had 42% of the United States' total growth. America's past has been one of steady centralization; its future is likely to be one of steady population deconcentration. People are moving to smaller, less-crowded communities, particularly those with a population under a quarter of a million.

Adults 65 years and older

Today's elderly, especially the young elderly (under 70 years) are a "marketeer's dream," says Arthur D. Little, Inc, a consulting firm based in Cambridge, Massachusetts. In 2025 there will be 64 million people over age 65, and the nation will have fewer than four working-aged individuals for every retirement-aged person. In addition to having more teeth, the elderly will be more affluent and better educated than in the past. Over the past few decades, the average years of education have increased from 10.3 years to 12.4 years and are still increasing. The 26% of the population over age 50 years controls three quarters of the nation's financial assets. With $130 billion in discretionary income, this represents one half of the spending power.

The over-age 75 population presents a special problem, and it is growing. Predictions indicate there will be 100,000 individuals over age 100 years by the year 2000. They have significant problems with ambulation, and for the dentist it will require greater knowledge of medicine and drug interaction because most adults over age 75 years are on multiple drugs. The care for our elderly citizens will demand changes in our education program and in practice. Thus, there will be more challenges for education to adequately prepare practitioners.

Society's emphasis over the next 20 years will shift from the needs of the young to the concerns and demands of Americans in the middle years, and to the elderly.

Retirement

There have been remarkable changes in the retirement ages of our citizens. The percentage of men in the workforce who are aged 65 and older fell from 46% to 19% in the past 30 years, and further decline in the percentage of the elderly employed is expected. In addition, the cost of time to the retired person is much less than for the employed. Therefore, there will be more demand for care. Equally evident is that dentists, as part of the population, also are retiring early. In view of the malpractice liability crisis, there appears to be a trend for more dental colleagues to retire earlier and also to discontinue their part-time practices as they reach retirement years. The decrease in the number of practicing dentists through retirement will also positively affect demand.

Dental economics

The recession of the late 1970s and the early 1980s had a significant impact on all sectors of the economy, including dentistry. But the economics of dentistry has significantly improved in the late 1980s. According to the Health Care Financing Administration (HCFA), dentistry was a $32 billion industry, growing at the average rate of about $1.6 billion each year since 1984.

For the last 3 years in a row, dentists' growth in net income has exceeded growth in the consumer price index (ie, income has risen faster than inflation). Real gross national product (which is gross national product adjusted for inflation) was in excess of a 2% increase each year for the last 6 years. The national expenditure for dental care is basically a function of national income and wealth. As wealth increases, dental care expenditures increase at an even faster rate.

Dental offices were the third highest ranking category of start-up businesses most likely to survive, according to a survey of nearly 1.5 million companies reported in the January 1988 issue of *Inc.* The study covered new business ventures started between 1978 and 1987 in 236 industry categories.

In 1987, the average net income of all general practitioners was $80,190; the mean net income of dental specialists was approximately $110,000. The average net income for a dentist under 35 years of age was $60,490 and for those aged 45 to 49 years it was $96,110 in 1987. Specialists in the 45 to 49 year age group averaged $128,600 a year net income. In 1987, college graduates aged 25 to 29 years earned an average of $28,240. Dentists under age 30 years averaged $44,480 in 1987, which was 1.6 times what college graduates in the 25 to 29 year age group earned. The average net income of a dentist in 1989 is expected to reach about $93,000.

Dentistry is an excellent example of free enterprise at its best. Dentists rank seventh in highest salaries, according to a book entitled, *Nine Highest Paying Careers for the 80's* by Anita Gates. Ranked above dentists were investment bankers ($100,000 plus); physicians ($100,000); security traders ($80,000); and security trade persons ($75,000). Law was 8th; optometry was 9th; veterinary medicine was 13th; engineering was 27th; architecture was 44th; computer programming was 55th; and commercial art was 80th.

In 1987, 100 million people were covered under dental benefit plans. Private dental insurance payments accounted for 37% of the nation's expenditures for dental care.

Dental practice

Solo/private practice will continue to be the predominant delivery system. Currently, over 90% of the dentists are in private practice, either owning their own practices or in partnership. Well over 70% are in solo private practice, and in 20 to 25 years solo private practice will still be the predominant mode for dental care delivery. The majority of dentists (93.1%) own their own practices. Of these, 56.3% are solo proprietors, 30.3% are shareholders in an incorporated dental practice, and 6.5% are partners. About 6.9% of private practitioners are non-owners; 4.5% are employed as an associate on a salary, commission, or percentage basis; and 2.4% are independent contractors.

The solo dental practice is the most typical type of practice. About 70% of the nation's private practitioners are working in a practice with no other dentist; 17.3% are working with one other dentist; and 12.6% practice with two or more dentists. Among dentists out of school less than 4 years, about 68% own their own practice. By 6 years after graduation, this figure increases to 82%.

As for time spent in practice, 88% of all dentists practice less than 40 hours a week and 10% practice 50 or more hours a week. The average number of dental patient visits per week in 1987 (including hygiene appointments) was 82, or an annual average of about 3,900. About 88% of dentists' time in practice is spent treating patients. On average, dentists work with and supervise about four staff members (three full-time and one part-time employee).

Dental workforce

For the academic year 1988 to 1989 there were 57 dental schools that had a 4 academic year – 4 calendar year program, whereas one school, the University of the Pacific (San Francisco), had a 4 academic year – 3 calendar year program and another, the Harvard School of Dental Medicine, had a 5 academic year – 5 calendar year program. Three private dental schools closed in the 1980s and two more announced future closure.

The 1988 first-year class in United States dental schools of 4,196 students represents a 4% decrease from last year's enrollment of 4,370 and a 33.4% decrease from the first-year enrollment in 1978. This year, for the eighth time, total enrollment in dental schools has dropped from 17,885 in 1987 to 1988 to 17,094 in 1988 to 1989, and first-year enrollment is down again for the tenth year. An analysis of the enrollment information on women students, though, indicates that the number continues to rise. The percentage of women in 1989 was 34%, a large increase from the percentage of just 10 years ago. Depending on their years in the labor force and their productivity in practice, the greater number of women dentists may have an affect on the supply of dental service. Also relevant is the retirement age of dentists and the greater number of women entering the dental profession. The age that dentists retire from practice may be declining. Also, with the increasing problems of malpractice insurance, fewer older dentists may find it financially rewarding to practice on a part-time basis. If this is true, the problems of excess dentists may be resolved sooner than expected.

The Human Resources and Services Administration has made predictions of dentists and dentists-to-population ratios to the year 2020. According to their predictions, the number of dentists will increase until the end of the century, peaking at 154,000. The number of dentists will decrease each year during the 21st century, falling to 135,800 in the year 2020. The dentists-to-population ratio will rise to 60.6 in the early 1990s then decline to 44.8 in the year 2020. Accordingly, the dentists-to-population ratio for the United States will fall to its lowest level since the end of World War I. From 1985 to the year 2000, the profession will increase by 16,000 dentists, but the population will grow by 30 million.

Medical workforce

The picture for the medical profession is quite different. The number of medical school applicants is just beginning to decline, and so far there have been minimal changes in the size of the entering class. A presidential task force estimated that by the year 2000 there will be over 100,000 excess physicians. Physicians are likely to see a major decline in their income and their relative negotiating power with fiscal intermediaries, hospitals, health maintenance organizations, and other delivery organizations. Their problems will be further exacerbated by the attempts of government and industry to control health care costs. Thus, just at a time when the medical workforce is expanding, the financial system is beginning to contract.

Dentistry is in a much stronger position than medicine to adjust to the new market conditions. As the decline in physicians' incomes accelerates (and the evidence is there already), applications to medical schools will decline, as they have in dentistry; however, dental school applications may benefit from this shift.

Numbers of specialists

A recent report from the Bureau of Health Professions of the Department of Health and Human Services predicted a rise in the ratio of specialists to active dentists from 13.9% today to over 20% by the year 2000. Specialty programs have been initiated and enlarged, usually at the expense of predoctoral teaching programs. Overspecialization in medicine has been responsible for the emergence of family practice as a new field of medicine.

Accreditation and licensure

Each of the 57 dental schools in the United States is accredited by a national accrediting agency. The accreditation of dental education institutions was established by federal legislation and is the responsibility of the United States Commission on Post Secondary Education. The responsibility for dental accreditation has been delegated to the Commission on Dental Accreditation. National standards, along with criteria guidelines, have been established by the profession and the educational community to which each dental school is measured. Each dental school undergoes a regular and vigorous accreditation process, which includes a site visit by a team from the Commission on Dental Accreditation.

In addition to the accreditation process, the passage of the National Board Dental Examinations is required as a partial fulfillment of the requirements for licensure in the 50 states of the United States. This is a two-part test, devised and administered by the Joint Commission on National Dental Examinations. Part I, taken after 2 years of dental school, focuses on the basic biomedical sciences; Part II, generally taken during the final year, focuses on clinical subjects.

An additional aspect of the private practice situation is state licensure. Formerly, all 50 states had their own didactic and clinical examinations. Didactic examinations have now been supplanted in almost all state boards by the National Board Dental Examinations.

In the United States, the licensure authority is vested with individual states. They verify competency by means of state or regional examinations. Currently, we have four regional examinations, each composed of a number of different states. These include the Northeast Regional Board, representing 15 states (including the District of Columbia); the Southern Regional Board, representing 4 states; the Central Regional Board, representing 10 states; and the Western Regional Board, representing 5 states. There are 17 states that do not participate in any of the regional board examinations; each has their own licensing examination. Passage of a regional or state board examination makes candidates eligible to practice in any of the states participating in the practical examination.

Twenty-seven state jurisdictions have statutory authority to recognize the licenses granted to a dentist by another jurisdiction and waive all theoretical and clinical licensing examinations for such dentists; however, currently only 18 states are exercising this authority. Licensure by credential is the policy of the American Dental Association. Licensure by credential involves awarding a license to a dentist who is already licensed in another state on the basis of his or her practice record, without examination, or without complete examination. In a 1986 survey, the American Dental Association found that 77% of its membership favored licensure by credential; hence freedom of movement and the licensure issue in the United States is a major concern of the association's membership. Regardless of the progress made with the National Dental Board Examinations for the didactic portions of licensure, the participation of 34 states in regional examinations, and the American Dental Association's policy on licensure by credential, there is still no national clinical examination that satisfies all of the 50 state jurisdictions.

Dentistry enters a new age of innovation

Dental health of Americans has been dramatically improved in the past 40 years. Decay rates in children have plummeted, edentulousness in middle-aged adults has nearly been eradicated, and older adults are keeping more of their natural teeth longer. That epoch included the advent of fluoride, research that identified tooth decay and gum disease as bacterial infections, and huge technological advances in devices and materials. The 1980s has signaled a new era that is changing the face of dentistry again.

In another 40 years we will look back and reflect that the 1980s and 1990s were unsurpassed in the development of dentistry. We have already seen dramatic advances in terms of the comprehensive care we are now able to offer each patient. One of the greatest things that will happen is the reduction of the restorative needs of our patients. Dental decay and periodontal disease, our major dental scourges, are now clearly controllable and essentially preventable.

As the turn of the century approaches, prevention and control of periodontal disease — which strikes 9 out of 10 adults sometime during their lives — will intensify. Efforts are already underway to develop tests that will identify patients at high risk of developing the disease. In periodontal disease control we continue to have some of our biggest breakthroughs. We are approaching prevention of periodontal disease with chemical as well as with mechanical means, and it all started with the identification of bacterial plaque.

The focus of restorative care will largely shift from children to adults, with dramatic gains in the control of decay around old restorations and on tooth roots. As adults keep more of their teeth, dentistry will develop more appealing and durable restorative materials. Tooth-colored, resin-based restorative materials have been improved at a rapid pace in the 1980s. As a result, esthetic dentistry is booming. Dental researchers have developed a simplified resin-based system that achieves a strong bond to dentin. Adhesive bonding to enamel and dentin will eliminate the concept of cavity preparation as we know it. This process could revolutionize the restoration of badly damaged teeth, preserving more tooth structure than is now possible while providing highly esthetic results.

The few teeth people lose will be increasingly replaced with dental implants. Implants will be used to replace single teeth or entire dental arches as legitimate alternatives to dentures and other restorative work. The use of implants is already booming as a result of improved design, materials, and techniques. There was a fourfold increase in implant procedures from 1983 to 1987; about 300,000 procedures are estimated by 1992.

Other new developments on the horizon include expanded use of computers, which are being used in experimental systems that can measure a tooth and direct a milling machine to precision cut a tooth crown. New computer software can provide dentists with immediate access to diagnosis and treatment options for dental procedures, and can be used for imaging, which allows patients to see a before-and-after picture of themselves. Although used quite successfully for other surgeries, dentists are now beginning to use lasers to cut inflamed or diseased gum tissue. A modification of the laser beam currently under review by the Food and Drug Administration will allow dentists to seal or remove decay, which may eliminate the dental drill in the future.

Dentistry will gradually evolve toward medicine, with an even heavier emphasis on prevention. The behavioral and psychological aspects of dental treatment will play increasingly important roles in patient management and motivation. There will be an increased emphasis on the development of strong communication skills, and oral health will be considered a part of general health. Geriatric care continues to be of ever-increasing importance to the dentist in the United States as the population continues to live longer and retain their natural teeth. The dentist of the future will need to know more about oral medicine and the treatment of elderly patients with major medical problems on multiple drug therapies. Advances in the development of synthetic bone point to continued improvement in the treatment of patients who have had periodontal disease or who have lost alveolar bone structure.

There is a new wave of optimism among the 143,000 dentists in the United States, and the profession is ready for a new golden age. The reasons for the optimism are primarily reduction of first-year class sizes from 6,301 in 1978 to approximately 4,000 in 1990; outstanding technological and scientific advances; and the increased longevity of the citizens of the United States. When you consider the demographics of the population and combine this with the technological and scientific changes and the decrease in dental graduates, there is an outstanding future for dentistry in the United States. All of this information, combined with the scientific and technical advances (which include implants, lasers, computers, surgical orthodontics, veneering, bonding, and sealants), strongly indicates that this is an exciting time for the dental profession. It is a time of change and challenge. The dental profession should welcome the change and savor the challenges, because they open up opportunities that shape the future. Let us forget about the anxiety and the doom and gloom — the best is yet to come. We all need to realize that we can adapt to meet the changes. Let us prepare our practices for the real world; develop practice patterns to handle the single parent and the elderly; prepare to move practices or to relocate them in rural areas; and expand practice skills to include periodontics, endodontics, orthodontics, cosmetic dentistry, prevention, implant therapy, facial pain, and oral medicine.

There are significant demographic statistics that provide a strong basis for a very positive future for the dental profession:

- There will be 52 million more Americans aged 17 to 65 years in the year 2000 than there were in the year 1975.
- From 1985 to the year 2000 the profession will grow by 16,000 dentists, but the country will grow by 30 million.
- There were 2.8 billion teeth at risk in 1972; there will be 5 billion teeth at risk in the year 2030.
- Americans place a high value on dental care — 60% of the adult working population now visit dentists annually. Adults over age 65 have increased their annual visits significantly from 25% in 1983 to 41% in 1986.
- Dentistry is an excellent example of free enterprise at its best. When you consider the demographics of the population and combine this with the technological and scientific changes and the decrease in dental graduates, there is an outstanding future for dentistry in the United States.

Further reading

American Dental Association: *Strategic Plan — Report of the American Dental Association's Special Committee on the Future of Dentistry.* Chicago: American Dental Association, July 1983.

Mandel ID: Looking towards the future of dentistry. In: *Block Drug Company Perspectives in Dental Science,* Vol. 1, No. 1, May 1985.

American Dental Association, Bureau of Economic and Behavioral Research. *Survey of Dental Practice.* Chicago: American Dental Association, 1983.

Health Insurance Association of America, 1982–1983, *Source Book of Health Insurance Data.*

American Dental Association, Division of Educational Measurements: *Annual Reports — Dental Education, 1970–1984.* Chicago: American Dental Association.

National Institute of Dental Research: *National Dental Caries Prevalence Study, 1979–1980.*

National Center for Health Statistics. Basic Data on Dental Examination Findings of Persons 1–74 years. Series 11, No. 214. BHHSDHHS Publication Number (PHS) 79–1662, issued May 1979.

Douglass CW, Gammon MD: The epidemiology of dental caries and its impact on the operative dentistry curriculum. *J Dent Educ* 1984;48(10).

Dugoni AA: Our future is fantastic. *J Am Coll Dent* 1984;51(1).

Peters IJ, Waterman RH Jr: *In Search of Excellence.* New York: Harper and Row Publishers, 1982.

Naisbitt J: *Megatrends: Ten New Directions Transforming Our Lives.* New York: Warner Books, 1982.

Further reading

US Department of Health and Human Services Public Health Services. *Report to the President and Congress on the Status of Health Personnel in the United States,* Vol. 1, May 1984.

Olsen E: Dental insurance, a successful model facing new challenges. *J Dent Educ* 1984;48:591–595.

Waldman HB: Spread the good news of dentistry's economy. *Dent Student* 1985;63:14–16.

Little RJ: *A Survey of Attitudes and Professional Activities of Graduates at the University of British Columbia and the University of Washington, Presently Engaged in General Dental Practice.* PhD Dissertation. University of Washington, 1974.

Haynes S: Orthodontic treatment in the British National Health Service: A quantitative study of the contribution of specialists and general practitioners in Scotland, 1966–79. *Eur J Orthod,* March 1981.

Barker BD: What Is the Question? Keynote Address, Annual Staff Conference, Division of Dentistry, Department of Human Resources, State of North Carolina, Raleigh, North Carolina, June 6, 1977 (Unpublished).

Morris AL, Bohannon HM: Oral health status in the United States: Implications for dental education. *J Dent Educ* 1985;49:434–442.

Dugoni AA, Chambers DW, Roberts WE: The role of orthodontics in the predoctoral education of a dentist. *Am J Orthod* 1981;79:564–571.

Dugoni AA: *Dento-Cranial Survey of Children Three to Eight Years of Age.* Unpublished Master's Thesis, University of Washington, 1963.

Dugoni AA: Future demands for dental care (guest editorial). *Am J Orthod Dentofacial Orthop* 1986;89:520–521.

Gotowka TD: Economic growth of the dental profession: Comparisons with other health care sectors. *J Am Dent Assoc* 1985;110:179–187.

Douglass C, Gillings D, Sollecito W, et al: The potential for increase in the periodontal diseases of the aged population. *J Periodontol* 1983;54:721–730.

McLain JB, Proffit WR: Oral health status in the United States: Prevalence of malocclusion. *J Dent Educ* 1985;49:386–396.

Chambers D: Changing dental disease patterns. *Contact Point* (University of the Pacific) 1985;63:11–17.

American Dental Association, Bureau of Economic and Behavioral Research: *Dental Statistics Handbook.* Chicago: American Dental Association, 1987.

Dugoni AA: The economics of dentistry. *Am J Orthod Dentofacial Orthop* 1986;90:78–80.

Fifth Report to the President and Congress on the Status of Health Personnel in the United States, March 1986, U.S. Department of Health and Human Services, Health Resources and Services Administration, Bureau of Health Professions.

Solomon E, Stoll DJ: Knee-deep in the hoopla: Predictions of manpower stability and economic prosperity. *J Dent Educ* 1986;50:327–329.

Council on Dental Education, American Dental Association: *Annual Report Dental Education (1970–1985).* Chicago: American Dental Association, 1985.

Bailit HL: Environmental Issues in Dentistry — Reflection on the Practice of Dentistry in the 21st Century. Presented at the Pew National Dental Education Program, Dean's Training Session, Houston, Texas, January 8, 1986.

Bureau of Economic and Behavioral Research, American Dental Association: *The 1988 Survey of Dental Practice.* Chicago: American Dental Association, 1988.

Council on Dental Education, American Dental Association: *Annual Report Dental Education, 1988–1989.* Chicago, American Dental Association, 1989.

Reinhardt JW, Douglass CW: The need for operative dentistry services: Projecting the effects of changing disease patterns. *Op Dent* 1989;14:114–120.

Vermette M, Doherty J: Economic growth in the U.S. dental sector, 1950-1986. *J Dent Educ* 1989;53:480–484.

Beazoglou T, Gual A, Heffley D: The economic health of dentistry: Past, present and future. *J Am Dent Assoc* 1989;119:117–121.

Chapter 6

The State of Dentistry in Japan: Predictions for the Future

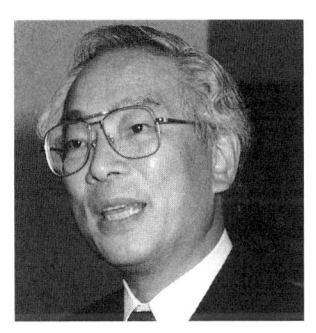

Sumiya Hobo
Tokyo, Japan

Abstract

The field of dentistry has changed dramatically in Japan as well as throughout the world. In Japan, there is still a high incidence of caries related to minimal use of fluoride-containing toothpastes as well as no water fluoridation. There is an increasing number of dentists, but at the same time, the number of patients visiting dental offices has also increased.

The cost related to tuition for dental schools has had an impact on the applicant pool. Clinical practice has been affected by socialized dentistry and the multitier system of insurance available in Japan. Technological innovations directly influence and improve the quality of care for patients related to adhesives, restorative materials, esthetics, implant treatment, and other areas of treatment. The key to survival for the dental professional during this time of rapid change is to stay current on new, advanced treatment modalities.

Decrease in caries incidence

In developed nations, the caries rate has decreased dramatically. In the early 1980s, the World Health Organization proposed a goal to decrease the DMF (decayed, missing, filled) index to less than 3.0 for 12-year-old children by the year 2000. This was achieved within the 1980s. In 1980, the DMF index for the United States dropped by 50% since the late 1960s to 2.6. For the United Kingdom it dropped to 2.55. The DMF index for Japan remains at 4.6, which is considered high. According to the results of an investigation done by the Ministry for Public Welfare, 86.7% of the Japanese population between 5 to 50 years of age have caries.

There may be an explanation for the decrease in the dental caries rate in western nations. One possible explanation involves the use of fluoridated water to help prevent caries. The fluoride creates a more resistant hydroxyapatite tooth surface and suppresses acid production caused by the obstruction of enolase.

The United States has seen an 80% decrease of caries in children who drink fluoridated water. In Japan tap water is not fluoridated.

Another explanation involves incorporating fluoride into toothpaste. Fusayama stated that the most effective way to prevent caries is through the use of a toothpaste that contains fluoride.[1] In nations showing a decrease in caries, the fluoridated toothpastes account for a high percentage of the market share. In Japan, fluoride-containing toothpastes have less than 15% market popularity, which probably relates to the poor caries incidence in Japan.

Besides the above-mentioned reasons, the use of resin sealants to fill fissures in the occlusal surface has been an effective method for decreasing the incidence of caries. Recent sealant materials show an approximate 5-year durability for effective prevention of dental caries. In the future, the prevention of dental caries may involve the use of a mouthwash and a vaccine. In Scandinavia, a mouthwash that contains 0.2% chlorhexidine with 1% peroxysulfate has been used to help eliminate *Streptococcus mutans*. If the patient rinses daily with this solution for 1 minute, the occurrence of caries can be prevented effectively. However, this mouthwash may affect taste sensation temporarily and may cause enamel discoloration with long-term use; hence clinical application of this mouthwash is questionable.

In the near future, the study of caries prevention will advance more rapidly. For example, Slavkin has identified a gene involved with enamel formation and has suggested the possibility of a new method of placing the gene along with yeast in a cavity preparation to produce new enamel.[2] If this method is successful, a cariously damaged tooth could be rebuilt with new enamel. The use of laser beams to treat caries is under study; the studies involve use of a laser beam to fuse enamel crystals to defective enamel. With all these advancements, the caries incidence in Japan should decrease noticeably in the near future.

Rapid increase of dentists

The problem of increased numbers of dentists is not limited to western nations; it also occurs in Japan. Newly graduated dentists have difficulty finding employment, which in turn causes a social problem. This phenomenon is serious but when considered from a broader perspective does not necessarily mean a tragic conclusion for dental practitioners.

Japan's population of 69 million in 1935 increased to 83 million in 1950 and now is approximately 120 million. The number of dentists totaled 26,000 in 1950, 56,000 in 1982, and 66,800 in 1989. The number of dentists has increased rapidly and at the same time the number of patients visiting a dental office has also increased. In the past 23 years, the number of visits to Japanese dental offices by patients over 65 years of age has doubled. With the rapidly increasing elderly population, the number of patients requiring dental treatment is increasing; therefore, the necessity for dental treatment remains important.

In Japan the number of dental schools has increased quickly from 7 to 29 within the past 25 years. Recently, the number of applicants to dental school has decreased. All private dental schools have decreased their enrollment by 20% beginning in 1989, following guidelines set by the Ministry of Education. By 1995, the number of graduating dentists will reflect this decreased enrollment. In direct contrast, the general population continues to increase. The actual number of dentists will therefore reflect a new balance between dentists and patients. The trend is changing, and although there appears to be an excessive number of dentists, there will not be a problem in the 21st century.

Japanese dental schools require 2 years of predental education and 4 years of dental courses; a total of 3,000 students graduate every year. There is a 1:3 ratio between the number of students graduating from government schools and the number graduating from private schools. The tuition for government dental schools is reasonable and about the same as that required for a liberal arts education. The tuition for private dental schools is extremely high because of the lack of financial support by the government: approximately $280,000 (US dollars) for a 6-year education. This economic fact alone accounts for a decline in the number of applicants to dental schools. In order to reduce operating costs, some Japanese private dental schools have eliminated the clinical practice exposure. This gives the new graduate dentist less sense of clinical competence upon completion of their education, however. Despite these problems, no Japanese dental schools have closed.

The wave of dental technology innovations

Adhesive materials

The biggest innovation in dentistry in the past 20 years has been the development of techniques to bond various restorative materials to natural tooth. Smith (1968) developed polycarboxylate cement, the first cement to have a chemical bond to a tooth surface.[3] Wilson and Kent (1972) developed a glass ionomer cement that also adheres to dentin in a manner similar to the polycarboxylate cements.[4] The polyacrylic acid contained in glass ionomer cement reacts with protein and blocks the dentinal tubules so that the cement does not irritate or stimulate the pulp adversely.

Buonocore (1955) developed an enamel etching technique whereby open pores produced in the etched enamel surface allowed formation of resin tags that resulted in a mechanical bond between the composite resin and enamel.[5] Bowen (1963) developed a BIS-GMA composite resin. A high percentage of an inert filler was dispersed throughout the resin to produce higher strength and lower coefficients of thermal expansion.[6] These developments have brought the adhesion of restorations into the forefront of clinical practice.

In Japan, Fusayama developed an indicator for carious dentin called the "Carious detector" to differentiate carious dentin from healthy dentin.[7] A more conservative preparation was developed and required a dentin bonding agent: the Clear-Fil Bond System F. This product now has the major market share among

Japanese practitioners. The 4-META bonding agent was developed by Masuhara (1978) for bonding to alloys. The development of bonding cements reduces the need for retentive preparations and changes the basic requirements for cavity and abutment preparations.[8] These new bonding agents have opened the door to adhesive dentistry in Japan.

Restorative materials

In Japan, the biggest change has been in restorative materials of choice; composite resin is becoming a popular material whereas amalgam has become unpopular. A possible explanation for this trend reflects the government regulations regarding sewerage and water drainage from dental clinics. Strict regulations have been issued to reduce the potential for mercury pollution of waste water systems. The Japanese have recognized the importance of controlling pollution, in particular the hazards of industrial mercury poisoning, that until recently affected many in the population. In the city of Kobe, the use of amalgam as a restorative material has been officially restricted, which in turn has influenced the curriculum in dental schools. Japanese dental schools have now eliminated amalgam preparation and restorations from their curricula and have replaced it with the use of composite resins. Although the social health insurance still reimburses dentists for amalgam restorations, the government regulates the waste water from the same dental clinics. The end result of this dichotomy will be the elimination of amalgam restorations from daily clinical practice in Japanese dentistry.

The previously popular restorative materials — acrylic resin and silicates — lack bonding characteristics. The light-cured composite resins are excellent in this regard and have superb esthetics. However, composite resin is not suitable for restoring the occlusal surfaces because strength and wear resistance are inadequate. The indirect composite resin inlay has been introduced in an attempt to improve the physical properties of resins used for direct restorations while minimizing the effects of curing shrinkage. The indirect resin inlays will be used more in clinical dentistry. In the future, composite resin will continue to be of value as a luting agent, but the film thickness obtained must be decreased and the resin must be less irritating to the pulp.

Porcelain occlusal inlays are also becoming popular as an alternative to composite resin restorations. Porcelain abrades opposing natural teeth, however. Thus there is a need for a porcelain with less abrasive qualities.

Fixed prosthodontics

The advancement in this field has been based on improved high-speed cutting instruments. More recently, the laser beam offers a possible future alternative to conventional high-speed instrumentation, but research is still in the early stages.

The materials used include metal, organic material, and inorganic material.

Metal has been used successfully although its color differs from natural teeth. High esthetic demands by today's patients make it difficult for dentists to use metal as a restorative material. Organic materials such as composite resins offer poor durability and water absorption properties and cannot be used as permanent restorative materials in fixed prosthodontics. The development of newer composite resins may offer an alternative with acceptable properties that could remain in use for 5 to 10 years at a low cost.

Porcelain, an inorganic material, is used extensively and has excellent esthetic qualities. Because it has a high fracture potential it is usually supported by a metal infrastructure. The development of porcelain-fused-to-metal (metal ceramic) restorations has offered esthetic alternatives to all-metal restorations. Currently, metal ceramic restoration methods offer the only way to fabricate a fixed, partial denture with high esthetic results and adequate strength characteristics. This method was introduced in Japan in 1965 and has been widely used since then. Several Japanese products, including porcelains and alloys, are available. The Renaissance crown, also introduced in Japan, uses four layers of foil pressed over a die and fused as the metal infrastructure. Nonprecious alloys are common, but the dentist trying to achieve an esthetic, artistic result uses precious alloys. Several renowned dental ceramists have come from Japan, including Kuwata and Asami.

Castable ceramics, an inorganic material, has been used for fabricating inlays and crowns. The glass is relatively simple to cast but breaks easily. A small amount of material that acts as a nucleus for crystal formation has been added to raw glass for use in making crowns following the lost wax method. Through a reheating process of the cast glass, crystallization occurs with the formation of mica and hydroxyapatite. This process makes the ceramic much stronger than the cast glass. In Japan, several companies are experimenting with castable ceramic materials, including the widely known Cerapearl castable apatite ceramic. Because glass ceramic material is monocolor, extrinsic stains are used to reproduce tooth colors, but this makes it difficult to obtain an esthetic result.

Currently, various types of porcelain jacket crowns are fabricated on a refractory model. Composite resin is used to adhere the porcelain jacket crown to tooth structure. The porcelain strength has been improved from 60 to 80 MPa to 420 to 560 MPa, but the strength also depends on the adhesive cement. These crowns have good esthetic qualities, but the composite resin can cause pulpal irritation and needs more research. With the stronger porcelains it is possible to make a crown entirely of porcelain, but this is not advisable for fabricating fixed partial dentures.

As previously mentioned, the development of adhesive cements has drastically changed conventional preparations. Good examples are seen in resin-bonded fixed partial dentures, which require minimal tooth reduction. Indications are still limited because the strength of the fixed partial denture depends largely on the physical property of resin. The other drawback to this restoration is that ideal use requires a nickel-chromium alloy, which could pose a health hazard.

The porcelain laminate veneer technique has provided another advance in fixed prosthodontics. This technique requires minimal tooth surface preparation 0.5 mm into enamel. The veneer is made from porcelain using a refractory investment die. A light-cured and chemically cured composite resin is used as an adhesive between the tooth surface and the veneer. The porcelain laminate veneer has advantages as a restoration in that chairtime, cost, and patient discomfort are all reduced. The adverse effects of composite resin on dental pulp are not usually a concern because the preparation for this restoration is contained within the enamel. There are high-quality products for the laminate veneer and bonding techniques, such as Cosmotech, which produce three-dimensional color instead of monocolor.

In Japan, esthetic dentistry has just begun to attract more patients and now draws more interest from dentists. Laminate veneers have been used by a small percentage of dentists. Recently, the Academy of Esthetic Dentistry in Japan has been established to promote esthetics, and esthetic dentistry will most likely gain popularity.

CAD/CAM is a new development for use in fabricating inlay crowns and fixed partial dentures. The system uses a three-dimensional milling machine that shapes a restorative unit using a video analysis of the actual tooth preparation. It is possible to prepare the tooth and deliver the prosthesis in the same clinical appointment. The computer system helps eliminate the human error in laboratory fabrication because it uses computer-controlled steps. At this time use of CAD/CAM systems is limited by the difficulty in finishing the occlusion of the resulting restorations and the monocolor appearance. CAD/CAM systems may be suitable for use in fabricating a framework for metal ceramic restorations or for an osseointegrated implant-supported denture. Presently, CAD/CAM systems have been used for fabricating inlays, with hope for further development and widespread use. Kanagawa University in Japan is now experimenting with the CAD/CAM system.

Dental implants

Implants provide an important new dimension in popular dental improvements. Dental implants are made mainly from titanium, alumina ceramics, and hydroxyapatite ceramics. From these materials, commercially pure titanium is recognized as an effective material for successful osseointegration of implants.

The Brånemark and IMZ implant designs and methods have been recognized as ideal in Japan. The titanium implants are embedded into bone for 3 to 6 months to allow osseointegration to occur between the bone tissue and the implant surface. After osseointegration, a second operation connects abutments to the integrated implant.

Brånemark's research studies on implant integration have been conducted for over 20 years with success rates in excess of 85%.[9] Because his implant design lacks a stressbreaking mechanism such as a periodontal ligament, the suprastructure is made of a resilient material, such as resin, which helps reduce stress from excessive occlusal forces. In the IMZ system, an intramobile element has been incorporated as a shock absorber. Both types of implants can be used in edentulous and partially edentulous patients. In the future, both implants may offer reliable alternatives in oral rehabilitation to help limit or eliminate long-span fixed partial dentures, conventional Kennedy Class I and II removable partial denture treatment, and complete denture treatment. Inorganic materials such as alumina ceramics or hydroxyapatite ceramics cannot be adapted to the two-stage surgical technique and fail to osseointegrate.

The two-stage technique in osseointegrated implants creates a difficult situation in Japanese dental practice. In Japan, the only established specialty is orthodontics; no other specialty is recognized. Hence, general practitioners cannot refer their patients to an oral surgeon. The surgical technique for osseointegrated implants requires a certain level of skill and knowledge and general practitioners must learn to do their own surgery. The future of osseointegrated implant treatment in Japan depends on whether or not general dentists are interested in doing their own surgery and are willing to pursue advanced training. It also depends on whether dentists have the space available in the dental clinic to remodel or build a surgical suite. Space is severely limited and is a rare commodity in Japan. Japanese plastic surgeons have expressed interest in performing surgery for dentists, which may help alleviate the current obstacles.

Periodontology

Periodontal treatment has advanced in diagnostic capabilities and treatment modalities. The key change has been in plaque control. Plaque forms the basis for calculus formation, and the bacterial toxin by-products irritate periodontal tissues and cause periodontal disease. Obviously plaque control is essential for controlling this disease. Another advance in periodontics is in the area of tissue healing. A periodontal ligament can reattach following the appropriate treatment to reproduce a gingival attachment.

The philosophical views concerning treatment in periodontics have also changed. Ramfjord stated that a pocket depth within 3 mm was sufficient and there was no need to pursue a more shallow depth. Scaling and root planing were adopted in patients with pocket depths ranging between 5 to 6 mm. Thus most pockets are treated without surgical intervention.[10] The future trend shows a decrease in periodontal surgeries.

A new achievement in periodontology is the development of bone implants. These bone implants consist of a granular type material, about 300 to 1,000 μm in diameter, made by burning hydroxyapatite ceramics. The material is used to replace lost alveolar bone due to periodontitis or traumatic occlusion. The concept is intended to support the tooth by regenerating new bone between the tooth, material, and surrounding bone. Because hydroxyapatite is made of the same inorganic material that is present in living tissue, it does not cause an antibody-antigen reaction by the human immune system. It is a bioactive material that allows osteoblastic activity, which in turn creates new bone.

Periodontology is ultimately a battle involving alveolar bone. It is a significant achievement to be able to use regenerative procedures to replace alveolar bone lost by periodontitis. If plaque control could be managed, periodontitis would decrease over the long term. However, it would possibly take another half century to eliminate periodontitis because study of soft tissue is more difficult than study of hard tissue.

The Japanese social health insurance system does not cover the entire costs of periodontal treatment; the total costs covered are approximately one tenth the average cost of the same treatment in the United States. The dentist may feel that this treatment requires much time and may not be monetarily productive for the office. This area is neglected, and because the patient does not perceive periodontal treatment as an obvious need, the importance of periodontal treatment is not widely recognized.

Endodontics

There have been no great changes in endodontic instrumentation over the last 70 years because the basic design of instruments such as reamers and files could not have been improved; the designs were perfected early. Improvements strive to develop instruments to reach apices of curved root canals, increase efficiency of canal preparation, and increase elasticity in sharper reamers and files. In early days, engine reamers had only 360 degrees rotation; they now have changed to partial rotation and the capability to rotate in reverse. The last 2-mm tip of the reamer is smooth to avoid shaving tooth material and changing the shape of the canal.

Progress has been made in electronics available for endodontic treatment. For example, the digital pulp diagnosis instrument and root canal length measurement instrument are two advances available for use. In the near future, an ultrasonic root canal treatment system should be available. Another element that is essential in endodontic treatment includes radiographs. Radiographs used today do not provide standardized information; thus it is difficult to compare them accurately during treatment. High-quality radiographs are essential to improvement of endodontic treatment.

Gutta-percha has been the material of choice for root canal fillings since 1867 and is still the most reliable root canal filling material. Several methods are available for filling the canals with gutta-percha, such as vertical condensation and lateral condensation. In Japan, several methods have been developed and used among general practitioners, such as the "Opian Carrier Method" developed by Ohtsu (1987).[11]

According to an American Dental Association report, 3,120,000 root canals were treated in the United States in 1950. The number increased to 4,100,000 root canals in 1959 to 9,200,000 root canals in 1969 and to 17,390,000 root canals in 1979, with similar increases seen in Japan. These results suggest that dentists have employed endodontic therapy over the years and have shown a high percentage of success because of technique innovations, thus preventing extractions. At present, root canal treatment will increase with easier methodology because of improvements in techniques and materials. However, the need for endodontic treatment will decline with the decrease in caries activity.

Temporomandibular disorders

Early treatment of temporomandibular disorders was based on a narrow perspective that "there is one cause and one treatment." This has fallen out of favor within the profession because the pathogenesis of TM disorders involves many fields of study. The approach to treatment involves cooperation within medical and dental fields. Temporomandibular syndrome is a multifactorial process that may present as pain in the masticatory structures and be defined by the onset of a unique symptom. After studying this syndrome, it appears to be more difficult to diagnose and requires more complicated and coordinated treatment.

The most conservative type of treatment for TM disorder is the use of an orthosis (splint), which is used to help relieve muscle tension, although it is not quite clear when the splint should be removed. To supplement this treatment, a portable Mandibular Kine-geograph (J. Morita Corp, Osaka, Japan) has been developed to estimate the silent period and level of muscle activity. Other developments include an instrument used to evaluate audible noises and x-ray machines. Diagnosis of articular disc problems is indispensable in treating a TM disorder. Arthrography is a valid instrument for diagnostic purposes, but it is often too painful for routine use. Nuclear magnetic resonance computed tomography will be used for diagnosing articular disc problems, but at this time the instrumentation and costs are prohibitive for the average dental practitioner.

The treatment of TM disorders in Japan is in a stage of confusion because of the different ideas and opinions that have evolved without solid underlying treatment principles. This in turn affects the average general practitioner who would rather not treat the TM disorder patient. With the current status of international influence experienced by the Japanese, stress levels have increased in everyday life. This creates greater need for further education and training by practitioners. It will probably take another decade before sound TM disorder treatment principles based on a thorough understanding of the problem are developed.

Occlusion

The importance of occlusion in prosthodontics has been widely recognized as a fundamental necessity in Japan. The facebow and semiadjustable articulator are standard equipment in dental education. A superior and anterior position of condyle in glenoid fossa is widely accepted as the optimal condylar position. Disocclusion is considered essential for eccentric movement. When fully balanced occlusion was accepted, the lingual inclination of the maxillary anterior teeth and the cuspal inclinations of posterior teeth were made parallel to the condylar path. However, when disocclusion was introduced as one of the schemes of physiological occlusion, the lingual inclinations of the maxillary anterior teeth should be set steeper than the condylar path. The ideal angular differences between the lingual inclination of maxillary anterior teeth and the condylar inclination is not yet known. Anterior guidance needs to be studied more scientifically.

The field of occlusion in Japan has produced outstanding basic research. Japanese dentists have shown keen interest in occlusion throughout the century. Occlusion has appealed to many having an interest in detailed, scientific research and is one of the strongest subjects in the Japanese dental sciences. The computer-aided pantograph — the Cyberhoby — is commercially available in Japan to measure condylar movement. A computer system can calculate adjustment values for the incisal table of an articulator based on preselected amounts of disocclusion from a patient's condylar path data. This computer system is called the Anteroputer and has been developed to give a sound treatment basis for advanced practitioners.

Other fields

There has been interesting progress in various other fields in dentistry. For example, a shape-memory alloy is expected to be a material that can be used ultimately for orthodontic treatment. Removable partial denture frameworks may possibly be made from titanium, which is a metal with high biocompatibility. An anti-herpes vaccine is possible but an anticaries vaccine will be difficult.

AIDS has become a big concern in dentistry. The number of patients suffering from this disease is approximately 150,000 worldwide, and people who are carriers of the virus number over 100 million throughout 100 countries. The dental practitioner can be one of the first health care providers that come into contact with an AIDS patient by noting swollen lymph nodes in the head and neck area or by evaluating hairy leukoplakia or Kaposi's sarcoma. This disease places dentists at a high risk of infection during treatment unless appropriate safeguards are used. This necessitates the use of masks, glasses, protective gowns, and surgical gloves that must be disposable or easily sterilized.

In Japan, the number of patients with AIDS or that are HIV positive is 1,117 (June 1989), which is extremely low. Therefore, dental infection control is not commonly used in daily practice. Japan has progressed rapidly and has become an international community, more so with a greater influx of foreign business and cultural interests. The typically homogeneous society will change and will confront new challenges. This is reflected in the need for better control of cross-contamination, which at present is poor. Few dentists sterilize handpieces and burs. In clinics that survive on larger numbers of patients and increased volume of treatment, it is economically difficult to sterilize the equipment. The government has not instituted control over this sector of dental practice; hence infection control has not been emphasized and the insurance system does not cover the added costs to the practitioner. With time, the importance of infection control will be recognized.

Dental practice

The fact that the rate and occurrence of dental caries has decreased does not mean that dentistry is declining. The fields involved with osseointegrated implants and esthetics provide different treatment options using newer dental technology. In order to catch up with these advancements, it requires continuous postgraduate education.

The total gross income of all Japanese dentists is 2 trillion yen, annually. Total income made from dental product sales such as dental units, artificial teeth, precious alloys, and composite resin are 200 billion yen. The cost expended by the profession for postgraduate education, including various continuing education courses, books, and journals, is only 1 billion yen. When a Japanese patient pays 100 dollars for treatment, the materials cost will be 10 dollars with only 50 cents spent for knowledge. In past times when advancements in dentistry occurred slowly, the information obtained during one's education in dental school could last throughout the entire professional career. Today, the technology learned in dental school may need updating by graduation time. It is the responsibility of each dentist to strive to learn up-to-date information to become an independent professional. The dentist must also be willing and prepared to learn and change to meet the challenge.

This is especially critical for the Japanese dentist because socialized dentistry controls the direction of dental practice. There is a multi-tiered system of insurance available in Japan. National- or government-sponsored insurance covers 70% of all costs incurred by the entire family. Social- or company-sponsored insurance covers 90% and 70% of costs incurred by the head of the household and family members, respectively. Professional-sponsored insurance (ie, organized by doctors or other professionals) covers 100% and 70% of costs incurred by the doctor and family members, respectively. Some organized unions sponsor insurance that can cover 100% of costs incurred by the union member. Every Japanese citizen is covered by the national insurance if he or she does not belong to another insurance system.

Since World War II, the number of patients seeking treatment has increased tremendously, bringing good incomes to medical and dental professionals through the social insurance system. During the last 10 years, the government has tried to tighten the budget for health care. The system itself is supported by a percentage deducted from each person's income. A higher income pays more whereas a lower income pays less, but there is a limit or maximum amount that can be deducted from any one person's income. The system cannot be supported further because it has reached the maximum limits deducted from all individuals' incomes. One result has been a change in the reimbursements to professionals. For example, in medicine, there may not be alternatives to a standard, accepted treatment. An appendectomy may cost on the average about $420 and a C-T scan of the brain about $180. Only 70% of the costs are paid by the insurance system to the physician, essentially setting the fees; any physician performing the same procedures receives the same income. The private-practice physician cannot offer a better alternative to the standard treatment so he or she may have difficulty surviving without treating large numbers of patients covered by the social insurance system.

In dentistry, a dentist has many alternatives to one treatment covered by the social insurance system; hence, dental practice offers two levels of service: one reimbursed by the social insurance and one reimbursed directly by the patient. The social insurance will pay set amounts for certain types of dental treatment such as $175 for a complete denture (one arch), $38 for root canal treatment (one canal), $17 for composite resin restoration (one surface), $120 for a partial denture (Kennedy Class I), $74 for a palladium crown, and $24 for a molar extraction. Recent trends show the government wants to set fees on alternative treatment options. There is an organized effort to limit government intervention into dental practice. Previously, dentists could survive in practice by treating a large volume of patients using the social insurance system, but with an increase in number of dentists, the patient population per dentist has decreased.

Another interesting aspect affecting dental practice in Japan is that the increased life expectancy for males is 75.54 years and for females is 81.30 — some of the longest life expectancies in the world. The development of geriatric dentistry fits ideally into the Japanese population, and dental treatment should change to fit the needs of the people.

Knowledge is the key weapon for survival as a professional. In the era of dentistry the Japanese are now facing, where technology and information are changing rapidly, the dentist who is current on newer, advanced treatment modalities has a better chance of attracting patients and being successful in private practice.

References

1. Fusayama T: The future of dental practice, education and research. *The Nippon Dental Review,* 1985; March No. 509.
2. Slavkin HC et al: Human and mouse cementum proteins immunologically related to enamel proteins. *Biochemica et Biophysica Acta* 1989;991:12–18.
3. Smith DC: A new dental cement. *Br Dent J* 1968;125(5):381–384.
4. Wilson AD and Kent BE: A new translucent cement for dentistry. The glass ionomer cement. *Br Dent J* 1972;132(2):133–135.
5. Buonocore MG: A simple method increasing the adhesion of acrylic filling materials to enamel surface. *J Dent Res* 1955;34:849–853.
6. Bowen RL: Properties of a silica-reinforced polymer for dental restoration. *JADA* 1963;66:57–64.
7. Fusayama T: *New Pathology and New Restoration.* Tokyo: Quintessence Publishing Co, Ltd; 1985.
8. Masuhara E: *A Dental Adhesive and Its Clinical Applications.* Tokyo: Quintessence Publishing Co, Ltd; 1982.
9. Brånemark PI et al: Osseointegrated dental implants in the treatment of the edentulous jaw. Experience from a 10-year period. *Scand J Plast Reconstr Surg* 1977;11:1–132.
10. Ramfjord SP: Surgical periodontal pocket elimination: still a justifiable objective? *JADA* 1987;114(1):37–40.
11. Ohtsu H: *Opian Carrier Method.* Tokyo: Quintessence Publishing Co, Ltd; 1989.

Chapter 7

Stomatology in the USSR: Yesterday, Today, Tomorrow

V. K. Leontiev
N. Bazhanov

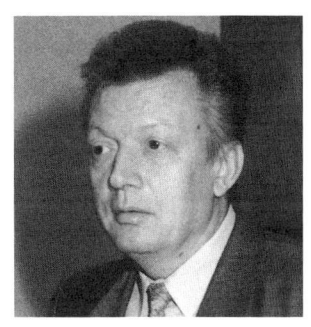

V. K. Leontiev
Moscow, Union of Soviet Socialist Republics

Abstract

Over 130,000 stomatologists and dentists and 60,000 other specialists have been trained in the USSR. Stomatologists are trained with a higher education qualification, and dentists, nurses, and technicians with a secondary education qualification. Dental care is free of charge, except for prosthetics. Dental clinics are open at schools, facilities, and in villages where oral sanitation and emergency care are rendered. Specialized and highly qualified aid is rendered to the population of the attached territory at dental polyclinics and dental departments of versatile polyclinics, where doctors render assistance according to their specialization. Scientific work is carried out in research institutes and at dental faculties of medical institutes. The USSR domestic industry manufactures all kinds of dental products, though their quality and quantity do not satisfy internal demand. The dentistry of the 21st century is expected to be mostly preventive.

Stomatology in the USSR today — what is known about it outside the country's borders? What exactly is this most important area of public health care in one of the world's most powerful countries? It is difficult to find answers to these questions in the pages of the foreign press, although the interest of specialists in this problem is both understandable and natural. In the era of "glasnost" and openness, "perestroika" and mutual trust, wider knowledge of this field is also necessary.

The basic principles according to which stomatological help is rendered to the Soviet population are accessibility; free treatment; proximity to the workplace, place of study, or residence; and specialization. Thus, priority is given to an active preventive approach to public health.

A stomatologist with a higher education qualification is a leading specialist who provides the population of the USSR with stomatological care. The prevention of stomatological complaints, the treatment of ailments of the teeth and mouth,

71

the organization of stomatological treatment for the whole population, and the direction of other specialists working in the stomatological field are all the responsibility of the stomatologist.

A significant number of Soviet stomatologists (about 30%), especially in rural areas, carry out the entire range of stomatological treatment — therapeutic, surgical, orthopedic, and pediatric. In addition, the majority of stomatologists carry out only specialized treatment. Here the stomatologist works either exclusively as a surgeon or in the field of general treatment and denture fabrication. A section of stomatologists also specializes in the treatment of children. This approach conforms with the aim of raising the quality and effectiveness of stomatological treatment and increasing the productivity of the work of doctors. Stomatological treatment is also carried out by specialists with an intermediate education qualification — dentists. They are responsible for preventive medicine, simple treatment, and for assisting the stomatologist.

Nurses are used as auxiliary medical personnel who prepare and sterilize instruments, give technical assistance, and fulfill other support functions. Specialists are trained at the intermediate education level in the technical preparation of dentures in specialized dental laboratories. These are dental technicians. They are not considered part of the medical profession and do not have the same rights.

Up until 1960, stomatological treatment in the USSR was carried out to a significant extent only by specialists with intermediate-level education because not enough stomatologists qualified at a higher level of medical training. Between 1956 and 1960 the decision to sharply increase the number of stomatologists trained at a higher level was taken, and the number qualifying only at the secondary level was limited. The figures for the training of stomatologists are shown in Figs 1 and 2.

In 1987 the number of stomatologists reached 4.7 per 10,000 population; only 1.5 had intermediate education qualifications. There are 91,000 stomatologists, 43,000 dentists, and more than 40,000 dental technicians.

The training of stomatologists in the USSR is carried out at two stomatological institutes (in Moscow and Poltava) and in 46 stomatological faculties at medical institutes, spread throughout the capitals of the Soviet republics and in many large cities (regional centers). At this time in the USSR, more than 7,000 stomatologists and approximately 1,500 intermediate-level specialists qualify every year. However, this is considered insufficient for the needs of the country, as a result of which new stomatological faculties are being opened. In fact, in Turkmenia, Uzbekistan, Tadzhikistan, and in several areas of the Russian Soviet Federated Socialist Republic, the number of stomatologists is only 3 per 10,000 persons, which is inadequate for the provision of stomatological treatment.

The training of stomatologists at a higher level is carried out in the stomatological faculties of the medical institutes. The period of training is 5 years, plus an additional year of practical training in the best clinics under the direction of experienced doctors (internship). On completion of study, the young stomatologist

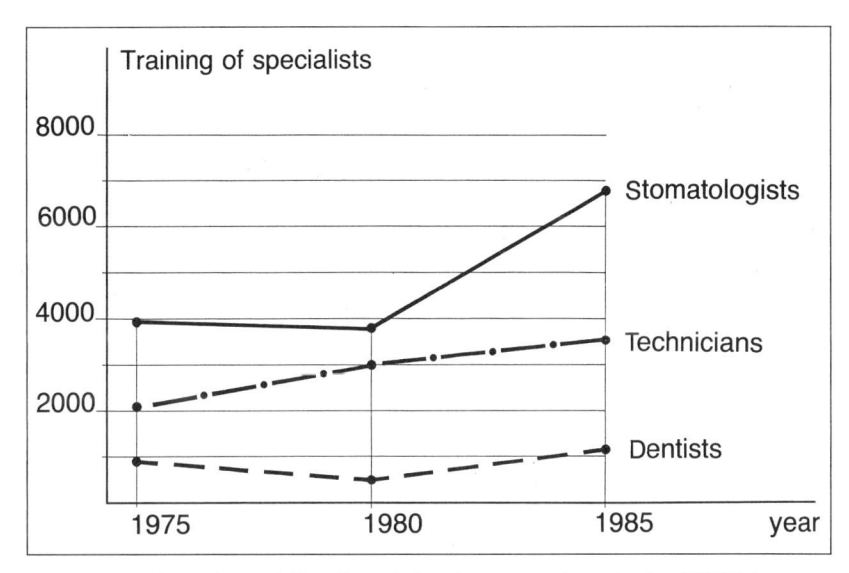

Fig 1 Number of specialists in training in stomatology in the USSR from 1975 to 1985.

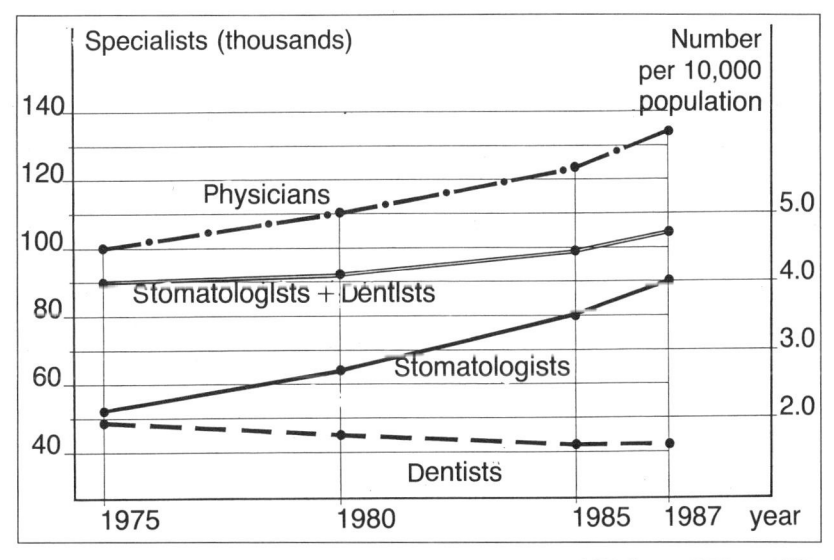

Fig 2 Number of specialists in stomatology in the USSR from 1975 to 1987.

must work for 3 years at the direction of the government, after which he or she may choose a place for future work. On completion of study at the faculty, every stomatologist must be competent in all the main areas of the specialization — therapeutics, pediatrics, surgery, and orthopedics — although the majority of students have already opted for one area of specialization during training. Apart from that, every stomatologist must be able to render urgent treatment in all areas of medicine.

The period of training of dentists, specialists qualified at an intermediate level, is 3 years. Nurses' study specifically for preventive work in stomatology has recently begun in the USSR. In total, over 200,000 specialists are working in various areas of specialization in the USSR; however, there remains a serious shortfall, particularly in the numbers with intermediate qualifications.

Postgraduate qualification of stomatologists in the country is carried out at medical schools that have a chair of stomatology. The government funds further qualification in individual fields of the specialization — therapeutics, orthodontics, oral surgery, and pediatrics. These courses last for up to 3 months, with a final examination. There are also short courses of training with specific objectives. Training is undertaken either on the initiative of the specialists themselves, or at the behest of the directors of the stomatological institutions, usually once every 5 years. The state encourages postgraduate training and further qualification.

Symposia, conferences, and postgraduate training of specialists are widely organized throughout the country; for example, there is short-term training for stomatologists (2 to 3 weeks) at leading clinics in concrete methodology and forms of work. On the whole, existing forms of postgraduate training of specialists in stomatology are not effective enough and require improvement.

The basic institutions that provide stomatological treatment (Fig 3) for the urban population of the USSR are the specialized stomatological polyclinics, the stomatological departments of general polyclinics, stomatological surgeries in factories and schools, rural doctors' surgeries, and mobile surgeries.

More than 1,700 stomatological polyclinics operate in the USSR. They are usually situated in a separate building or part of a building, in which 10 to 150 stomatological installations are situated. Between 15 and 300 stomatologists work in these clinics, giving treatment to the population of a defined area. A standard stomatological polyclinic structure is shown in Fig 4. The structure of the polyclinic includes departments for specialized therapeutic, surgical, and orthodontic treatment, treatment of children, and the fabrication of dentures. A stomatological polyclinic is headed by a chief doctor, who is aided by a medical and an administrative deputy. Stomatological departments are headed by experienced managers who are responsible for the direction and organization of treatment in their departments. The entire medical staff — stomatologists, dentists, nurses, attendants, dental technicians, etc — is immediately subordinate to them. A senior nurse is in charge of the department's auxiliary staff. The administrative deputy to the chief

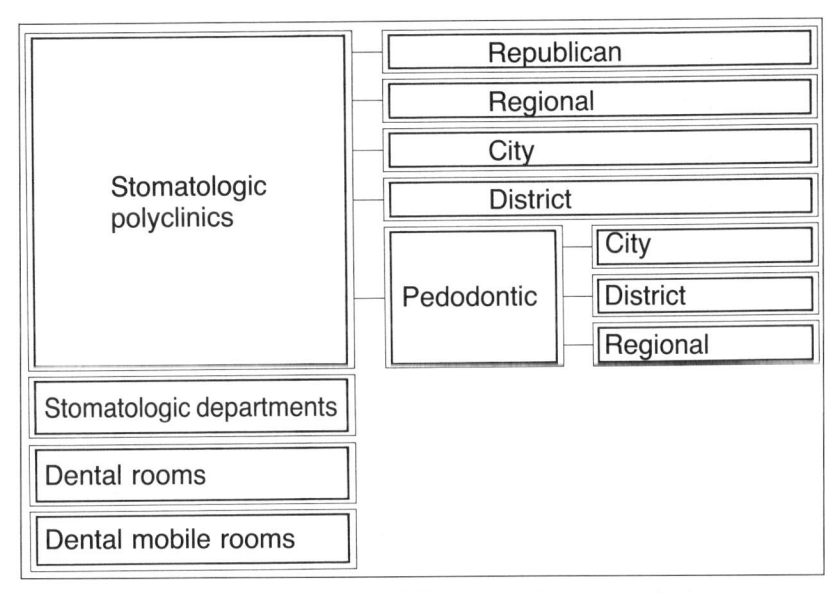

Stomatology in the USSR: Yesterday, Today, Tomorrow

```
Stomatologic polyclinics
├── Republican
├── Regional
├── City
├── District
└── Pedodontic
    ├── City
    ├── District
    └── Regional

Stomatologic departments
Dental rooms
Dental mobile rooms
```

Fig 3 Types of institutions in the USSR that render stomatological treatment to the population.

STOMATOLOGIC POLYCLINIC

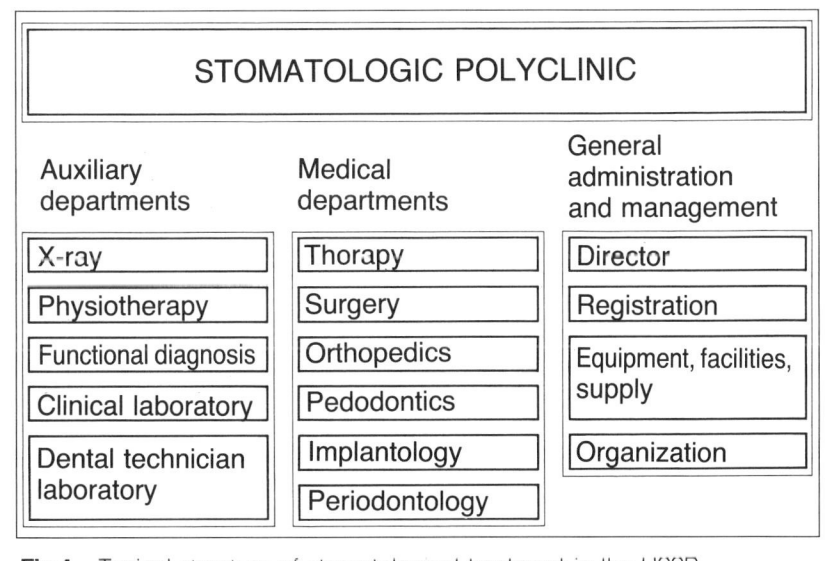

Auxiliary departments	Medical departments	General administration and management
X-ray	Thorapy	Director
Physiotherapy	Surgery	Registration
Functional diagnosis	Orthopedics	Equipment, facilities, supply
Clinical laboratory	Pedodontics	
Dental technician laboratory	Implantology	Organization
	Periodontology	

Fig 4 Typical structure of stomatological treatment in the USSR.

doctor organizes the administration and supply of the polyclinic.

Patients going to the polyclinic are met at the registry, where the case history is kept. They are then transferred to the duty doctor in the examination room. The duty doctor inspects the patient, makes a preliminary diagnosis, establishes a course of treatment, carries out urgent treatment, and sends the patient to be treated in the specialist departments, where the exact assistance necessary will be given. Often the patient requires a complex course of treatment and therefore is sent to two or three specialized departments, which are not always convenient to the patient but which provide efficiency and the highest quality of work from the doctor. In stomatological polyclinics there are radiology, physiotherapy, and anesthetic departments, a department of functional diagnostics, a laboratory, and other departmens, which enable the quality of investigation and treatment of patients to be increased. Many polyclinics have sub-departments of periodontology and implantology and an emergency outpatient department open around the clock. The majority of stomatological polyclinics are designed to give treatment to a population of between 30,000 and 300,000 inhabitants (regional polyclinics). There are also city, republic, and children's polyclinics, which apart from treating the population of a specific area, provide wide consultative, methodological, and organizational assistance.

A significant volume of stomatological treatment of the population is carried out in the stomatological departments of general polyclinics for adults and children. Normally this comprises one or more stomatological surgeries with 2 to 20 stomatological installations, where 6 to 70 stomatologists receive therapeutic and surgical patients (including children) and prepare dentures. A number of the doctors will provide more complex stomatological treatment.

In order to achieve the maximum level of accessibility of stomatological treatment to patients in the USSR, a significant volume of treatment is carried out in stomatological surgeries in schools, kindergartens, factories, and villages. These surgeries are equipped with one stomatological installation, and the stomatologist receives the patients. The stomatologist can give complex courses of treatment to patients. Urgent treatment is given in stomatological surgeries, and patients are also received at a mutually convenient time for prophylaxis, examination, treatment of stomatological ailments, prevention of complications, and constant monitoring of the health of all patients allotted to the stomatologist. This is done on the basis of active invitations to the surgery. For complex or specialized stomatological treatment, the patient is sent to a stomatological polyclinic or the stomatological department of a general polyclinic. In the USSR there are more than 25,000 stomatological departments and surgeries, the growth rate of which is shown in Fig 5. An insignificant amount of stomatological treatment in the country is carried out by stomatological cooperatives and doctors working on part-time schedules.

Surgical treatment of stomatological patients is also carried out in conditions of hospitalization. More than 10,000 hospital beds are allocated for patients who require surgical treatment by a stomatol-

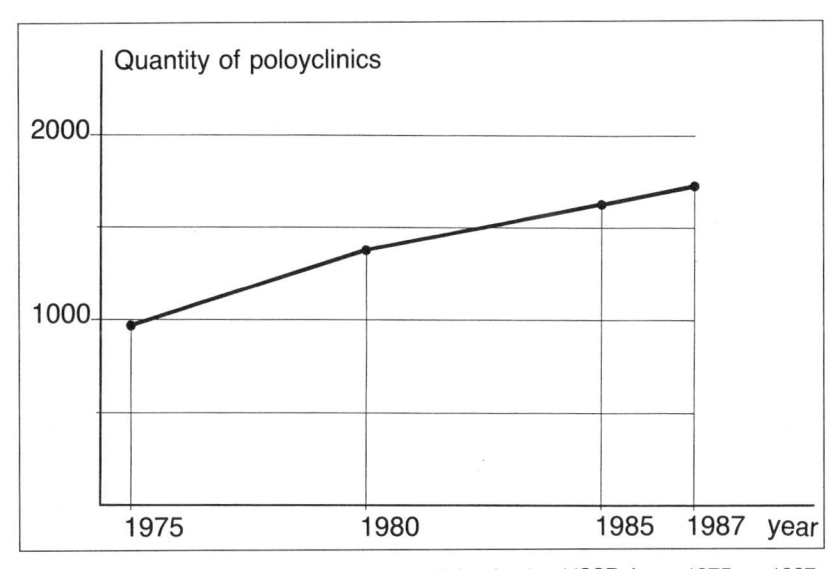

Fig 5 Number of stomatological polyclinics in the USSR from 1975 to 1987.

ogist. In the USSR, facial and maxillary surgery, trauma, inflammations and infections, surgical reconstruction of the face and jaw, plastic surgery on the soft tissue of the face, and the treatment of congenital or innate facial deformities or disfigurements are normally treated by stomatologists specializing in these areas. Oncologic problems are normally dealt with by oncologists, often working together with surgical stomatologists. Surgical clinics for stomatological patients are often situated in general hospitals, though in some cases independent clinics exist exclusively for the treatment of stomatological patients. The treatment of patients with congenital facial or maxillary problems is the task of stomatologists. A wide regional network of clinics is spread throughout the country, organized on the basis of stomatological faculties where treatment and observation of children is carried out.

The Ministry of Health, which includes the Department of Stomatology, is in charge of all stomatological treatment in the country. There are counterparts in the health ministries of the Soviet republics. They are together headed by the Senior Stomatologist of the Ministry of Health of the USSR. There are also regional senior stomatologists in the regional health departments. These positions are filled by leading specialists in the cities and regions of the country.

The administrative structure described above is responsible for the systematic improvement of the organization of stomatological treatment; for work to optimize the network of stomatological institutions and to provide new economic and organizational planning of their operation; for growth-planning; and for the development of stomatological treatment. Experience has shown that the administrative system described above is not sufficiently effective.

In 1988, the All-Union Scientific Production Association "Stomatology" was founded in the country. Its members included several scientific research institutes and laboratories, a faculty for the qualification of stomatologists, a network of stomatological treatment centers, a series of branches from the Soviet Republics, and several enterprises concerned with the manufacture of stomatological products. The association was called upon to raise the effectiveness of stomatological treatment by means of an acceleration in the development of modern prophylactic methods and treatment of ailments of the teeth and mouth cavity, and in the development and production of modern stomatological materials; by satisfying demand for these materials; by concentrating scientific research on longer-term development trends in stomatology; and by raising the standard of qualification of stomatologists. One of the main tasks of the association is to increase the effectiveness of the administration in stomatology by means of a unified scientific and technical policy in the branch of specialization. Such efforts would utilize achievements in science and technology and new economic and organizational methods based on computerization of the administration and the creation of a regional network in the form of branches of the association.

Intensive scientific research is conducted by specialized organizations. These are the Central Scientific Research Institute of Stomatology (in Moscow) and the Odessa Scientific Research Institute of Stomatology (in Odessa); two stomatological research laboratories (in Kharkov and Leningrad); countless stomatological institutes and faculties in various cities throughout the country; and chairs of stomatology at the medical schools and institutes.

Scientific research is financed by the Ministries of Health of the USSR and the Soviet Republics, by enterprises, and by medical institutions. Scientific research and developments are coordinated by the Academy of Medical Sciences, on the basis of which scientific advice is given to the field of stomatology.

The science of stomatology has long traditions in the USSR. I. G. Lukomskii was one of the first scientists to preach the preventive role of fluoride in preventing dental caries. Entin was a legendary scientist who introduced a physicochemical theory of dental caries. Interesting scientific advances in stomatology were made by A. I. Yevdokimov, Limberg, A. R. Rybakov, and others.

The leading scientific stomatological institution is the General Scientific Research Institute of Stomatology (CSRIS), founded by the academic Rybakov in 1962. About 700 people work at the institute. It has clinical and research divisions, including three polyclinics, two clinical departments (for inflammations and for facial plastic surgery) and a radiology department, a physiotherapy section, and departments of functional diagnostics, anesthesiology, child stomatology, and stomatological surgery for children. In the research division there are laboratories for biochemistry, microbiology and immunology, prophylaxis, pathomorphology, pathophysiology, illnesses of the mucous membrane of the oral cavity, endodontology, periodontology, complex methods of prosthesis, metal and ceramics, materiology, and social methods of research and prognosis. The basic scientific concerns of the institute are epidemiological and social research in stomatology; etiology and pathogenesis of dental caries; periodontal diseases; diseases of the mucous membrane of the oral cavity; new methods of diagnosis, treatment, and prevention of diseases; development and trial of new techniques and materials for stomatology; and the approbation and development of medical preparations. In CSRIS there is also a scientific council for the defense of dissertations.

The organizations that are carrying out intensive scientific work in the field of stomatology include the medical institutes in Kiev, Alma-Ata, Kemerovsk, Omsk, Kalinin, Pesh, and Kazan. Great successes have been achieved in this country in the fields of diagnosis and treatment of preliminary forms of dental caries; in the development of preventive measures that do not employ fluoride; in the development of surgical procedures in facial and maxillary reconstruction; in laser and ultrasonic stomatological apparatus; in the use of computers for diagnosis and treatment of stomatological complaints; in new stomatological materials; and in functional diagnosis of stomatological complaints.

Weak links in scientific research are the problems of materials, new technology, dental prosthesis, anesthesiology, and fundamental research. There are insufficient links between research and the production of stomatological products, and between stomatology and general medicine. These weak links pose problems for the further improvement of mutual contacts between research and practical stomatology, and production is among the most important factors for the further development of specialization in the country.

Equipment, materials, and instruments for stomatology are mainly provided by internal production within the USSR. Only a small percentage of stomatological products are imported.

The main manufacturers of stomatological products are the medical instrument factory in Kazan, the medical equipment factory in Volvograd, the All-Union Scientific Production Association "Stomatology" factory in Kharkov, the Mozhaisk medical instrument factory, and the medical polymer factory in Leningrad.

The Kazan factory is a well-equipped modern enterprise, producing various types of burs, small stomatological instruments, and ferrules for the USSR and for export. The Volvograd factory produces a variety of stomatological appliances and dental chairs. The factories in Kharkov and Leningrad produce an assortment of stomatological materials — molding, restorative, and kaolin-based substances, dentures, stomatological plastics, and secondary materials. The factory in Mozhaisk produces stomatological instruments. A significant proportion of stomatological products is produced by other factories.

On the whole, there are insufficient stomatological products to satisfy the demands of doctors and the needs of the patients. It has been necessary to reconstruct factories, introduce new technology into them, and develop new products and raw materials. For a long time this work has not been carried out with the necessary intensity, and as a result, provision of stomatological products does not meet the demand. This is the case particularly with restorative and molding materials, porcelain substances, dental laboratory equipment, and stomatological appliances. In addition to this, a range of products (burs, molding substances, silver amalgam, etc) are of high quality but are not produced in sufficient volume. As far as quality is concerned, the Soviet Union is without doubt among the leading countries in the world in some stomatological products — lasers for treatment and for the making of parts, ultrasonic apparatus, and equipment for functional diagnosis. However, a whole range of stomatological products, including ovens for firing porcelain, composite resin materials, ionic cements, moldable ceramics, etc, are not produced in the USSR at present. There are insufficient products and insufficient variety.

Currently measures are being taken to modernize the stomatological industry. Contacts between the producers and consumers are in hand. In this respect the All-Union Association "Stomatology" has the main role: it includes a department concerned with industrial operation. The association has become the customer, tester of products, and the medical consumer. Measures are being taken to increase both the quality and quantity of products for stomatology and to attract new factories to participate in this task. The production association "Stoma" in Kharkov is an experiment in this field, producing stomatological products. In this way, a single chain has been created by the "Stomatology" association: investment/scientific/development planning — industrial production/training. This is intended to improve development of stomatological products in the country.

The All-Union Scientific Society of Stomatologists (ASSS) is also engaged in intensive work in the USSR. More than 70,000 stomatologists, dentists, and dental technicians are members of this public organization. The society exists in all republics and regions of the country and publishes the scientific journal *Stomatology*. Its task is to develop stomatology, solve the professional problems of stomatologists, work out recommendations in various fields of the profession, direct and organize stomatological treatment, and collaborate with the state and regional health organs on professional problems. The society organizes the stomatological congresses of the USSR and the republics, scientific conferences, symposia, and seminars. It maintains international links with the societies of stomatologists from other countries.

In the 1960s, an intensive study of stomatological diseases was carried out among the Soviet population. At present, epidemiologic research is being carried out in much of the country.

A varied picture of illness in the Soviet Union can be observed — from low or very low incidences in Central Asia and other regions, to very high in the Baltic Republics, particular regions of Russia, and Siberia. In the USSR the caries index in children wavers between 4.0 and 5.0. The level of illness in the population is defined by the character and volume of stomatological treatment. On average, throughout the country every person visits a stomatologist approximately twice a year, and this index is steadily increasing.

The ideology of the provision of stomatological treatment in the USSR is based on the active position of the stomatologist in relation to the population for which he or she is responsible. The activity lies in the fact that the stomatologist does not wait until a patient comes to him or her; the stomatologist must himself actively detect and treat illness.

In the USSR, this principle is embodied in the system of oral hygiene maintenance. This consists of active exposure of all problems to stomatological treatment, medication, and active observation of the patient's state of health by means of periodic evaluations and necessary stomatological treatment. The frequency of visits is determined by the level of activity of stomatological diseases, and they are carried out at intervals that do not permit stomatological complications to arise (one to four times a year). This system is especially effective for those organizations involved with the infant population (schools and kindergartens), and also for some groups of blue- and white-collar workers. In the USSR, stomatologists actively examine approximately 90 million people annually, of whom 27% are adults and more than 45% children. In this way, 70 to 75% of those requiring stomatological treatment receive it in full after planned examinations. In some republics this treatment is received by 80% of the population (Estonia, Latvia, Lithuania), in some by less than 50% (Turkmenia, Tadzhikistan, Uzbekistan).

Professional oral hygiene maintenance is an effective method of treating the population, although it does have shortcomings in that it does not contain the primary measures for prevention of stomatological complaints.

The average number of stomatologists in different regions of the country ranges from 4 to 5 per 10,000 of the population. Some of them work in schools, kindergartens, factories, and places of education, where stomatological surgeries can be organized in order to bring treatment closer to the workplace or place of study. A governmental decree has been passed requiring a stomatological surgery to be set up in every school; about 40% of the country's schools currently have them. The principle of bringing stomatological treatment to the patient allows necessary treatment to be given at the place of work or study, which is convenient and leads to a minimal loss of time. However, it is not possible to obtain highly qualified or specialized treatment in these surgeries because they are not adequately equipped or staffed for such treatment. Therefore, a system of treatment also exists in the form of regional stomatological polyclinics or stomatological departments at general polyclinics, as has been mentioned above. In these, the patient can obtain all forms of stomatological treatment. Large factories have their own hospitals and polyclinics, where only workers and their families are treated. Stomatological treatment of children is provided on a territorial basis as well as directly in surgeries at the place of study.

A lesser number of patients try to obtain stomatological treatment from part-time practitioners or from cooperative practices for a higher fee. Paid stomatological treatment can also be obtained at special polyclinics, where treatment is provided for a small fee to all those who go there, regardless of their place of residence.

Of all the types of stomatological treatment in the USSR, only prosthetic treatment must be paid for; however, the cost of treatment, with the exception of dentures made from precious metals, is very low and is totally free for pensioners. Most fixed prosthodontics in the USSR are made from stainless steel and precious metals; removable dentures are made largely from plastics. On average, 7 to 8 million sets of dentures are prepared every year, although demand is not met. The equipment of dental laboratories and the quality of materials requires improvement. In recent years there has been a great increase in orthopedic treatment using implants. The manufacture of dentures using integral metal castings, metal and ceramics, and metal and plastics is not sufficiently widespread.

The basic materials for restoring carious lesions are amalgams and cements. Composite resin materials are not produced. Imperfect restorative materials and instruments lead to a significant loss of work time, both on the part of the stomatologist and on the part of the patient, and to the premature loss of teeth. This problem is one of the most important in the USSR.

Periodontal complaints are treated mainly by a complex method involving therapeutic, surgical, and protective approaches, although the demand for this type of treatment is also not met in full.

The main trend in the development of stomatology in the USSR is toward prevention. There has been wide scientific research into this problem, and in various regions successful experiments showing the great effectiveness of preventive programs have been carried out. In various cities, more than 200 fluoride appliances have been set up, although not all are functioning satisfactorily. There is not enough toothpaste in the country, and only 15% to 20% of that contains fluoride. Prophylactic and educational measures are carried out, but in insufficient volume and quality. A system of preventive medicine is beginning to take root in schools and kindergartens. The lack of participation of teachers and middle-ranking medical staff in preventive work is a serious shortcoming. Among the means of preventive stomatological treatment in the USSR, fluoride-based tablets, fluoride lacquer, and various mouth-rinsing preparations containing fluoride are produced. Education of the population in how to clean teeth is widely employed. The fluoridation of salt is being studied. However, on a national scale, prophylaxis of stomatological diseases is insufficient. Development programs are only weakly implemented, and not only in the country's regions. Governmental organizations are not participating in these programs, and social aspects are poorly implemented.

Thus, stomatological treatment in the USSR shows serious shortcomings alongside its undeniable successes. A system of stomatological treatment of the population with a strong material base, a defined system of training specialists in stomatology, and an industry working for stomatology have all been created. However, the material provision of stomatology is unsatisfactory with regard to both quantity and quality, trends toward preventive treatment in stomatology are completely inadequate, and serious problems exist in the organization and administration of stomatological treatment of the population.

The last 2 to 3 years have seen great efforts to improve stomatological treatment of the population in several directions. In order to strengthen the organization of stomatological treatment and administration, maximum autonomy and rights have been given to the heads of stomatological institutions. To maintain a unified policy in the specialization, the All-Union Scientific Production Association "Stomatology" has been created, a stomatological department has been set up at the Ministry of Health, and a series of positive normative documents concerning economic, organizational, and administrative problems have been published.

In order to strengthen the material and technical provision of stomatological treatment, joint enterprises with foreign companies have been, or are in the process of being, set up for the production of composite resin materials, dental burs, and prophylactic materials. A series of contracts has been signed with industrial enterprises in the country for the design and construction of stomatological appliances, equipment, and instruments. The association is assisting factories to undertake the production of stomatological materials and instruments, and new economic and organizational mechanisms are being formulated for work with industry. Scientific resources are being concentrated in this direction, and first-class scientific development is being attracted.

In order to develop preventive stomatology in the USSR, the supply of prophylactic substances is being increased, a sharp rise in the output of toothpaste is projected, and the volume, level, and effectiveness of education is being extended, with the involvement of the state and social system, teachers and educators, and middle-ranking medical personnel. It is projected that by the year 2000 stomatology in the USSR will be raised to a modern level in both the preventive and the curative treatment of the population.

Prospects for the development of stomatology in the 21st century may be seen in the solution of problems of etiology and pathogenesis of fundamental stomatological complaints — dental caries and periodontal diseases — and the creation on that basis of highly effective etiologically and pathenogenetically based preventive methods. The solution of these problems will probably lead to a sharp decline in the prevalence and intensity of stomatological illnesses within the next 30 to 40 years. The most promising trend is toward antenatal prophylactic treatment, which will ultimately result in the resistance of oral and maxillary tissues to stomatological problems. Methods of immunization and positive shifts in the human diet are also seen as promising.

It seems that many problems in stomatology in the next century will be connected with the negative role played by the reduction of the human dental-maxillary system. The significance of the part played by this process in the appearance of dental and maxillary abnormalities, a series of other stomatological ailments and their prevention, in all processes connected with the formation, growth, and development of the face and jaw against the background of the elimination of other etiological factors, is growing sharply. This is because reduction is an epoch-making process, and the problems connected with it will be very difficult to solve.

Very complex problems remain in the field of maxillary and facial traumatology, although solutions are improving sharply. It is quite possible that the focus of treatment of congenital deformations and maxillary and facial disfigurement will shift to the preventive sphere as a result of increasing knowledge about the principles of this pathology.

However, it would obviously be false to maintain that stomatological problems will disappear completely. They will remain at a certain level for a long time, but the methods of their treatment will be determined by early detection of disease and its connections with other diseases. Therefore, it is doubtful whether they will remain actual problems, connected with prosthetic treatment, restorations, and the extraction of teeth.

Thus, stomatology in the 21st century will not be left without work to do, but its focus, following today's tendencies, will shift into the field of prevention. One can imagine the stomatologist's patient in the 21st century as a person with a full set of teeth and a wide smile, who takes great care to prevent — and therefore is not greatly troubled by — stomatological diseases.

Chapter 8

Prospects for Dentistry in 21st-Century China

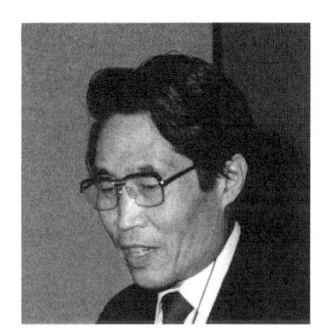

Zhang Zhen-kang
Beijing, China

Abstract

Following the establishment of a new China, dentistry has been developing rapidly; however, the ratio of dentists to the general population is still very low. China faces the problem of providing dental care for a population of 1.1 billion; hence, the only direction for China to take is the development of preventive dentistry. Recently, under the Ministry of Health, the National Committee for Oral Health has been established, and the targets to be attained by the year 2000 have been worked out. This paper mentions that following government approval of private practice, group practices and private clinics will play an important role in dental health care.

A precise prediction on 21st-century dentistry in China is very difficult because of the huge population and imbalance in economic development in China. It is also impossible to discuss all aspects of development in dentistry. Therefore, I will limit myself to a discussion on the general trend of the development of dentistry in China.

In the history of ancient Chinese dentistry there have been proud achievements. For example, records of dental diseases can be traced back to the 14th century BC in oracle bone inscriptions; use of arsenicals for dental pulp devitalization is described in a famous medical book written in the 2nd and 3nd centuries; in the 7th century amalgam was used to restore teeth; in the 10th century bristled toothbrushes using horsehair had been invented.

Unfortunately, the development of dentistry in China lost its impetus in the past centuries. In 1949, the founding year of The People's Republic of China, there were only 656 dentists and six dental colleges operating on a limited scale. Supported by the government, dentistry has been developing rapidly since then. At present there are more than 10,000 dentists and 30 dental colleges. However, with a dentist-to-population ratio of 1:100,000, the coverage of dental care is still very small and dental services are mainly limited to curative therapy. According to statistics, in provincial capitals the filled teeth make up 0.3% to 21.5% of the total DMFT. In Shanghai and Guangzhou, two large cities of China, the proportions are 44.8% and 39.7%, respectively. Rates of caries restorations in primary teeth are below 10%; however, Shanghai and Beijing have higher rates: 36.3% and 11.6%, respectively. The lowest rates are in Huhehot, the capital of Inner Mongolian Autonomous Area (0.07%) and Lhasa (0.1%). Another example of the shortage of dental services is evidenced by the fact that the Department of Orthodontics at the School of Stomatology, Beijing Medical University, opens once a year for patient registration. In 1980 more than 3,000 people registered and it took the orthodontists 4 years to treat them. People in rural areas complained, "Before the founding of New China, we had teeth but had no food to eat. Now we have plenty of food but have no teeth to eat it with." This ironic remark expresses the eager demand for oral health care in China.

Current disease status

Dental caries

According to a national survey on 130,000 students in 1983, the mean DMFT of 12-year-old students was 0.67. The mean DMFT in five age groups (7, 9, 12, 15, and 17 years) was 0.66 and caries prevalence rate was 30.43%. The caries prevalence is regarded as very low according to the World Health Organization classification. However, following the increase of sugar consumption in recent years, the caries incidence has increased. From 1982 to 1987, a longitudinal study on primary and middle school students in the northeastern city of Shenyang shows that the DMFT of 12-year-olds had increased from 0.9 to 1.2, and the caries prevalence from 36.7% to 52.5%.

Periodontal diseases

According to the 1983 national survey among 130,000 students using the Community Periodontal Index for Treatment Needs (CPITN), the prevalence rate of gingivitis was 63.93%, detection of dental calculus was 41.8%, mild periodontitis was 1.7%, and severe periodontitis 0.08%. However, the prevalence of periodontitis in adults of various age groups was reported to be 50% to 69%, and dental calculus was present in 98% of adults examined.

Preventive dentistry

The World Health Organization has set an ambitious goal for the year 2000: "Oral health for all!" This illustrates that the general trend of oral health services should face the community and bring benefit to the public. To enjoy a high level of health is regarded as one of the basic human rights. However at present, dental service in China is basically curative treatment and is only enjoyed by a small portion of the population. Fortunately, dental caries and periodontal diseases, despite their high prevalences, are preventable. It is wise to emphasize prevention of dental diseases because it is less expensive and more effective. China, as a developing country, should not repeat the experiences of western countries.

Today, preventive dentistry in China is at the initial stage of development. It was only in early 1989 that the National Committee for Oral Health was established in the Ministry of Public Health. Not all the dental schools and dental hospitals have a department of preventive dentistry. The number of qualified professionals in this field is estimated to be less than 200. The three-leveled dental prevention network has not been widely established. In most of the Chinese cities and countries, school health programs do not include oral health care.

Several months ago at the first meeting of the committee many famous dentists and experts on preventive dentistry, deans of the dental schools, and officers of the Ministry of Public Health discussed the goals and targets for oral health care in China by the year of 2000. A project outlining the desired results of achievement and plans for a national epidemiologic survey on dental diseases in some major cities have been worked out. The goals of the project are: *(1)* to further reduce the caries incidence; *(2)* to develop dental prevention at a primary level; *(3)* to launch a community dental health education movement; and *(4)* to achieve a status that everyone will be consciously involved in dental prevention. The targets to be attained by the year of 2000 are as follows:

1. 50% of 5- and 6-year-old children are to be caries free.
2. The DMFT in 12-year-olds should be 1.5 or less.
3. In 60% of all 18-year-olds, at least 3 sextants of teeth in each mouth should be periodontally healthy (CPITN = 0).
4. 70% of the population should brush their teeth at least once a day.
5. 80% of kindergartens, primary schools, and high schools are to be provided with oral health programs aimed at preventing dental caries and periodontal diseases.
6. Oral health education should reach 90% of the population; at least 80% of school teachers, students, and parents should be aware of the main causes of dental caries and periodontal diseases, as well as home care measures.
7. The ratio of dentists to the population should reach 1:10,000 and that of high-, middle-, and primary-level dental personnel 1:2:4.
8. A national data bank should be established for dentistry and should include information on epidemiology, workforce, and resources for dental prevention and treatment.

China has a population of 1.1 billion; 800 million people reside in the countryside. About 220 million people are illiterate. Many people do not seek dental treatment until they have a severe toothache. It is estimated that only 40% of the population brush regularly. Generally speaking, people have poor knowledge about their teeth and poor oral hygiene. Therefore, it is a tremendously arduous job to educate and motivate the public to improve their oral health. Their unhealthy habits can only be altered when everyone participates in oral health activities. In recent years, an activity named "Love Your Teeth Day (Week)" has been carried out annually in some cities with good results. A powerful alliance has been formed by dental professionals and government officers to organize various cultural activities, including seminars, exhibitions, popular science books, and entertainment. These activities have been well received by the public. Recently some noted dentists proposed that September 20th of each year be the national "Love Your Teeth Day." This proposal has been approved by the Ministry of Public Health, and the activity will be jointly planned and hosted by four ministries and five public organizations.

The key to successfully providing oral health for all lies in the countryside, where cultural and medical facilities are insufficient. Additionally, the necessity of preventive dentistry and primary oral health care has not been realized by the local authorities; therefore, it is imperative that dental health programs be a part of the overall primary health care project worked out by the Ministry of Public Health. The goals of oral health care should be listed in the socioeconomic development plans of different levels of government administration, especially in the countryside. Primary dental care will be provided by "country doctors" who have been trained for a short period of time with fundamental dental knowledge and skills.

Organization of personnel

The prospective achievements for the next century are impossible if great importance is not attached to dental education. It is the only way qualified personnel, strategies, and technology can be provided.

Dentists are seriously lacking in China. In 1984, the ratio of qualified dentists to the population was 1:100,000 for the whole nation; in Hunan Province, 1:270,000. According to the present status of dental education we need 30 years to reach the planned ratio of 1:10,000. This is obviously too slow.

In the past few decades, the training of primary- and middle-level dental personnel has been overlooked. Data from the Ministry of Public Health shows that the ratio of high-, middle-, and primary-level medical personnel is 1:1.82:1.09, and the ratio of high- and middle-level dentists (the latter are also called dental therapists) is 1:1, which is also unreasonable. Among over 1 million country doctors, most are incapable of doing dental health work. Therefore, it is of utmost importance to put the training of primary- and middle-level dental personnel as a priority. An ideal ratio of personnel structure would be 1:2:4 (high:middle:primary). With this structure, dental health service with a different function can be formed. In the next 10 years the dental education system must be adjusted to meet this purpose. The strategy is to steadily develop college education, to rapidly develop the 3-year professional training programs, and to speed up the development of middle- and primary-level trainings.

More private practices

For a long time the policy of the Chinese government was to gradually eliminate private practice. By the end of the cultural revolution there were only a few private dental clinics. The number of private practitioners was about one or two thousand, and most of them had only been trained as apprentices. The clinics were poorly equipped, and backward techniques were used. The majority of the clinics were located in rural areas where regular dental service was lacking. They have played a small role in dental health care and never enjoyed a good reputation. People usually seek treatment in dental hospitals or dental departments in general hospitals, where the personnel are employed by the government.

Consistent with the open-door policy of our government, private practices are now allowed. Private dental clinics and group practices have developed quickly, and the number of dentists "moonlighting" has increased.

It must be pointed out that the health care portion of the state budget constitutes only 3.25%. No money has been earmarked for dentistry. At the current rate of economic development, it is unlikely that the government will invest heavily in building a large number of dental hospitals or dental departments. It is also unrealistic for all the graduates from either dental colleges or middle-level dental schools to be employed by the government. On the one hand dentists are badly needed; on the other hand not all the trained personnel can be employed. This results in a "pseudosurplus" of dentists. Therefore, it is predicted that the "surplus" dentists and dental therapists will be encouraged to practice privately or collectively. This might be a trend in dentistry in China in the next century. There will be various forms of coexisting dental clinics and private offices. The private practice might become popular and play an important role in dental health care, as it does in western countries.

The development of dental health care relies on the level of the nation's socio-economic and cultural development as well as the demand of the people. Both conditions are serious in China. The economy needs to be strengthened. In some remote regions people still live in poverty. The average level of education is only at the fifth year of primary school. The public has very little elementary knowledge of dental hygiene and diseases. There is still a long way to go to catch up with developed countries. We are determined to spare no effort to achieve the goals set for the year 2000 and to ensure that all people learn to take care of their teeth. Meanwhile, we need international support and cooperation; we need advanced knowledge and technology.

Chapter 9

Dentistry in the 21st Century: Austria

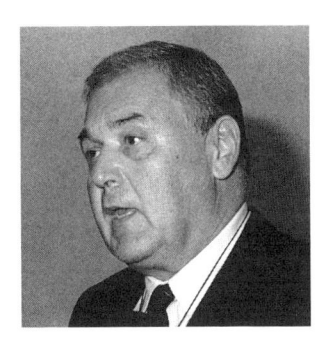

R. Slavicek
Vienna, Austria

Introduction

In Austria dentistry is considered a medical specialty and thus requires a medical degree followed by a 2-year course in dentistry. Because of the country's glut of physicians, there are regular waiting periods of 8 to 10 years at the three dental university teaching hospitals.

The social structure of the country causes the curative branch of preventive dentistry to be part of the social security scheme and thus is included in the insurance benefits schedule. This also applies to dental surgery and the provision of full dentures and metal partial dentures. Orthopedics and orthodontics are only covered to a qualified and limited extent by social insurance contracts. Fixed crowns and bridgework, precision partial dentures, vast areas of orthodontics, and implant therapy are not covered under social insurance contracts but under private insurance schemes. Out of the total range of medical branches that also comprise dentistry, only curative treatments are covered under social insur-

All illustrations from: Ludwig-Boltzmann-Institut für Gerostomatologie, Vienna ance schemes, not in general preventive therapies. There are some qualified exceptions as far as obstetrics is concerned.

On account of this policy but also undoubtedly due to the still prevailing reluctance of the population to take preventive measures on their own initiative, the rate of common dental diseases is still very high. The present DMF rate in 6-year-old children lies, with regional differences, between 3.5 and 5.0. On the basis of this information, extensive curative service is expected at least for the first third of the 21st century. The service of auxiliary personnel within the field of prevention is controversial in Austria and, at present, not covered by law.

Science and education must meet the challenges of the 21st century. In the view of all responsible people concerned, the present specialized training proves to be inadequate and too short at the university and at professional levels. Political pressure due to a rather manufactured need driving from ill-serviced regions necessitates keeping up an inappropriate training period.

A policy regarding future development should concentrate on extending the training period to at least 3 years. The crucial question for all future structures is, however, whether the basic training in general medicine in its present form should or can be retained, which is particularly important in view of the present developments regarding membership in the European Community. In my opinion, dentistry will clearly shift back from the mechanistic isolation of pure dentistry to general medicine. An about-face from the present system and adaptation to the training system within the EC is therefore not necessary. However, with regard to future structures, the main points of basic medical training for the branches of dentistry will have to be individually and specifically elaborated. The focal points within the specialized branches of dentistry, the development of which will also be dealt with, will undoubtedly clearly shift.

An essential factor in the elaboration of projections is the population structure to be expected in the future. The age distribution is particularly relevant not only in the field of general medicine but also in dentistry. It is therefore highly interesting to compare past and present with the future. Based on the data provided by the Austrian Central Statistical Office, the following comparison may be made.

Population structures and age distribution

What are the consequences for dentistry? In view of the increase in the number of elderly, dentistry will need to give more attention to geriatric issues. To this end, gerostomatology and also the related medical and health care issues will take up a significant part of the overall capacity of this branch. The service of trained auxiliary personnel specialized in preventive medicine will be channeled to the first fifth of the age distribution. It will be especially important to provide groups handicapped by age or disease with specially trained health care personnel and also with specialized dentists. The problem of the extended family arising from the inclusion of the elderly needs to be

Population structures and age distribution

Austrian Population, 1869

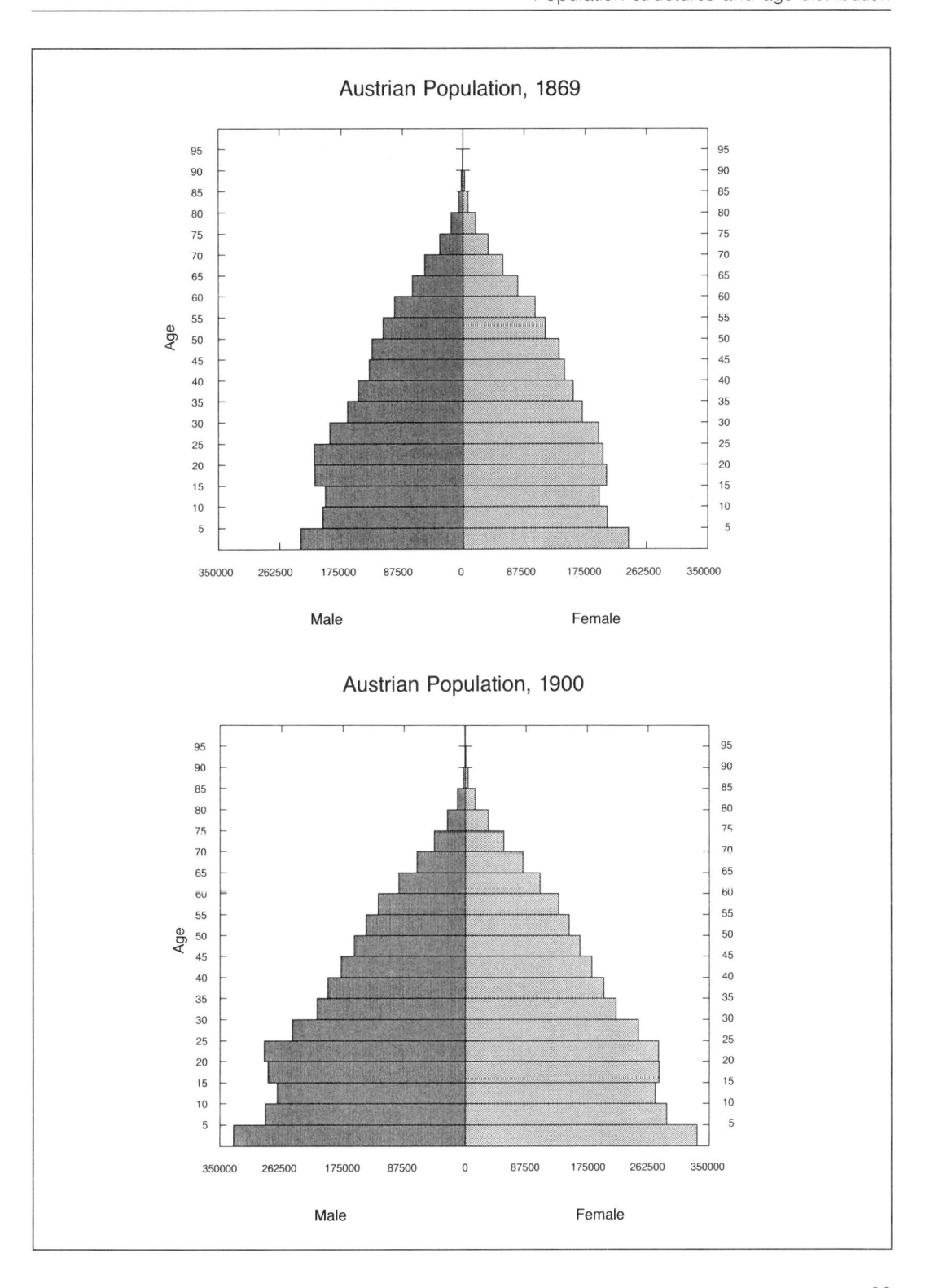

Austrian Population, 1900

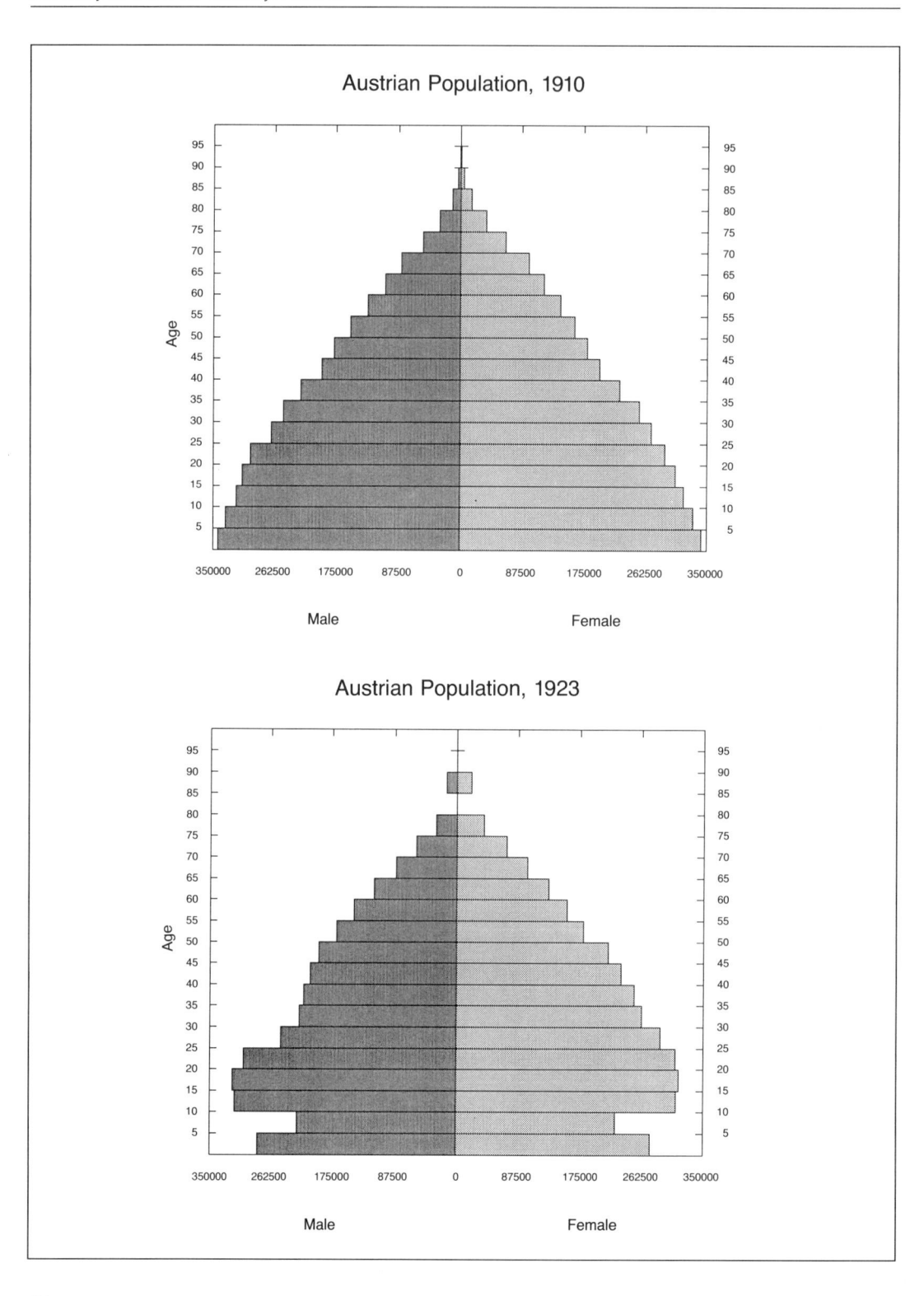

Austrian Population, 1910

	Male					Female		
350000	262500	175000	87500	0	87500	175000	262500	350000

Austrian Population, 1923

	Male					Female		
350000	262500	175000	87500	0	87500	175000	262500	350000

Population structures and age distribution

Austrian Population, 1934

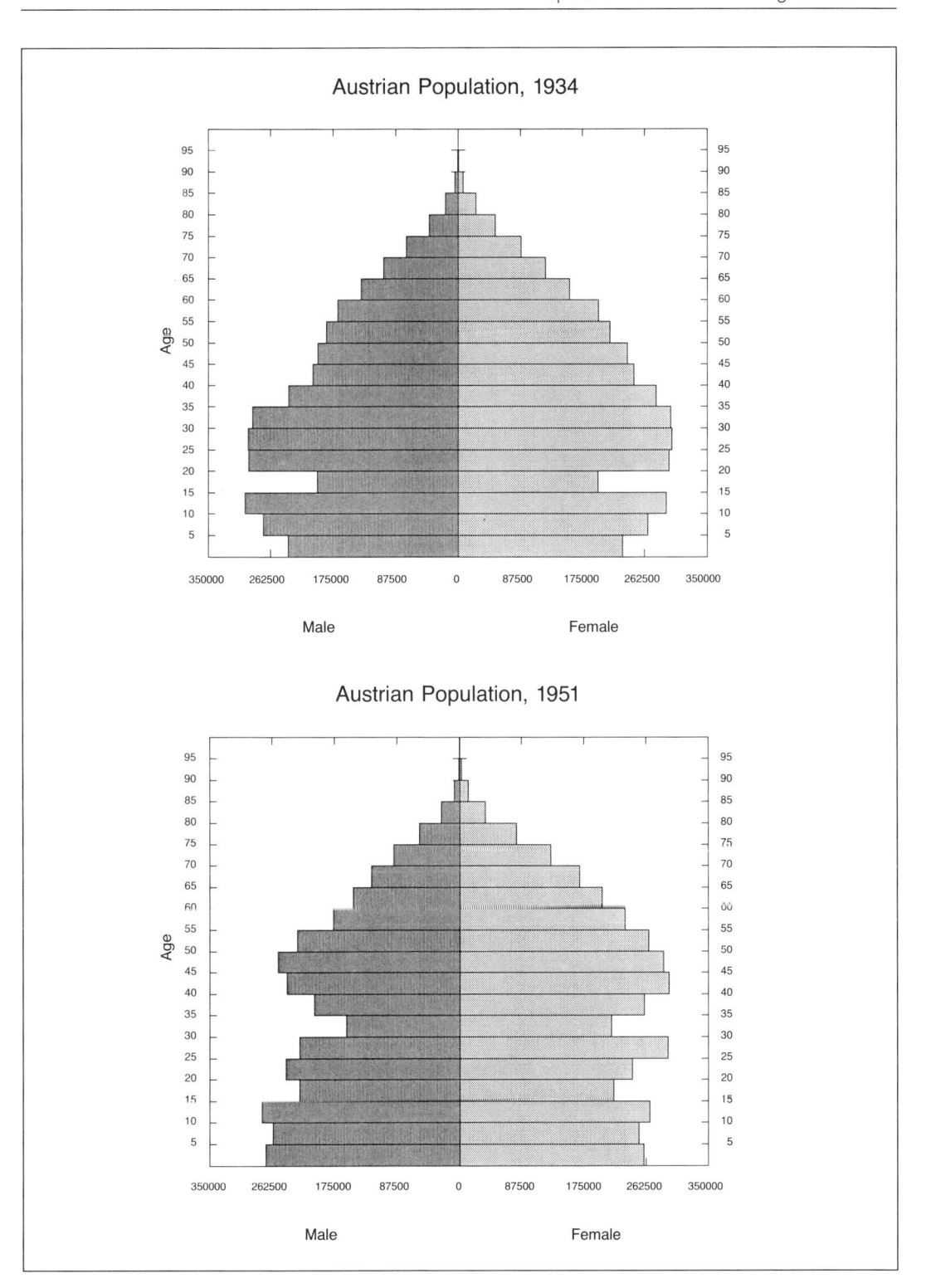

Austrian Population, 1951

Austrian Population, 1961

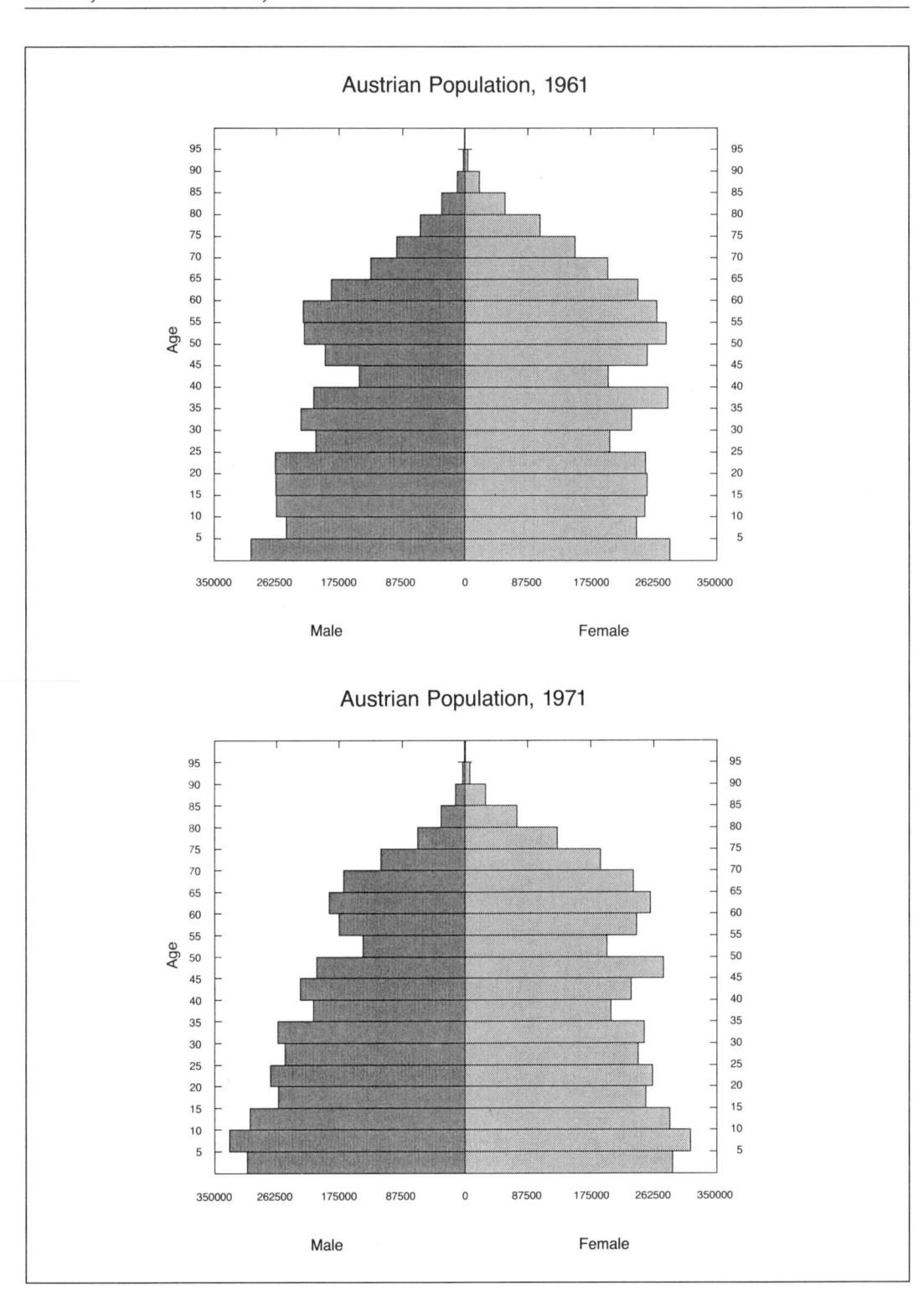

Austrian Population, 1971

Population structures and age distribution

Austrian Population, 1981

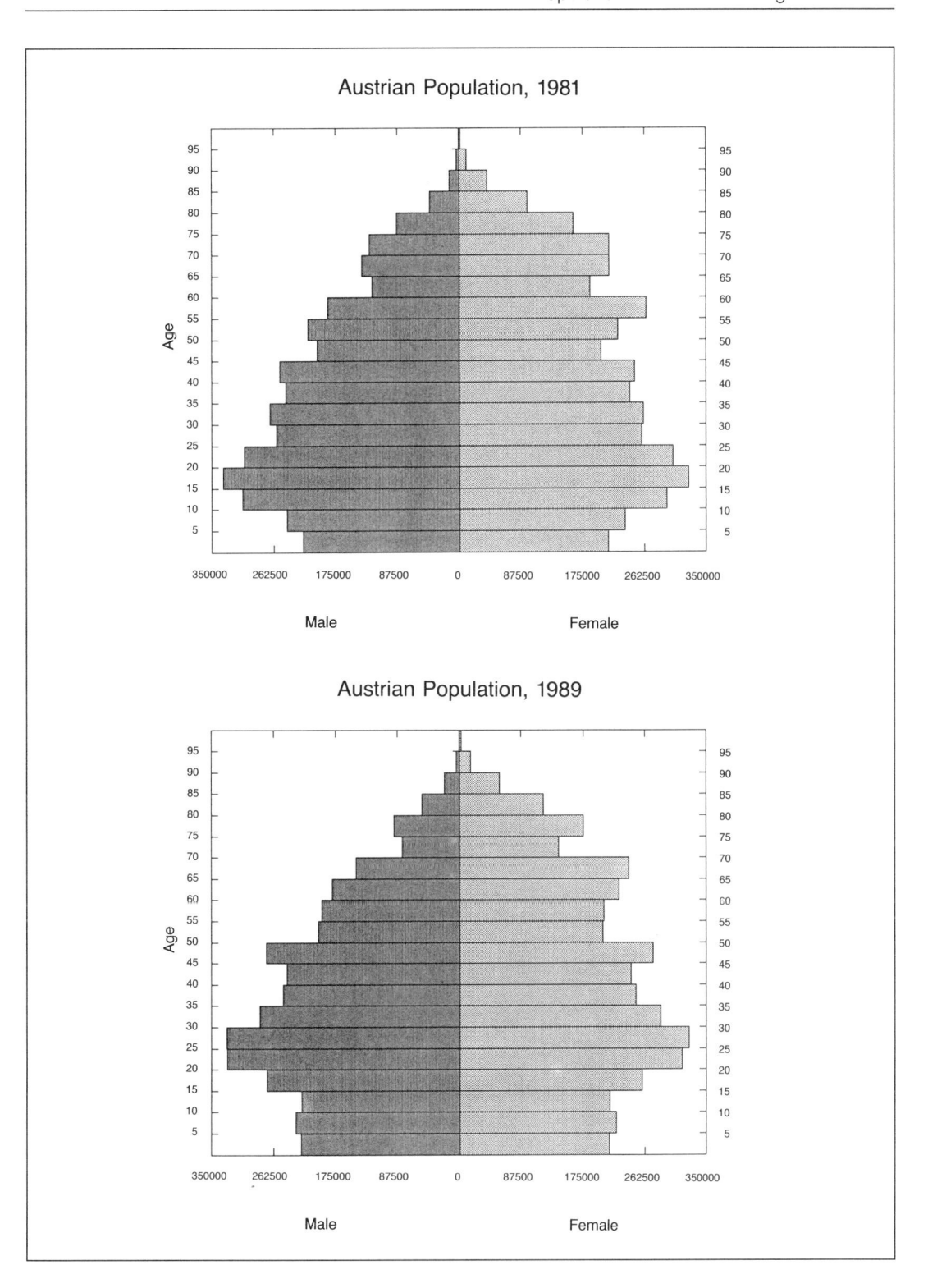

Austrian Population, 1989

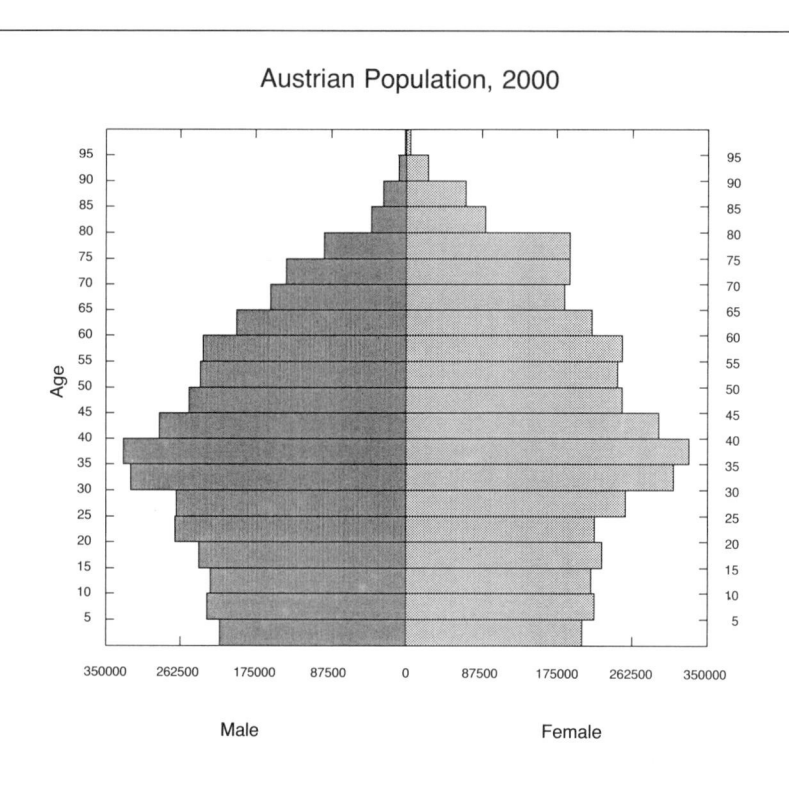

Austrian Population, 2000

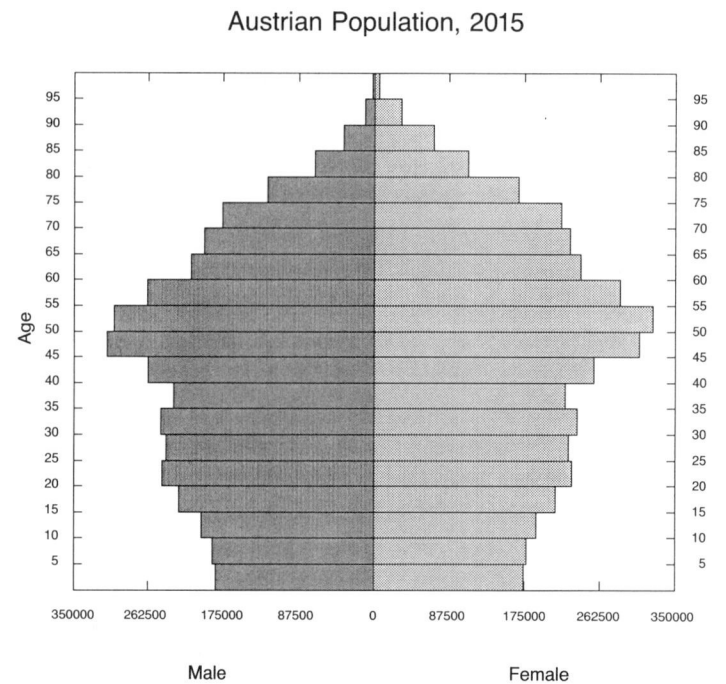

Male | Female

Austrian Population, 2015

Male | Female

Austrian Population, 2030

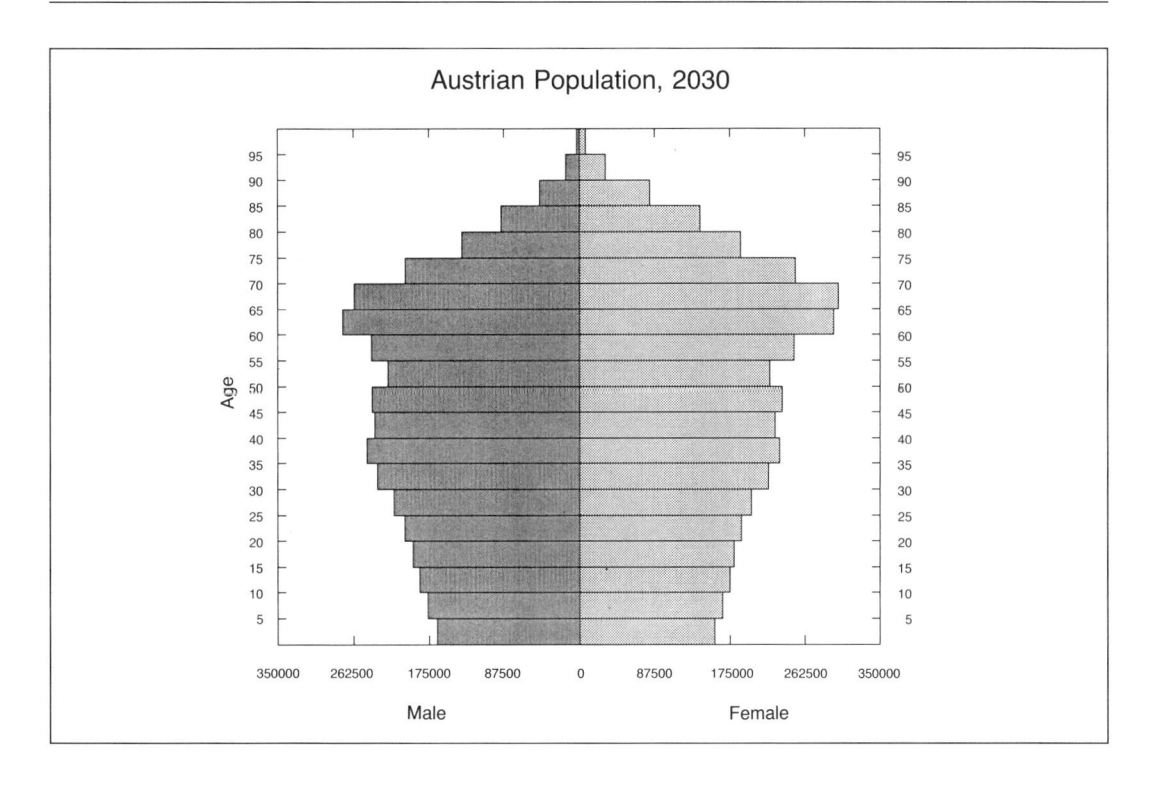

specially highlighted. It must be recognized that today, and to an increasing extent in the future, the family will include one more generation than families did 50 years ago if there is no artificial segregation of the elderly to retirement homes.

This is becoming increasingly important also from the dentist's point of view. In today's family structure we expect the onset of dental problems in children to be prevented by well-informed and active parents, which will be the only means to minimize common dental diseases. The main elements of such a strategy are instructions in dental hygiene, supervision, and especially the introduction of better dietary practices. Those in the generation behind these elderly patients, however, will be responsible for their care and supervision within the extended family structure. In this respect, conditions are similar to those prevailing among infants. Nursing training must be provided as well as education in nutrition, which varies according to the individual age groups. The dentist of the 21st century will need to give increased attention to science and research in general and particularly with regard to gerodontic concerns.

Infant mortality has been reduced as the result of medical achievements. Because the most important functions of the masticatory organ are developed within the first 3 years, dentistry has to concentrate on this early period of development. I believe that one development will be directed towards pediatric dentistry, which will mainly concentrate on diagnostics and prevention. In this respect, studies of the development of the general functions of the masticatory organ and its hierarchical links to the organism as a whole will be particularly relevant. Pediatric dentistry and orthodontics will certainly undergo great structural changes.

A main task to be dealt with and one that constitutes an uncertain factor within prognosis is the surveillance and care of those population groups who, for various reasons, are outside the "normal" social structure. Material and economic factors, social environment, drug addiction, AIDS, and psychological and mental segregation may all contribute to certain groups not being included in the normal social structure. For the curative field of social dentistry, these groups will constitute a particularly intensive field of work well into the 21st century. A global social concept dealing with the care of these groups will be mandatory because it is these groups in particular that will challenge many of the more optimistic projections regarding the elimination of caries and periodontopathies.

Development and tasks of the sub-branches

Restorative dentistry

With shifts in time, restorative dentistry will be greatly reduced. The exceptions have been discussed previously. Changes in the material sector are foreseen for the beginning of the 21st century. Also, amalgam will no longer be used as a restorative material as a result of the concern about mercury and for other reasons. However, it should be ensured that the future generation of materials shows at least the same favorable qualities as amalgam. Emphasis must be placed on the vast area of application to be expected within the social sector.

Periodontics

Periodontics will no longer deal with the field of prophylaxis and will mainly concentrate on the research, science, and general medical aspects of diseases of the oral cavity and the periodontal support structures. The future periodontist will be an expert in general medicine rather than in dentistry.

Prosthodontics

The prosthodontist of the future will be more specialized than today. Computer-based prosthodontics will be used increasingly, primarily with regard to planning and fabrication. The dental laboratory of the future will operate mainly on the basis of computer-controlled prosthodontics. A possible exception may be the esthetic sector, though this has to be viewed with scepticism, too.

Orthopedics and orthodontics

There will be a great increase and reorientation in orthodontics and orthopedics: indications will depend on functional considerations. Preventive measures will have to be coordinated with pediatric dentistry. It is expected that present dog-matic objectives of a uniform occlusion concept will be abandoned in favor of a more individual and functional concept. Great changes are foreseen in the treatment of skeletal dysgnathia. Orthodontic efforts will develop from an empirical, reactive craft into computer-controlled orthodontics. A growing cooperation with dental surgery is to be expected as well.

Summary

Projections for the development of dentistry are evidently based on the analysis of the current situation as seen from a worldwide but also — and probably more importantly — from a regional standpoint. An assessment of the priorities can be attempted only after a global and regional evaluation of the present fact situation. The predicted changes concern all structural units related to dentistry, such as science, research, postgraduate medical education, professional policy, public health policy, and last but not least, the dentist.

In each case, however, consideration must concentrate on the dental needs of people within the period of prediction. Because the center of attention has to be focused on humankind, all projections must be based on developments within the population groups and, above all, on the age distribution of the population. Here, too, there will be a strong upward trend, again differentiated by regions, based on the achievements of general medicine. From this standpoint, there will be a clear shift of emphasis, but changes in therapy will also occur.

Following a significant decrease in incidence of the two main dental problems of the 20th century, caries and pathological conditions of the periodontal support structures, there will be a shift of emphasis in curative activities.

A significant unknown factor in the projections exists for a group of individuals who, to an increasing extent, swerve out of the normal social structure of the population. These would include, for example, the large group of drug addicts, who in the 21st century will constitute a main variable in all medical branches. For these people, the trends and therapies of 20th century dentistry will remain.

The general medical aspects of dentistry will become more important, just as the services for the ordinary sector will decrease. the crucial role of the masticatory organ, at present embodied in the curative, mechanistic field, will, in a strongly altered form, be transferred to the preventive field. However, new issues will arise as a consequence of the successful preservation of teeth and concurrent strong interferences and changes in the functions of the masticatory organ.

In the field of materials development, bold innovations are to be expected, mainly with regard to biocompatibility, esthetics, and also immunology.

Another aspect deals with the new problems deriving from the aging of the population. In this connection, it is not so much the curative sector that will be affected, but problems of nursing and care arising in consequence of aging and diseases of the elderly.

Chapter 10

Dentistry in the 21st Century: An African Perspective with Special Reference to South Africa

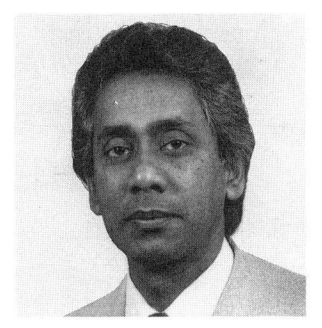

Jairam Reddy
Durban, South Africa

Abstract

The paper locates dental services and treatment in the context of general health as influenced by social, political, and economic factors. Critical determinants such as tuberculosis, malnutrition, and infant mortality rates indicate that health is a development problem. Fragmentation of health services, minimal expenditure on primary health care, and urban/rural imbalances are inherent defects in the South African health care system. While the prevalence of dental caries is declining in the developed countries, it is increasing in the developing world. Gingivitis is common. Universities and the state should train and employ larger numbers of auxiliaries. Opportunities must be provided for black health personnel. A National Health Service with emphasis on primary care, health education, prevention, and fluoridation should be promoted. There is an urgent need to develop a vision in planning and implementing a health care system that is affordable and accessible to the population.

This paper will attempt to locate dental services and treatment in the 21st century within a broad framework of general health as it is influenced by social, political, and economic factors.

The doctrine of race discrimination as practiced in the Republic of South Africa comprises several crucial strands that have a bearing on the health of that nation. The consequences of discriminatory legislation have contributed to poor housing, educational, and health standards for the majority of its population. Its current economic growth rate of around 1% to 2% in the face of growing and sustained economic sanctions is unlikely to provide levels of employment to attain reasonable living standards for its burgeoning population, estimated to be some 50 million by the turn of the century.

To illustrate the impact of apartheid on health, three well-known indicators can be considered: tuberculosis, malnutrition, and infant mortality rate.

While tuberculosis has been wiped out among the white community, it remains unacceptably high among blacks. Of the over 5,000 deaths from the disease in 1984, over 80% occurred among the black community. At the present time it is estimated that there are 8 million infected persons in South Africa (100,000 with active disease) and six or seven deaths from the disease per day.[13] Crowded housing conditions, malnutrition, unemployment, poor sanitary conditions, and lack of water lie at the root of the problem.

With regard to malnutrition, the Second Carnegie Inquiry into Poverty and Development in Southern Africa (1984)[41] revealed that approximately one third of black, colored, and Asian children below the age of 14 years are underweight and physically stunted for their age.

The infant mortality rate for whites falls within the range of most developed countries (12.3 deaths per 1,000 live births), whereas the rate for blacks, some ten times that figure, is closer to that for Third World countries.[27]

Conceptual understanding of health

Health in an underdeveloped society is primarily an outcome of politically determined structural and economic social relations. Health is therefore a problem of development rather than disease.[28]

Fragmentation of health services in South Africa

Historically, much of our health service developed in disparate bits and pieces. Among the contributors to this process were the colonial authorities, mines, missionaries, and local government structures.

The Constitution of the Union of South Africa in 1910 allocated responsibility for hospital services to the four provinces. In 1919, after a great influenza epidemic, a department of health was established to take responsibility for environmental matters bearing on health and infectious diseases.

During the 1960s and 1970s the implementation of the grand vision of apartheid resulted in ten homelands, each with its own health department. At the time the 1983 constitution was implemented, health services were fragmented along the following lines:

1. Provincial services, comprising public sector hospitals and clinics
2. Municipal authorities, responsible for public sanitation, preventive health services, and ambulance services
3. National Department of Health and Welfare, which oversees psychiatric services, medicolegal services, infectious disease control, and medical services in certain rural areas
4. Ten Bantustan Health Services, which are responsible for all health services in the territories
5. The private sector, including general practitioners, specialists, private hospitals, and medical aid schemes
6. Mines, which have their own medical services and hospitals

The 1983 constitution created three more health departments under the "own affairs/general affairs" concept. All hospitals for whites, coloreds, or Indians of which more than 95% of the patients come from any one group will be governed by the respective "own affairs" department of health.

Each of the 14 health departments has its own bureaucracy and ministry. This health system has an incoherent structure, vague lines of authority, and established vested interests, which combine to make adequate coordination extremely difficult.

The National Plan for Health Service Facilities of 1900, which divided health services into six levels, has a reasonably sound theoretical framework. However, fragmentation, bureaucracy, inadequate funding, and political factors have rendered it ineffective. In the Kwa Zulu area of Natal, for example, some rural hospitals have had to either close down or reduce their service significantly because of the lack of qualified staff.

A national health service

While a dual (public/private) system of health care is likely to prevail in South Africa in the foreseeable future, a compelling case for a united national health service to cover the health needs of the entire population can be advanced.

The private medical sector, as part of the free market system, operates on the premise that consumers are able to choose between competing health care providers. By choosing the better product at the lower price, the consumer keeps prices down while encouraging quality.

This model is inappropriate for medical care for a number of reasons: *(1)* consumers do not have the expertise or the necessary information to make an informed choice of medical services; *(2)* the range of choices is limited, especially in certain areas and in certain specialties of medicine; and *(3)* price competition hardly exists in the medical profession.

The National Health Service in the United Kingdom utilizes a smaller proportion of national resources than does the United States, which has greater privatization. Yet infant mortality and life expectancy data favor the United Kingdom over the United States and Germany.[11] A recent study has shown that the introduction of a nationalized health program in the United States not only will improve access to health care but will also reduce costs significantly without affecting care of patients.[23] Further, a recent local study has shown private care to be more costly.[51]

Medical Aid schemes cover the employed, wealthy, and privileged in South Africa. For example, although over 80% of whites are covered, less than 5% of blacks are covered. Even for those covered, studies have shown that the claim rate is related to income.[12] Also, the method of remuneration of medical aid schemes is heavily biased in favor of curative medicine.

No one knows the extent of the colossal waste resulting from the fragmentation of services. Recently the retiring governor of the S.A. Reserve Bank estimated this to be about 48 billion rand since the inception of apartheid.

What is needed in South Africa is a single national health service, with planning and execution of health care delivery in decentralized regions and policy laid down by one coordinating authority.

Changing patterns of dental disease

Dental caries

In a number of western countries, dental caries has declined appreciably since the 1970s.[3,7,14] The following factors have been suggested as reasons: increased use of fluoride, improvements in oral hygiene, dietary changes, and microbial, host, and salivary factors.

The prevalence and severity of dental caries is rising rapidly in many developing countries.[50] The DMFT rate increased from 0.4 to 1.5 between 1966 and 1982 in Uganda; 2.8 to 6.3 over 18 years in Chile; and 1.2 to 3.6 in Lebanon. Barmes[5] reported large increases in caries of 0.1 to 7.1 over 21 years in Kenya; 0.2 to 1.6 over 17 years in Ethiopa; and 0.7 to 4.5 over 15 years in Thailand. These changes have profound implications for treatment needs in these countries with scarce resources. Barmes calculated that an increase in DMF rate of 0.7 to 3.5 would require an additional 700 dental operators per 1 million children.

There is overwhelming evidence that refined sugars, especially sucrose, are the principal cause of dental caries.[40] Sugar consumption not only is increasing in underdeveloped countries but is predicted to exceed the use in industrialized countries, where sugar consumption is falling.[47] Soft drinks are an important factor in the sharp increase in sugar consumption.[29]

Periodontal disease

The prevalence and severity of periodontal diseases are relatively high in Africa.[2,20] Studies also show a marked variation between geographical areas and socioeconomic groups. In most of the above studies it was found that there was a positive correlation between poor oral hygiene and the distribution of periodontal disease.

Recently Manji[33] reported that 26.9% of 5- to 19-year-old children were free from gingival disease, 53.8% had mild gingivitis, 18.1% had moderate, and 1.2% severe in Nairobi. In an examination of 5- to 19-year-old schoolchildren in Tanzania, Mosha and Jorgen[35] found that despite the widespread presence of soft deposits and inflammatory changes of the gingiva, only 2% of the examined teeth exhibited pocket formation of between 3 and 6 mm.

In developed countries, acute necrotising ulcerative gingivitis is largely a disease of adults. In contrast, in Nigeria it afflicts children aged 2 to 10 years.[21,45] Its etiology is unkown but is thought to be related to stress, malnutrition, and certain microbial species.[21]

Dental workforce training

It is estimated that 90% of South Africa's dentists are white. Despite this, less than one third of the country's dental students are nonwhites. The dentist/population ratio for the various population groups is shown in Table 1.

The Inter-dental Committee of Dental Services and Training (1981)[26] found that there was a tremendous backlog of treatment in the black, colored, and (to a lesser extent) Indian populations.

The Committee of Inquiry on Possible Further Facilities for Medical and Dental Training (1984)[38] reported that "among the Black and Coloured population groups there are shortages of general dental practitioners, dental therapists and oral hygienists. The shortages of Black and Coloured dentists exceed the shortage of Black and Coloured doctors."

The Brown Commission of Inquiry into Health Services (1986)[6] stated, "There is therefore a great need for more Asian, Coloured and particularly Black doctors, dentists and other health personnel, and the Commission recommends that this matter should receive the attention of the Education authorities."

There is not only a serious shortage of dental specialists but also of academic staff for the dental faculties. Further, with the exception of the University of the Western Cape, the staff in the other dental faculties are predominantly, if not exclusively, white.

There is growing demand for sophisticated dental service from the black population groups. Evidence for this comes from private dental practitioners in the black areas, the University of the Western Cape, and the University of Durban Westville. In 1985 there were waiting lists of 150, 300, and 500 patients in the departments of conservative dentistry, prosthetics, and orthodontics, respectively, at the University of the Western Cape. Of the 82,937 patients treated at the University of Durban Westville in 1986, nearly a quarter were for restorative and preventive treatment and this is rising steeply. Louw[31] found a significant demand for restorative treatment among the colored population in the Western Cape. A survey by Wilding et al[49] found that growth of dental practices is significantly greater among Indian, colored, and black practices compared to that of white practices.

It is significant that both the quality and number of applicants have dropped in the predominantly white schools, whereas it has increased in the black schools, especially at the University of the Western Cape. It is also significant that the Faculty of Dentistry of the University of Durban Westville has been inundated with several hundred inquiries even before the announcement of the date of intake of students.

Moreover, it has been established in South Africa and other parts of the world that dental disease rates are static or declining in the developed population, while they are rising rapidly in developing populations. Cleaton-Jones et al[9] compared

Table 1 Dentist/population ratio

Population	Ratio
White	1:2,000
Indian	1:7,500
Colored	1:30,000–50,000
Black	1:2,000,000
Total	1:11,000,000

data on dental caries in the primary dentition between 1976 and 1981 in Transvaal, South Africa. Urban white children reflected a decrease in caries prevalence and in the DMFT score. On the other hand, children of urban blacks, rural blacks, and Indians showed an increase. Of these groups the most rapid rate of increase was seen in the Indian children.

The most reliable way to calculate dental workforce estimates is to examine the oral and dental disease status of the population. One such study carried out by Louw,[31] showed that for a population of 427,000 colored subjects aged 2 to 19 years there was a need for 909,290 amalgam restorations and 273,200 extractions. On the basis of this epidemiological data, he recommended the following workforce requirements for the colored population (11- to 19-year-olds of the Western Cape): 20 dentists; 20 oral hygienists, 172 therapists, 100 dental prevention assistants, and 200 dental surgery assistants. He suggested that by training 25 dental therapists per year it would take 9 years to reach the ideal figure of 172.

The requirements for dental services for the developing population will increase rapidly because of both increasing disease and increasing numbers in the population.

Dental prevention assistants

In order to reinforce the preventive dental team, "dental preventive assistants" should be trained. Their duties would be to assist the oral hygienists in their task of education, motivation, and preventive methods like supervised toothbrushing, the use of fluoride tablets, and rinsing programs.[15,25] This category could comprise people such as volunteers from the nursing and teaching profession and could be trained in 1 to 3 weeks.[43] Sheiham[44] estimated that 50 dental prevention assistants could be trained for the cost of one dentist in a much shorter time. It is estimated that there should be one such person for every 5,000 people. This category of dental workforce has been instrumental in reducing oral disease significantly in Sweden.[1] In a recent paper[32] Magri showed that mothers and homemakers, employed in schools after brief training in preventive dentistry, were able to reduce caries prevalence significantly.

This analysis has shown that based on national, regional, and racial needs in 1989 there is a serious shortage of dental specialists, therapists, oral hygienists, and to a lesser extent dentists. If the output is not increased, the shortage will worsen. The requirements for dental services among the developing population will increase rapidly within the next 10 years as a result of increasing disease and an explosive increase in the population.

The number of white dentists in training should be reduced. Although in the developed countries such reduction has resulted in the closure of a number of dental schools, in South Africa this could be made up from the other ethnic groups, which have a severe shortage of dental care personnel.

As we move toward the end of the century a critical determining feature of peaceful change in South Africa will depend on the extent to which educational opportunities can be extended to deprived and discriminated communities.

The educational milieu of the black student in South Africa

Black education is in a perilous state, especially in the secondary schools, the source of future university students. Overcrowding, the lack of qualified teachers and laboratory facilities, poor discipline, etc, are the characteristics of these schools. The estimated per capita expenditure (in rand) per annum on school pupils in South Africa (1987/1988) was as follows[37]: whites 2,299; Indians 1,714; coloreds 887; and blacks 368.

A further aggravating factor is that by the turn of the century there will be some 80,000 black matriculants and less than 40,000 white.

There is little doubt that our students will face enormous problems of adjustment and ability to cope in universities. An academic support program (ASP) should complement an admissions policy that looks for potential and sensitivity in our dental students. Central to the ASP should be psychological empowerment; ie, it must assist students in mobilizing their cognitive skills and infusing their own life experiences into their academic work. The effect of ASPs would assist students to become effective and independent learners. Environmental support such as bursaries, accommodations, and transport are crucial to the success of our disadvantaged students.

It is unfortunate that some African countries have opted for expensively trained dentists rather than auxiliaries. One example of this is Kenya.[22] Yet other countries such as Zambia and Botswana have chosen an appropriate primary health care model in training dental auxiliaries with expanded functions and a sound community orientation.

Most African countries should consider adopting this model; the few dentists and specialists required could be trained in the developed countries in the near future. Preference should be given to dentists trained in public health planning, community dentistry, and primary dental health care.

At a more basic level, in countries like war-torn Mozambique, with scarce resources and virtually no dentists, students have been trained to provide emergency care, oral hygiene, diet control, and fluoride use.[24]

Curriculum

Present dental curricula in our dental schools emphasize high technology dental restoration. Minimal exposure is given to prevention, community dentistry, and primary dental care. Dental training should be based increasingly in community settings.

Dental schools must set out aims and objectives in biomedical and behavioral terms and should include the following:

1. Promotion of attitudes toward dental patient/community that do not rein-

force common forms of prejudice such as racism, sexism, and elitism
2. Communication skills
3. Skills to promote interdisciplinary activity among different categories of health workers
4. Understanding of social sciences, epidemiology, and primary health care
5. An integrated curriculum
6. Student involvement in curriculum development

In considering a dental health policy for the developing populations of Africa, the following theoretical framework in the form of a dental charter is proposed:

Dental charter

1. All people shall have the right of access to dental health care at a cost they can afford.
2. Free dental care should be provided for the indigent, handicapped, unemployed, mothers, and preschool and primary schoolchildren.
3. The country should have a single comprehensive health service of which dentistry should be a part. Such a health service should be under the control of one department of health with as much regional autonomy and community participation as possible.
4. The Primary Health Care Approach (Alma Ata Declaration, 1978) should be pivotal in restructuring the health service, including dental care.
5. Preventive measures promoting self-care to improve the quality of life should receive priority in the professional dental services.
6. School dental services should be restructured with emphasis on preventive care.
7. Well-controlled and scientific epidemological studies should be undertaken to ascertain the patterns of dental diseases in the South African population. This will form the basis of dental workforce planning.
8. Appropriate numbers and types of dental health care personnel should be trained. Emphasis must be placed on primary dental health care workers — dental health educators, oral hygienists, and dental therapists.
9. All dental health care workers trained at state expense should be expected to participate in the state dental services for a mandatory period.
10. Strategies to eliminate fragmentation, duplication, and control of health services on racial lines should be given priority.

Dental health education

Studies have shown that the emphasis on restorative care is inadequate to maintain the dental health of the population.[10,16] Greater attention to prevention and control of disease would be more effective.[30,42] Further public health approaches to health promotion are more effective than those based on individual responsibility.[4,8]

In the African context dental health educators can be trained in a variety of settings and include a range of personnel — village health workers, traditional healers, nurses, homemakers, oral hygienists, etc. Short courses from several weeks' to several months' duration should be offered.

Dental health education should be imparted with the following objectives:

1. Adopt public health approaches rather than individually oriented programs
2. Utilize supportive health education as opposed to authoritarian mode
3. Change from prescriptive health education to health promotion
4. Change from professional dominance to lay competence
5. Combat influence of those interests that stand to profit from ill health, eg, sale of sugar and sugar products
6. Promote fluoridation of public water supplies
7. Integrate dental health education with general health education
8. Practice health education in a social rather than solely a biomedical context

Maintenance of standards

National standards of dental practice should be set by integrating training/research institutions with the national health service (including academics, planners, users, and practitioners). The forum would identify standards for good practice in light of current knowledge. As a minimum the following areas should be covered:

1. Caries and periodontal disease diagnostic procedures
2. Use of radiographs
3. Use of topical fluorides and fissure sealants
4. Cavity preparation principles
5. Basic standards for materials and equipment
6. Use of therapeutic agents
7. Methods of management of periodontal disease

A central supply organization for drugs, materials, and equipment should be set up as a cost-containment exercise.

Restorative dentistry in the 21st century

It is important to remember that the removal of carious tissue and replacement with a suitable material does not cure the disease; the cause remains and it may progress at other sites or even cause secondary caries at the restored site. The ideal therefore is to remove the cause and remineralize the destroyed tooth surface. A further problem arises in the inconsistency of caries diagnosis.[34,39]

Even under optimal conditions the durability and quality of restorations leaves much to be desired. The British health service estimates the life-span of amalgam restorations to be no more than 5 to 10 years,[16,17] and as the restorations are replaced they become more complex. Evidence is accumulating that patients are becoming dissatisfied with the cycle of repetitive restorative dentistry[36] and are likely to demand a more preventive approach in the 21st century.[18]

Scientific research coupled with increasing preventive demands from patients will reduce the clinical intervention approach to a minimum. Dentists who adhere to the maxim "if in doubt, fill or refill" will take pride in adopting the philosophy "if in doubt prevent, wait, and reassess."[19]

With the decline in caries prevalence and increased prevention there will be a decreasing demand for restorative care in the next century in the developed countries. On the other hand, if present caries trends continue there will be increased restorative demands in developing countries. Restorations that are conservative and of high quality would become routine. The extent of the cavity form will be determined by the extent of the carious lesion and not some preconceived outline form.

A search for the best materials will continue and amalgams and composite resins of superior quality are likely to be available. The discarding of amalgam because of toxicity and its replacement with glass-ionomer – based restorative materials is likely. The use of sealants to treat small carious lesions in fissure areas without cavity preparation will become common.

Conclusion

The following remarks are cogently and succinctly stated in a document by the College of Medicine of South Africa.[48]

The effective delivery of health care in modern context, in a developing country, requires:

I. A well-planned, well-structured, well–co-ordinated and adequately funded health care system. This must include primary, secondary and tertiary facilities and a considerable degree of unification in their functions and future development.
II. Mechanism for equitable and efficient access to these services.
III. Training (academic) centres of excellence which will serve a major role in providing and co-ordinating training and education of health care personnel throughout the health care system.
IV. Conditions of service and remuneration (at the various levels within the system) commensurate with the levels of expertise and responsibility required at each level.

There is an urgent need for the public, the medical profession and governing bodies to put aside some of their own self-interests and desires and to have vision in planning and implementing a health care service which we can afford and which will retain the best features of the divergent health care systems currently in operation.

An equitable and affordable health care system can only result if South Africa and other African countries can resolve their sociopolitical problems and transform to a democratic, nondiscriminatory society where human rights are protected and where all citizens have the opportunity to participate fully in the affairs of the country.

The world community can play a role in its attainment.

References

1. Ahlberg JE: *Dental care delivery in Sweden,* in International Dental Care Delivery Systems (ed Ingle), J.I & Blair p 1978.
2. Akpabio SP: A public health service in East and West Africa. *Den Pract Dent Rec* 1966;16:412–421.
3. Anderson RJ, Bradnock G, Beal JE and James PMC: The reduction of dental caries prevalence in English schoolchildren. *J Dent Res* 1982;61:1311–1316.
4. Anderson R: *Health Promotion.* WHO Regional Office, Copenhagen, 1983.
5. Barmes DE: Epidemiology of dental disease. *J Clin Periodontol* 1977;4:80–93.
6. *Brown Commission of Inquiry into Health Services 1986* – Final Report, Pretoria, South Africa Government Printer.
7. Brunell JA and Carlos JP: Changes in the prevalence of dental caries in U.S. schoolchildren. *J Dent Res* 1961–1982;61:1346–1351.
8. Burt BA (ed): The relative efficiency of methods of caries preventing in dental public health. *Proceedings of a Workshop,* University of Michigan 1979; June 5–8, 1979, Ann Arbor.
9. Cleaton-Jones P, Richardson BD, Setzer S and Williams S: Primary dentition caries trends, 1976–1981 in four South African populations. *Community Dent Oral Epidemiol* 1983; 6:312–316.
10. Cohen L: International Comparisons in the Provision of Oral Health Care. *Br Dent J* 1980; 149:347–351.
11. Coovadia HM: *The Case for a National Health Service: A Framework For Discussion.* Proceedings of the NAMDA Annual Conference 1987; pp 11–21.
12. Counihan FH: Facts and Figures Experience of a Medical Plan. *S Afr Med J* 1980; 57:962–967.
13. De Beer: *The South African Disease – Apartheid Health and Health Services, South African Research Service.* Johannesburg, 1984.
14. Downer MC: *Changing patterns of disease in the Western world. In Cariology Today.* International Congress, Zurich 1983, 1984; pp 1–12 (Kotze, Basel).
15. Driscoll WS, Heifetz SB and Bruinelle JA: Treatment and post treatment effects of chewable fluoride tablets on dental caries findings after 7 years. *J Am Dent Assoc* 1979;99:817–824.
16. Elderton RJ: Longitudinal study of dental treatment in the general dental service of Scotland. *Br Dent J* 1983;155:91–96.
17. Elderton RJ: *The quality of amalgam restorations. In Allred H (ed). Assessment of the quality of dental care London.* London Hospital Medical College, 1977:45–81.
18. Elderton RJ: Longitudinal study of dental treatment in the General Dental Service in Scotland. *Br Dent J* 1983;155:91–96.
19. Elderton RJ: Restorative Dentistry and Prospects for the Future. *Dental Update* 1989;2:21–31.
20. Enwonwu CO and Edozien JC: Epidemiology of periodontal disease in Western Nigerians in relation to socio-economic status. *Arch Oral Biol* 1970;15:1232–1255.
21. Enwonwu CO: Epidemiological and biochemical studies of necrotising ulcerative gingivitis and noma (cancrum oris) in Nigerian children. *Arch Oral Biol* 1972;17:1357–1372.
22. Gilmore ND: Dentistry in Kenya. *J Public Health Dent* 1984;44:19–21.
23. Himmelstein DU and Woolhandler S: Socialised medicine: A solution to the cost crisis in health care in the United States. *Int J Health Serv* 1986;16:339–354.
24. Hobdell MH: Dental Health Services in Mozambique. *Br Dent J* 1981;151:161–162.
25. Hope T: Results of 10 years of supervised fluoride toothbrushing in Rygge, Norway. *Community Dent Oral Epidemiol* 1979;7:330–334.
26. *Inter-dental Committee of Dental Services and Training* 1981, Pretoria, South Africa Government Printer.
27. Joubert G, Bradshaw D, Odendaal HJ and Yach D: Improving child survival. *In South African Medical Research* 1988; pp 96–103. Owen Burgess Publishers, Pinetown.
28. Jinnabhai CC, Coovadia HM and Abdool Karim SS: Socio-medical indicators of health in South Africa. *Int J Health Serv* 1986; 16:163–175.
29. Lappe FM and Collins J: *Food first. The myth of scarcity.* Souvenir Press, London; 1980.
30. Löe H: *Principles and progress in the prevention of periodontal disease* 1980; pp 225–268. In Letiner T and Cimasoni G (eds). *The borderline between caries and periodontal disease.* New York, Grune and Stratton.
31. Louw NP: *Essential dental health needs of the coloured population in the Cape Peninsula.* PhD thesis, University of Stellenbosch, 1982.
32. Magri F: Dental health education by dental preventive workers in Swiss communities. *International Association for Dental Research, 64th General Session.* The Hague, Netherlands, 1986; Abstract 491.
33. Manji F: The dental health of children aged 5–14 years in two primary schools located in the industrial area of Nairobi. *Trop Dent J* 1983; 6:35–44.
34. Merrett MCW and Elderton RJ: An in vitro study of restorative dental treatment decisions and secondary caries. *Br Dent J* 1984;157:128–133.
35. Mosha HJ and Jorgen L: Dental caries, oral hygiene, periodontal disease and dental fluorosis among school children in Northern Tanzania. *Odontstomatol Tropic* 1983;6:215–219.

36. Nuttall NM: Characteristics of dentally successful and dentally unsuccessful adults. *Community Dent Oral Epidemiol* 1984;12:208–212.
37. *Race Relations Survey, South African Institute of Race Relations,* Johannesburg, 1988.
38. *Report and Recommendations of the Committee of Inquiry on Possible Further Facilities for Medical and Dental Training* – 1984.
39. Rytomaa I, Jarvinen V and Jarvinen J: Variation in caries recording and restorative treatment plan among university teachers. *Community Dent Oral Epidemiol* 1979;7:335–339.
40. Screenby LM: Sugar availability, sugar consumption and dental caries. *Community Dent Oral Epidemiol* 1982;10:1–7.
41. *Second Carnegie Inquiry into Poverty and Development in Southern Africa,* 1984.
42. Sheiham A: *An analysis of dental care system in Western Europe 1983;* Ch 4, pp 11–20. In Global Problems in Dental Health. Ed. Nyssonen, V. Centre for Continuing Education, University of Kuopio, Finland.
43. Sheiham A, Effendi I and Bei Kien Noi: Assessment of dental needs: Pilot studies in Indonesia. *Trop Dent J* 1979;11:45–53.
44. Sheiham A: An evaluation of the success of dental care in the United Kingdom. *Br Dent J* 1973;135:271–279.
45. Sheiham A: An epidemiological survey of acute ulcerative gingivitis in Nigerians. *Arch Oral Biol* 1966;11:937–942.
46. *South African Institute of Race Relations Survey* 1987/88.
47. Third World Sugar Forecast. *Afr Bus.* January 1981.
48. *Transactions of the College of Medicine of South Africa. The Future of Academic Medicine in South Africa* 1988; pp 14–19.
49. Wilding RJC, Reddy J, Owen CP: Dental manpower needs in South Africa – A survey of practices. 1986;41:469–475.
50. World Health Organization. Oral health global indicator for 2000. Dental caries level at 12 years. *WHO Oral Health Unit,* Geneva 1982.
51. Zwarenstein M, Dorrington RE, Budlender D, Frankish J and Bradshaw D: *Expenditure on Medical Care in South Africa (1978–1982).* Proceedings of the 1987 NAMDA Annual Conference, pp 24–34, 1987.

Chapter 11

Dentistry and Science in the 21st Century: Developing New Paradigms

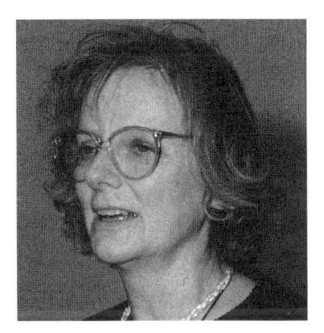

Birte Melsen
Århus, Denmark

Abstract

The future is a product of the past and the present. Within dentistry in Denmark, the effort focused on prophylaxis has to a large degree succeeded in preventing dental disease in the young population. The adult population, however, still present us with problems of partial edentulism and complicated dental problems.

In the future, research will change its focus from prevention for the young to a deeper fundamental understanding of the etiology and pathogenesis of dental diseases seen in relation to increasing age and related changes in the "host's" biology.

A view into the future will show us a dentist who, through a computer, will have access to a global range of recent scientific reports. The wide range and the quality of new information forces dentists to make choices based on their special priorities. Difference in priority based on ethical, esthetic, and emotional values will generate subcultures among dentists.

Dentistry cannot be seen as an isolated phenomenon as it is related to the development of both the local and global communities. In the following I will briefly survey the local background from which Danes look to the future and describe our expectations of the profession as we move into a new millenium.

Dentistry in Denmark, as throughout Scandinavia, is influenced by the strong organization of public dentistry offered to the younger generation, and ongoing research has focused on the etiology and prevention of dental disease.[1–5] Basic to understanding our view on the future in dentistry in Denmark is, however, a fundamental knowledge of its present state and history. The first school of dentistry was established in 1912 in the town of Svendborg, and schools in several provincial towns soon followed. Nevertheless, it was not until 1971 that the law on public dentistry was passed.[6] This law gave all children below the age of 18 the right to receive dental care free of charge. This care included necessary orthodontics to ensure the development of a healthy and well-functioning occlusion for the physical and psychological well-being of the individual. The program came into effect gradually, starting with the children first entering school in 1971. From the beginning a strong emphasis was placed on prevention. Passive prophylaxis, including regular cleaning, topical application of fluoride, and regular rinsing with fluoride solutions, was one part of the preventive regime.[7] Other measures included active prevention and were intended to influence the attitudes of the children and their parents and encourage better dental hygiene and eating habits. Brushing instructions, self-care programs, and regular visits to the dentist were among the components stressed.[8] All efforts were based on research on the natural history of dental diseases, caries, and periodontal disease, as well as the results of numerous epidemiological studies.[9–12]

The result of this massive effort was that dental health among the young population improved: the DMFT rate in 12-year-old children dropped from 9.9 in 1976–1980 to less than 4.2 in 1986. Of all 18-year-old Danes today, 42% leave the public system without any caries experience. The improvement of dental health has also been reflected in the adult population. The number of patients with full dentures has dramatically decreased and the expectations of adults for their dental development are changing as well.[13,14]

This trend toward an improved dental health seems to be the same in a large number of countries and was recently confirmed by a major epidemiological study carried out among different age groups in the United States.[15]

With this information in mind, it is obvious that the dentist of the future has to deal with two different populations: the young population characterized by healthy dentition — little if any caries, a healthy periodontium, and minor malocclusion — and an elderly population, many of whom have had an extremely high treatment experience and lost one or more teeth with complications. The number of edentulous patients, however, will decrease.

The treatment required for the non-edentulous patient will involve various aspects of the most recent technological developments if we are to improve the prognosis for maintaining the remaining dentition for the patient's lifetime. The dental rehabilitation that many of these patients need must, however, be paid primarily by the patient; it is thus a matter of time, resources, and economic priority whether such treatment will be carried out. The priority adult patients give to dental treatment will be a reflection of the patient's attitude to dental health, which is a direct result of how well the dental profession is able to sell its "products."

It is striking how much developments within dentistry seem to reflect those of society. As in society, progress within dentistry comprises two separate but closely related components: "hardware" and "software."

Within dentistry, developments in hardware have resulted from advances in high technology, especially those made within the last decade. These include composite resin materials, which can be bonded directly to the tooth (including dentin), and the development of implants, which have contributed to changes in treatment planning and in the prognosis for complicated cases. New restorative materials continue to be introduced. Preparation and impression techniques using lasers are just being developed and in the future we shall see restorations being produced by computer-guided technology. Implants will be used not only as bases for reconstruction but also as anchorage for tooth movement and reconstruction of alveolar processes in partially edentulous patients.[16,17]

Current hardware development concerns treatment. However, much of dental research is changing its focus from a preoccupation with caries prevention in young children to better understanding disease development in and around the oral cavity and its relation to age. Age-related changes in predisposition to disease, changes in the immune system, and the capacity for tissue repair must be studied through epidemiologic, clinical, and basic molecular biological studies. Because this type of research must be carried out by scientists with different specialties working in collaboration, interdisciplinary projects will become more common.

As a result of scientific efforts, "software" is produced. Software development in dentistry, as in all of society, is characterized by an exponentially growing stream of information. One can further imagine that the results of progress within most areas of dental science will be readily available to the individual dentist and that the lag between obtaining laboratory data and actually applying these data in the clinic will be shortened.

Recently the director of the (US) National Institute of Dental Research, Harald Löe, emphasized the importance of bringing to dental schools, to health policy makers, and to those who control financial resources for dental health services the message that the transfer of science and technology for oral disease prevention must be facilitated.

The dramatic increase in availability of information within dentistry will, however, not necessarily generate homogeneity in the dental services offered to the public. Through his or her personal computer the dentist will obtain easy and rapid access to scientific literature. Instead of being limited to a few journals received by mail subscription, it is likely that in the future, through an electronic subscription, a dentist will have access to a major data base. The ability to access such a wide range of sources, however, increases the responsibility of the dentist. It is one thing for a dentist to feel confident that he or she is keeping current by subscribing to a few well-respected journals. However, in the future the practitioner will have many scientific literary sources available, and choices will be determined by personal interest. It will be impossible for the individual dentist to keep completely up to date within even a specialty area. Thus, the dentist will need to define a set of priorities. The priorities may be influenced by certain "schools" or groups of researchers, and because it is likely that more than one group will emerge with some degree of popularity, factions will invariably arise and communication among these factions will become more difficult. This has already occurred in orthodontics, where the specialist trained in functional appliances has great difficulty in understanding the dentist working only with the straight wire technique.

Until now, science was regarded as having provided objective information. This meant that science was expected to be uniform and lead to the best solution to a problem. With the explosive growth of available information, however, such uniformity is giving way to a diversity of scientific "truths," and it will be the dentist's responsibility to select the one in which he or she has the most faith.

At the same time we must realize that it will no longer be reasonable to expect our treatment models to stand forever. Further, information on new developments within dentistry will, in different publications, be available to the public; patients will thus no longer accept their dentist's solution as the only method of treatment but may come up with alternative solutions or consult different dentists for the same problem. Because no one will be able to possess a reasonable survey of all developments within all treatment modalities, a "decentralization" will take place.

The classic picture of science as the one way of reflecting nature in an objective manner has been replaced with acceptance of the fact that so-called scientific truth exists only temporarily, until rejected or modified by new experiments. The separation of subject and object, the basis of modern science, is no longer possible. The object will be described under influence of certain norms, ethical, esthetic, and emotional, each of which will determine specific factions.

As a consequence, we must realize that the last century has been characterized by a development that has been perceived as a crisis: products and knowledge are being thrown into the market faster than they can be accepted by the average consumer. This is occurring in dentistry as well and may have to be accepted as a state of normalcy. The hardware as well as the software, as discussed above, will be subject to selection by the individual dentist, and many will be left with the impression that the time of turnover of the products of science, hardware or software, is rapidly decreasing. It is possible that most of our resources will, in the future, be focused not on production itself but on public relations. Marketing strategies will be needed to promote new products. Within dentistry this means that the public's level of tolerance of dental imperfections must be lowered in order to generate more demand for esthetic dentistry, orthodontics, and orthognathic surgery. Treatments are becoming more sophisticated, and as a result the need for general dentists will probably drop dramatically, because most preventive therapies for both caries and periodontal disease can be handled by a hygienist. Dentists will have to collaborate in order to make the most advanced products available to the public.[18]

Monitoring of the demand for treatments will be handled by dental associations. The practice of creating a demand for treatment has been seen in other disciplines and may not be far ahead for dentistry. Scientific results will be brought to the public in a popularized version, thereby generating a demand for dentists who keep up to date in treatment developments. Put bluntly, dentists will be sharpening the consciousness of their target group. Still more treatment approaches will be marketed, thereby creating some degree of frustration in that one method of treatment may be replaced by another. The most important factor in development may be the generation of demand.

The dental profession has been largely successful in preventing major dental diseases. However, instead of being content with these achievements, the dentist of the future may generate a new basis for existence by producing a public demand for ideal esthetics and perfect masticatory function. In the extreme, this would mean that most of the population would have indications for major treatment.

In response to this trend, the so-called green movement is developing. Its followers believe that the explosion of new information no longer provides a true reflection of an object, and they therefore generate their own reality based on individual needs set by the norms of their subculture. They select a weighed, perhaps biased, picture of a reality created through internal communication within the subgroup. Each subgroup will be characterized by a set of common norms regarding ethics, esthetics, and emotion according to which they act. The pluralism described will also result in various types of dental offices. While some will focus on high technology, others will take a more holistic approach, collaborating with borderline disciplines within medicine and homeopathia.

In Danish society the lack of having to fight for the most basic material items has resulted in the development of many varied lifestyles. Such diversity will eventually be answered creatively to produce a reasonable survey among the different areas. As scientific "truth" will be more closely related to the subject than the object, solutions to problems will be the products of norms, values, and emotions: art and science will no longer be incompatible. The rhetoric, the sales ability in establishing the importance of specific scientific results will become an acceptable part of science. Science will no longer simply reflect the "truth" but create its own truth as defined by a specific faction. Of the three classical areas – knowledge, ethics, and esthetics – esthetics will be elevated. Historically, esthetics has been perceived as the playground for artists, the sensitive souls of society. As art has been characterized as generating its own reality, so too will science in the future reflect the same characteristics.

In conclusion, one may predict that the need for a new set of paradigms will develop. These will be chosen based not necessarily as result of the state of art within the dental profession but on "whose" truth will gain most interest. We are at an edge and have the possibility to chose our future, for better or worse. It is frightening; it is exciting.

References

1. Gröndahl H-G, Hollender L, Malmcrona E, Sundquist B: Dental caries and restorations in teenagers. *Swed Dent J* 1977;1:45–50.
2. Axelsson P, Lindhe J: The effect of preventive programme on dental plaque gingivitis and caries in school children. Results of one and two years. *J Clin Periodont* 1974;1:126–138.
3. Helm S: National statistics on caries and oral hygiene derived from the Danish child dental health recording system. *Community Dent Oral Epidemiol* 1973;1:1221–1226.
4. Holst D: *Third party payment in dentistry: An analysis of the effect of a third party payment system and of system determinants.* Oslo: University of Oslo, 1982. Thesis.
5. Hamp SF, Lindhe J, Fornell J, Johansson LA, Karlsson R: Effect of a field program based on systematic control on caries and gingivitis in school children after 3 years. *Community Dent Oral Epidemiol* 1978;6:17–23.
6. Ministry of Internal Affair's Announcement no. 666, 22nd December, 1977.
7. Melsen B, Agerbæk N, Rölla G: Topical application of 3% monofluoride phosphate in a group of schoolchildren. *Caries Res* 1979;13:344–349.
8. Melsen B, Agerbæk N: Effect of an instructional motivation program on oral health in Danish adolescents after 1 and 2 years. *Community Dent Oral Epidemiol* 1980;8:72–78.
9. Anerud A, Löe H, Boysen H, Smith M: The natural history of periodontal disease in man: Changes in gingival health and oral hygiene before 40 years of age. *J Periodont Res* 1979;14:526–540.
10. Cohen LK, O'Shea RM, Putnam WJ: Toothbrushing: public opinion and dental research. *J Oral Ther* 1968;4:229–246.
11. Craft M, Croucher R: Factors that influence dental visiting among young adults 16–20 years old. *Community Dent Oral Epidemiol* 1980;8:347–350.
12. Carlos JP: Epidemiological trends in caries: Impact on adults and the aged, in: Guggenheim B (ed) *Cariology today*. International congress in honour of Hans R. Mühlemann, Zürich, Sept 2–4, 1983. Basel: Karger, 1984; pp 24–32.
13. Kirkegaard E, Borgnakke WS, Grønbæk L: *Oral Health Status, Dental Treatment Need, And Dental Care Habits in a Representative Sample of the Adult Danish Population. Survey of Oral Health of Danish Adults*. Department of Child Dental Health & Community Dentistry, Royal Dental College, Aarhus, and Department of Community Health and Postgraduate Education, Copenhagen Dental College, 1987.
14. Melsen B, Hørup N, Terp S: Factors of importance for maintenance of teeth. *Community Dent Health* 1987;4:11–25.
15. Löe H: The changing face of dentistry. *Periodontology Tomorrow*, June 115–117, 1989, Aarhus.
16. Tatum OH: Maxillary and sinus implant reconstructions. *Dent Clin North Amer* 1986;4:207–229.
17. Roberts WE, Smith RK, Zilberman Y, Mozsary PG, Smith RS: Osseous adaptation to continuous loading of rigid endosseous implants. *Am J Orthod* 1984;86:95–111.
18. Melsen B: *Orthodontic Treatment of the Degenerated Dentition*, in *Orthodontics in an Aging Society*, DS Carlson (ed), Monograph 22, Craniofacial Growth Series, Center for Human Growth and Development, The University of Michigan, 1989, Ann Arbor, pp 105–136.

Chapter 12

21st-Century Dentistry in Canada

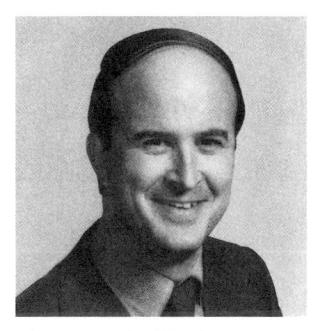

George A. Zarb
Toronto, Ontario
Canada

Abstract

Dental education, practice, and research are integral parts of our profession's future currency. Individual fluctuations may occur and are bound to affect the entire future context of dentistry. Societal needs must lead to changes in practice patterns, which in turn will influence the entire educational process. This is a particularly compelling challenge for the dental educator. Furthermore, dental research has always been the practitioner's silent partner, but its continued viability may be compromised by changes in funding patterns and reduction of dental school numbers.

The late Marshall McLuhan compared assignments such as ours — that is, predicting the future of dentistry — to riding the automobile of progress as it headed uncertainly and sometimes recklessly toward the future. The driver's eyes were fixed upon the horizon ahead, but McLuhan cautioned that such a journey would probably be far more relevant if the rearview mirror was studied once in awhile. As a transplanted European, I have pursued a clinical academic career profoundly influenced by forward-looking new-world vistas, while not losing sight of traditional old-country concerns usually expressed by the observation "when in doubt don't do it." I have therefore chosen to heed McLuhan's advice as I attempt a synthesis of some ideas that relate to the concerns of practice, education, and research in the dentistry of the future. The three concerns are inseparable. They are integral parts of the same currency, and all fluctuate in response to changing societal needs. However, at the risk of oversimplifying my remit, I will address each concern separately. My ob-

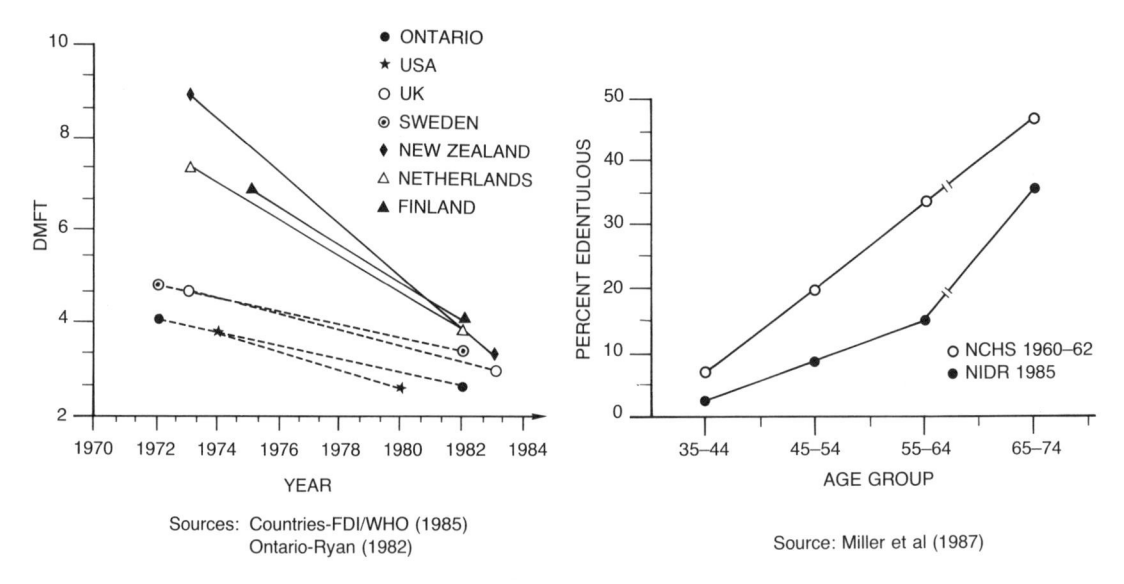

Fig 1 Trends in dental caries prevalence 1972–1983 DMFT at 12 years in various countries.

Fig 2 Percent of edentulous US adults and seniors.

servations will of course run the risk of sounding somewhat parochial in the larger global context. However, I believe that Canadian concerns in the three areas of practice, education, and research are similar to those confronting my colleagues in industrialized countries.

Dental practice

The notion that patterns and styles of future practices will be automatically based in the knowledge, equipment, and philosophy that are available today is clearly an untenable one. It may be tempting to suggest that the advances of the past 25 years — caries control, understanding of biological processes, biomaterials, osseointegrated implants, etc – have been so profound that future developments will only occur in smaller increments. If this is the case, the greater temptation will be to concentrate more on strategies of patient needs and not to be swept away by the desire for more mechanics and technological refinements. This is indeed a salutary approach, because the twin concerns of patient care and technical performance have sometimes run the risk of being mutually exclusive, particularly in dental school environments.

On the other hand, equally dramatic advances in prevention and treatment of disease processes could very well occur, with very professional implications on the workforce and practice pattern fronts. A lingering look at the rearview mirror reveals that dental practice has been dominated largely by the need for tooth repair and replacement. This pattern has already changed and will change even more profoundly as the decline in caries is reflected in a significant decline in operative treatment needed by children and young adults. The increase in the number of retained teeth in adults is evidenced by the fact that over the past 25 years, edentulism has been reduced by half in 35- to 64-year-old employed persons. To a lesser extent this has also occurred in the over-65 group (Figs 1 and 2). In addition, the average number of teeth retained per dentate individual has increased. Although comparable Canadian data are not available, the trend is probably similar.

The greater retention of teeth in the 30- to-64 age group has increased the need for replacement restorations, as well as for crowns and fixed and removable partial dentures. The apparent significant increase in replacement therapy in this patient age group has largely offset the significantly reduced requirements of juveniles and young adults. The adult population, with its improved dental awareness but compromised dentitions, is now the major user of operative, endodontic, and prosthetic services. As this group ages, it is likely to continue to require very high levels of replacement/reparative dentistry.

Root caries has been cited as occurring in epidemic proportions and is likely to place enormous demands on the dental profession. It is conceded that the incidence of root caries increases with age and that its management is clinically demanding. However, data from several US studies indicate that its prevalence among individuals over age 65 is equal to or less in magnitude than the prevalence of coronal caries (Fig 3). It is also

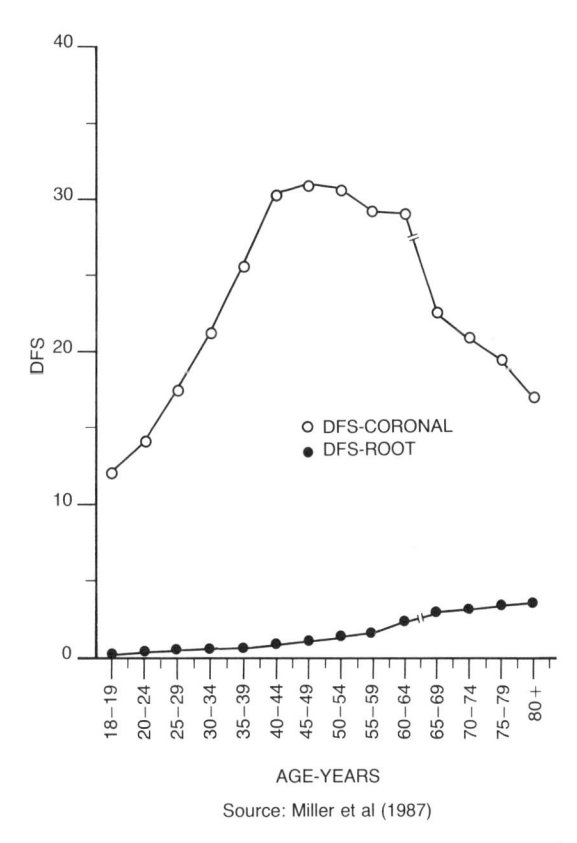

Fig 3 Decayed and filled coronal and root surfaces (DFS) in US employed adults and seniors.

expected that greater attention to oral hygiene and widespread use of fluoride toothpaste by the adult population will decrease the rate at which new root surface lesions occur and will more than offset the increased number of teeth now at risk. It is anticipated that an overall increased restorative need in adults over age 50 may largely counterbalance the progressive decrease in the reparative requirements of the under-50 population. However, the next decade should produce a reduction in both overall need and demand for restorative treatment.

With the decline in dental caries, periodontal disease has emerged as the primary dental health problem and the major cause of tooth loss. Fortunately, the public has become increasingly aware of the problem and for the most part has the necessary dental insurance to cover, at least, preventive and sensitive periodontal care. In addition, the dental workforce has been rapidly augmented by dental hygienists who are skilled and motivated to provide these services.

Recent research indicates that gingivitis, while prevalent in a high proportion of the population, comes and goes in individual sites and is probably not the initial stage of periodontal disease in most instances. Earlier studies included gingivitis as a component of periodontal disease indices and generally found a high prevalence of periodontal disease. The recent 1987 study by the National Institute of Dental Research[1] used separate indices for gingivitis, attachment loss, and periodontal pocket depth and found much lower prevalence and severity of periodontal disease than was formerly reported. Attachment loss of 4 mm or more was found in only 20% of working adults, a result similar to that obtained in a North Carolina study by Hughes.[2] The NIDR study also found that pocket depth of 4 mm or more (most severe pocket per individual) was observed in only 15% of working adults and seniors. These and other data suggest that the periodontal health of the great majority of adults, including seniors, can be maintained by a combination of personal oral hygiene and periodic sanative care.

The greatest unknown factor regarding future demand is the degree to which people not currently getting periodontal care will begin to seek it. The extent to which this potential demand will be realized is difficult to estimate because much of the unmet need is centered in the low socioeconomic groups, and these groups are not readily motivated. In any case, the largest part of this need is for sanative and preventive care, which is provided largely by dental hygienists rather than dentists. Page[3] concluded that "periodontitis is not a universally prevalent disease in adults, as previously thought, nor is it an unmanageable problem in the American population. The population seems to have a relatively small high risk group."

Further research is needed to permit identification of these high-risk individuals at the early stages of periodontal disease. This would allow the application of intensive preventive and control measures, including thorough subgingival scaling and root planing and selective antibiotic or anti-inflammatory therapy, or a combination of these, before significant periodontal breakdown has occurred.

Nevertheless, periodontal disease is likely to remain the major dental health problem for many years to come. The primary responsibility for the prevention, detection, and control of this disease rests squarely on the shoulders of the general practitioner. There is no doubt that the average dentist must devote considerably more attention and time to this problem than has been the case in the past.

Malocclusion that severely interferes with function or presents a serious esthetic problem affects approximately 14% of the child population. An additional

Table 1 Studies of oral health status of seniors in Ontario*

Investigator (year)	Location (year of study)	Site	Sample size*	Age range (% ≥ 80)	% visiting a dentist in the past 1–2 years[†]
Lightman, Thompson, and Grainger (1969)	Toronto (1966–1969)	Home for aged	491 (467)	50–99 (38)	Not reported
Martinello and Leake (1971)	London (1969)	Homes for aged	517 (510)	50–99 (63)	9.1 (13.2)
Leake and Martinello (1972)	London (1970)	Seniors' apartments	502 (497)	50–99 (18)	15 (24)
Banting (1972)	Hamilton (1971)	Private residences	288	65–90+ (13)	19 (31)
Martinello (1976)	Chatham (1974)	Home for aged	208 (203)	50–100+ (54)	5 (9)
Leake and Howley (1982)	East York (1981)	Home for aged	86	62–99 (57)	13 (24)
Main (1983)	North York (1983)	Recreation centres	219	65–89	– (47)
Ellis, Hyduk, and McFarlane (1983)	Toronto (1982)	Private residences	213	65–85+ (16)	29 (36)
Armstrong (1984)	Kenora-Rainy River (1984)	Collective living centres (CLCs)	215	Not stated	20 (–)
Ryan, Ontario Public Health Branch (1985)	Ontario (26 Health Units, 1985)	CLCs	1,082	65–85+ (56 est.)	20 (–)
Johnston (1985)	Oxford County (1985)	CLCs	201	Not stated	Not stated
McIntyre, Jackson, and Shosenberg (1986)	Scarborough (1985)	CLCs	345	60–102 (65)	Not reported
Leake, Price, and Schabas (1987)	East York (1985)	CLCs and seniors' apartments	234	65–104 (57 est.)	25 (42)
Adams (1985–1986)	Waterloo Wellington Counties (1985–1986)	Nursing homes	697	Not stated	Not stated

* From Leake, JL and Otchere, D: Planning for the Future, Ont Dent 27–32, March 1988.
[†] Excluding persons aged <60 years.

Table 1 continues on following page.

Table 1 (continued)   Studies of oral health status of seniors in Ontario*

Investigator (year)	Location (year of study)	Site	Sample size*	Age range (% ≥ 80)	% visiting a dentist in the past 1–2 years[†]
Locker, Leake, Price, Schabas, and Chao (1987)	East York (1986–1987)	Private residences	246	50–91 (9.7)	60 (64)

* From Leake, JL and Otchere, D: Planning for the Future, *Ont Dent* 27–32, March 1988.
[†] Excluding persons aged <60 years.

Table 2   Percent distribution of edentulism among the elderly in Ontario*

Sample location (year)	Age group				
	60–69	70–79	80–89	90–99+	Total
CLCs, Toronto (1969)	63.6	83.8	85.4	70.4	80.7
CLCs London (1971)	61.1	80.4	77.0	79.8	77.0
Seniors' apartments, London (1972)	65.1	76.9	80.0	66.7	74.1
Private residences, Hamilton (1972)	–	–	–	–	66.0
CLCs, Chatham (1976)	64.7	71.6	83.3	79.4	76.4
CLCs, East York (1982)	–	62.2[†]	80.6	100.0	76.0
Seniors' recreation centres, North York (1983)	–	–	–	–	25.0
Private residences, Toronto (1983)	–	–	–	–	51.2
CLCs, Kenora-Rainy River (1984)	–	–	–	–	71.7
CLCs, Ontario (1985)	–	–	–	–	61.0
CLCs, Oxford County (1985)	–	–	–	–	66.6
CLCs, Scarborough (1986)	–	–	–	–	70.0
CLCs and apartments, East York (1985)	50.0a	55.0b	62.0c	82.0d	57.0
CLCs, Waterloo (1985–1986)	–	–	–	–	70.5
Private residences, East York (1986–1987)	25.6a	30.4e	–	–	27.5

a, 65–74 years, b, 75–109 years, c, 85–94 years, d, 95–104 years, e, 75–91 years.
* From Leake, JL and Otchere, D: Planning for the Future, *Ont Dent* 27–32, March 1988.
[†] Includes persons aged 69 years ≤ including 69 years.

20% have moderate malocclusion, although it is not clear whether treatment is really necessary for the latter group. A modest but increasing demand for adult orthodontics has also been reported, with Swedish studies suggesting an urgent need for treatment in 9% of adults. It is doubtful whether the average general dentist could devote sufficient time to develop and maintain competence in the advanced clinical skills required for difficult orthodontic treatment.

The implications of changing patterns in health care as well as better information about the demand for it appear to be twofold. First, those who seek care regularly will require on average less dental treatment and therefore less care. This assumes that the facilitative effect introduced by dental insurance on utilization or dentist overservicing will not be extensively applied. Second, those who seek care as symptoms arise will tend to have fewer problems and therefore will require less care. However, an increasingly dentate population will have dental care needs for a longer period of time. It is therefore unlikely that over a lifetime the demand for dental care due to improved oral health will automatically be lower.

Furthermore, a depressed birth rate indicates that over time an increasingly larger proportion of the population will be elderly. Historically, older people have used dental services less than younger age groups, although the former are likely to have more retained teeth, so that treatment demand will probably increase somewhat above present low rates of utilization.

Age-specific cross-sectional studies on oral health in elderly patients also reveal that edentulism is higher with older age groups. There also appears to be a marginal decline in edentulism in elderly patients living in collective living centers. These patients, whether dentate or edentulous, have significant untreated dental disease and additionally need significant maintenance treatment for new or previous prosthetic services. Independently living elderly who participated in a survey showed significantly decreased rates of edentulism. These studies identified the need for care accumulated at the time of the survey and do not specify continuing maintenance or incremental care needs. Standard survey techniques are required to help determine whether the levels of dental disease in the elderly are the result of previous lack of care, high incidence of disease, or both.

Acceptable, agreed-upon criteria or standards for making precise decisions about whether the dental workforce supply for a region is adequate, inadequate, or excessive are not available. However, the strong general impression supported by some research indicates that the supply of dental care exceeds the demand for it. This is a signal for an oversupply situation, and several schools have responded to this reality by scaling down the size of the undergraduate programs.

The practice outlook for the future will be one that evolves in the context of a virtual prevention of dental diseases of bacterial origin in a significant segment of the population. Greater treatment time will be spent diagnosing and assessing risk factors and their sequence, particularly in the longer-living medically compromised patient.

Table 3 Dental health status of dentate elderly persons in Ontario*

Site (year)	Number	% of persons with teeth			Mean no. of teeth		
		Decayed (% dentate)	Periodontal disease	Need extraction	Decayed	Need extraction	Filled
CLCs, Toronto (1969)	90 (19)	–	–	–	–	–	–
CLCs, London (1971)	116 (23)	–	–	–	1.2	1.3	3.1
Seniors' apartments, London (1972)	130 (26)	–	–	–	1.0	0.2	3.7
Private residences, Hamilton (1972)	98 (34)	35.7	60.2a	21.4	1.3	–	4.5
CLCs, Chatham (1976)	49 (24)	–	–	–	1.0	1.4	1.2
CLCs, East York (1982)	21 (24)	–	28.6	–	1.8	–	1.4
Seniors' recreation centres, North York (1983)	165 (75)	31.0	33.0b	29.0	–	–	–
Private residences, Toronto (1983)	104 (49)	66.3	49.0c	–	2.0	1.0	–
CLCs, Kenora-Rainy River (1984)	56 (18)	–	88.0d	–	1.7	1.2	2.0
CLCs, Ontario (1985)	426 (39)	–	53d	–	1.0	1.2	3.6
CLCs, Oxford County (1985)	67 (33)	15.0	–	54.0	–	–	–
CLCs, Scarborough (1986)	91 (30)	71.4	24.2e	–	–	–	–
CLCs and apartments, East York (1987)	101 (43)	51.0	18.0e	29.3	1.4	–	–
CLCs, Waterloo (1985–1986)	205 (29)	23.4	72.6a	51.7	–	–	–
Private residences, East York (1987)	100* (72)	60.0	60.0e	14.0	1.3	0.6	5.2

a, Need periodontal treatment, b, need major periodontal treatment, c, need sealing, surgery, and possible extractions, d, tissues inflamed, e, has periodontal pockets.
* From Leake, JL and Otchere, D: Planning for the Future, *Ont Dent* 27–32, March 1988.
† Includes persons aged 65 and over.

Table 4 Prosthodontic and other reported needs of the elderly in Ontario*

Author (year)	Prosthodontic needs	Other needs
Lightman, Thompson, and Grainger (1969)	5% new dentures per year needed	
Martinello and Leake (1971)	281 complete new dentures (0.6 per person); a further 243 to be considered for replacement; 94 for needed repairs	In 116 dentate, 362 teeth had gingivitis and pocket formation; 82 teeth had loss of function
Leake and Martinello (1972)	168 new dentures (0.3 per person); a further 265 to be considered for replacement	In 130 dentate, 240 teeth had gingivitis and pocket formation; 45 teeth had loss of function; 21.8% had TMJ symptoms
Banting (1972)	112 new dentures (0.4 per person) and 109 relines/repairs	Surgical excision of soft tissue lesions in 5 cases; estimated per capita cost of treatment of $75.00
Martinello (1976)	167 new full dentures (0.8 per person); a further 95 to be considered for replacement; 45 for relines/repairs	Periodontal care needed for all dentate; 26% had TMJ symptoms
Leake and Howley (1982)	36 new dentures (0.4 per person)	22% needed immediate care; 44% needed professional care
Main (1983)	72 new dentures (0.3 per person) and 87 relines	33% of dentate needed major periodontal treatment
Ellis, Hyduk, and McFarlane (1983)	65 new dentures (0.3 per person) and 55 relines/repairs	49% of dentate needed periodontal treatment; 45% needed only hygienists' services
Armstrong (1984)	52 (41%) people had unacceptable dentures; 43 (40%) people needed denture repairs	40% with soft tissue lesions
Ryan, Ontario Public Health Branch (1985)	252 (25%) people had unacceptable dentures; 187 (19%) people needed denture repairs	14% with soft tissue lesions
Johnston (1985)	15% of total sample required denture fabrication or relines	
McIntyre, Jackson, and Shosenberg (1986)	226 new dentures (0.6 per person)	30% with soft tissue lesions
Leake, Price, and Schabas (1987)	71 new dentures (0.3 per person); 65 repairs or relines	9.3% needed urgent care; 23% had chewing limitations; 5% had TMJ symptoms; 40% wanted advice; 86% periodontal needs to be treated by hygienist
Adams (1985–1986)	163 new dentures (0.2 per person); 98 relines	72.6% of 205 dentate needed periodontal care
Locker, Leake, Price, Schabas, and Chao (1987)	103 new dentures (0.4 per person); 56 relines or repairs (n = 246)	15% needed urgent care; 26.8% had chewing limitations; 5.2% had TMJ symptoms; 29.7% wanted advice (includes only people aged 65 and older)

* From Leake JL and Otchere D: Planning for the Future, *Ont Dent* 27–32, March 1988.

Dental education

As an educator, I would like to think that dental practice is the tail that is wagged by the education dog. This has not necessarily been the case in the past, but I surmise it must be the case in the future.

Traditionally the dental school's mission has been as a provider of the workforce. This was achieved largely by placing major value on patients who satisfy the technical requirements established by each clinical division, with a resultant piecemeal approach to dental health care. It was all very well for dental deans to wax eloquent over their description of a dental school's objective: "The development of biologically oriented, technically capable, socially sensitive dental practitioners who are keenly aware of the significance of their potential contribution of the total health of their patients." The end-product reflected the inherent educational conflict of clinical treatment idealism versus pragmatism. While all clinical departments strove to teach ideally, the pragmatism of realistic treatment planes with options to the ideal proved elusive. The emphasis on developing the necessary technical skills to carry out treatment frequently precluded the right cognitive or behavioral skills to think through the diagnosis and treatment, posing challenges for an increasingly complex society. Service as an integral part of education, like the two inseparable sides of a coin, has not been de rigueur, and the need for reconsidering the relationship between teaching and the delivery of a dental health care service has become glaringly apparent. Dental education has not been alone in this predicament: medical education has struggled with the same questions.

A changing scientific and organizational ladscape has been paralleled by changes in the social and economic climate in which dentists practice. This has resulted in inflated expectations on the part of patients, along with consumerist attitudes with their implied risk of legal confrontations. Dentists have been largely successful in avoiding the sort of harsh sentiment expressed by George Bernard Shaw about another health profession: "I do not know a single thoughtful and well-informed person who does not feel that the tragedy of illness at present is that it delivers you helplessly into the hands of a profession which you deeply mistrust." In fact, dentists appear to by and large enjoy public trust; eg, an early 1980s Gallup survey revealed that nearly 83% of those interviewed thought that both the technical quality and personal manners of their dentists were good. It must not be overlooked, however, that dentists as health professionals remain vulnerable to harsh criticism by both individuals and consumer groups. Society's legitimate demand for equal treatment with respect and dignity, for accountability for our services, has created an all-encompassing level of concern for public welfare. Furthermore, the information void about efficacy of treatment protocols has raised concerns and doubts about the scientific certainty usually associated with dental treatment planning.

Dental schools can no longer identify their objective of patient care as a by-product of their educational and treatment roles. Patient care will be dominated by a service-first philosophy. A reconcili-

Table 5 Number of licensed dentists and dental hygienists in Canada and Ontario, 1961–1988*

Year	Canada			Ontario		
	Dentists (a)	Hygienists (a)	Both	Dentists[†] (b)	Hygienists[†] (b)	Both
1961	5,906	89[‡]	6,056	2,398	57	2,455
1966	6,532	303	6,835	2,732	189	2,921
1971	7,664	849	8,513	3,241	423	3,664
1976	9,401	1,929	11,330	3,733	703	4,436
1981	11,484	4,125	15,609	4,452	1,853	6,305
1986	13,164	6,064	19,228	5,075	2,784	7,859
1988	–	–	–	5,285	3,115	8,410

* From Burgess RC, Holmes BW, Macdonald JB and Watson P: Future Undergraduate Dental Education at the University of Toronto, Report of the Working Group, April 1989.
[†] Does not include out-of-province or life members.
[‡] Directory of Canadian Dental Hygienists 1964 was used to estimate this figure.
Sources: (a) – Health and Welfare Canada:
Canada Health Manpower Inventory 1972, 1974, 1985
Health Personnel in Canada 1987
(b) – Royal College of Dental Surgeons of Ontario: Annual Proceedings 1961 to 1988

Table 6 Ratio of dentists or/and dental hygienists to population in Canada and Ontario, 1961–1988*

Year	Canada			Ontario		
	Dentists (a)	Hygienists (a)	Both	Dentists (b)	Hygienists (b)	Both
1961	1:3,088	1:121,586[†]	1:3,011	1:2,600	1:109,400	1:2,540
1966	1:3,064	1:47,000	1:2,928	1:2,548	1:25,000	1:2,383
1971	1:2,814	1:25,405	1:2,534	1:2,377	1:18,210	1:2,102
1976	1:2,463	1:12,005	1:2,044	1:2,227	1:11,830	1:1,874
1981	1:2,134	1:5,935	1:1,570	1:1,948	1:4,680	1:1,375
1986	1:1,937	1:4,205	1:1,332	1:1,805	1:3,291	1:1,166
1988	–	–	–	1:1,773	1:3,014	1:1,116

* From Burgess RC, Holmes BW, Macdonald JB and Watson P: Future Undergraduate Dental Education at the University of Toronto, Report of the Working Group, April 1989.
[†] Estimated figure.
Sources: (a) – Health and Welfare Canada:
Canada Health Manpower Inventory 1972, 1974, 1985.
Health Personnel in Canada 1987
(b) – Royal College of Dental Surgeons of Ontario: Annual Proceedings 1961 to 1988

Table 7 Number of dentistry and dental hygiene graduates per year in Canada and Ontario, 1961–1988*

Year	Canada			Ontario		
	DDS/DMD	Hygiene	Both	DDS/DMD	Hygiene	Both
1961	174	8[†]	204	72	8[†]	87
1966	296	82	378	118	43	161
1971	363	125	488	139	47	186
1976	465	359	824	175	80	255
1981	479	382	861	174	182	356
1986	536	503	1,039	172	198	370
1988	–	–	–	140[‡]	215[‡]	355[‡]

* From Burgess RC, Holmes BW, Macdonald JB and Watson P: Future Undergraduate Dental Education at the University of Toronto, Report of the Working Group, April 1989.
[†] Directory of Canadian Dental Hygienists 1964 was used to estimate this figure.
[‡] Royal College of Dental Surgeons of Ontario: Annual Proceedings 1988.
Sources: Health and Welfare Canada:
Canada Health Manpower Inventory 1972, 1974, 1985
Health Personnel in Canada 1987

Table 8 Ontario dentist manpower projections for 1981–1996 (when the number of graduates is lowered)* †

Year	Number of Dentistry Graduates from U of T and UWO		
	Same as 1976–1980 n = 173/year	20% reduction beginning 1987 n = 140/year[†]	Further 32% reduction beginning 1993 n = 95/year[‡]
Number of licensed dentists			
1981	4,504	–	–
1986	5,073	–	–
1991	5,624	5,470	–
1996	6,165	5,858	5,698
2001	6,635	6,235	5,875
Population per dentist			
1981	1,925	–	–
1986	1,806	–	–
1991	1,709	1,758	–
1996	1,616	1,701	1,749
2001	1,543	1,642	1,742

* Adapted from the dental manpower projections of Lewis (1981, 1985, 1986). The extrapolation of his projections to 2001 was made assuming steady attrition and migration rates.
[†] From Burgess RC, Holmes BW, Macdonald JB and Watson P: Future Undergraduate Dental Education at the University of Toronto, Report of the Working Group, April 1989.
[‡] This is the track that Ontario has been on since the enrollment reductions of 1983. The smaller graduating class sizes began in 1987.
§ This is the track that will be followed if class sizes at U of T and UWO are reduced to 64 and 36 freshmen per year, respectively, beginning in 1989.

ation of technical skill acquisition with the ability to manage complex treatment plans based on medical and societal factors will increase in importance.

Recognition of the potential for diagnostic and technical skill acquisition away from the traditional, albeit not always practical, chairside systems could catalyze profound and exciting initiatives in dental education at both the undergraduate and postgraduate level.

Dental research

In the past, support for dental research has been provided by a number of sources: government agencies and industry in the main, together with some level of support from university global budgets. In North America, dental research has been given a reasonable priority rating, which is probably a fair reflection of the impact of dental diseases and their consequences on human welfare. In the United States, research problems related to the oral cavity have been carried out in colleges of dentistry, as well as in a separate National Institute of Dental Research, which was set up by that country's National Institutes of Health. In its 40-year history the NIDR has compellingly demonstrated the advantages of special identity for dental research, particularly with its established expertise in the disciplines of mineralized tissue and corrective tissue research. Its director recently pledged "commitment to an increase in fundamental knowledge about the growth, maintenance, repair, and regeneration of oral tissues that will improve the oral health of peoples of the world."

In Canada, dental and oral sciences research is carried out exclusively in faculties of dentistry. Our government agency responsible for health research is the Medical Research Council, which has a dental sciences committee. This committee does not command a separate budget but is provided recognition and distinction for dental research by having grant applications rated by those with special knowledge of dental problems.

The Canadian MRC is currently contemplating the abandonment of its dental sciences committee, which may be interpreted as reflecting a belief that dental research no longer requires distinction from the general field of biomedical research. Two apparent arguments account for this stance. The first is the decline in the number of grant applications from the dental research community. The second is that dental research no longer warrants special consideration because it is now of such a nature that it can be reviewed by other committees.

The first argument reflects the alarming predicament that results when the numbers game is applied to the dental research community. In the Netherlands, for example, the reduction of dental schools from five to two has been identified as having resulted in disastrous side effects for dental research. In the United States the equivalent of 26 dental schools have closed in the past 3 years, and the president of the American Association of Dental Schools has noted that "the number of dental researchers has dropped precipitously." This can only lead to the conclusion that the amount of dental research activities will diminish.

The absence of an apparent favored status might very well be a fair reflection of changing societal needs. It does, however, place dental research activities in a nondistinct and therefore unprotected position. It is all very well to argue that as dental research becomes stronger it will become accepted as a legitimate and valued component of the medical research effort. Political reality, however, suggests that the efforts to retain representation as equals in councils of biomedical research, and to maintain the highest and even improved qualities of dental research, can only become more difficult. Change appears to be inevitable and perhaps even desirable, but change without some form of protectionism or alternate funding mechanism could very well suggest a bleak future for Canadian dental research.

Conclusion

Dentistry is justifiably proud of its ongoing contributions to coping with society's oral health needs. The recognition and control of dental diseases, the ingenious techniques of intraoral salvage operations, the contributions to orofacial esthetics, the control and avoidance of dental pain, are only some of the very impressive contributions that our profession has made. Although we as dentists do not have as our professional remit the prolongation of our patients' lives, we have certainly fulfilled our commitment to the enrichment of those lives. In fact, few health disciplines can claim the same safe and predictable success in enhancing our patients' life quality. We look forward to an ongoing future of pursuing this mission and applying it even more universally than we have in the past.

References

1. Miller AJ, Brunelle JA, Carlos JP, Brown LJ and Löe H: Oral Health of United States Adults. The national survey of oral health in US employed adults and seniors 1985–1988. US Department of Health and Human Services, NIH Publication No. 87–2868, p 168.
2. Hughes JT, Rozier RG, Ramsay DL: *Natural History of Dental Disease in North Carolina 1976–1977.* Durham, Academic Press, 1982, p 275.
3. Page RC: Discussion paper on the NIDR 1985 Survey: Oral Health of US Adults. *J Public Health Dent* 47:200–202.
4. Burgess RC, Holmes BW, Macdonald JB, and Watson P: Future Undergraduate Dental Education at the University of Toronto, Report of the Working Group, April 1989.

Chapter 13

Dentistry in Singapore

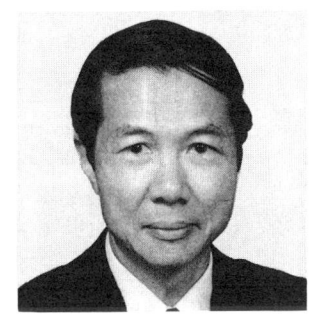

Yii Kie-Mung
Republic of Singapore

Abstract

Information relevant in planning and providing dental care is introduced. Dental care services are provided by the government and private sectors, the latter being the dominant sector.

Payment for service is largely "fee for service" type. But some form of dental insurance scheme is emerging.

The number, categories, and profile of dentists are given. Training of dental personnel is described. The role and programs of the national Singapore Dental Association are highlighted.

Today in Singapore, there is no shortage of dentists but there is need for more trained dental auxiliaries; accessibility to dental care service is easy and the cost is within reach of most people; training facilities are good; the oral health status of Singaporeans is comparable to the best in the world.

Singapore is a young nation, having gained independence in 1965. Its total land area, including the islets, is 662.6 square kilometers. Singapore's immediate neighbors are Malaysia (Peninsular Malaysia to the north, Sabah and Sarawak to the east) and Indonesia to the south. It occupies a strategic geographic position in Southeast Asia. It has a population of 2,647,100: 76% Chinese, 15.2% Malays, 6.5% Indians, and 2.3% others.

People below 15 years of age form 23.4% of the population, 15 to 60 years 68.5%, and those above 60 years comprise 8.1%. Singapore's life expectancy was 73.6 years in 1986. Singapore's population in the year 2000 is expected to number 2.93 million. The proportion of people in the age group 30 to 59 years will form 46.5% in the year 2000. In the oldest age group, 60 years and above, the population is expected to reach 10.4% by the same time.

Singaporeans enjoy a high standard of living. The labor force comprises 62.6% of the population aged 15 years and above. The per capita Gross National Product was $15,720 in 1987.

Dental care

Dental service in Singapore is provided by governmental and private sectors.

The Ministry of Health provides a wide range of dental services through its school, hospital, and community dental services. In 1988, these services were manned by 84 dentists, 25 therapists, and 234 dental nurses. There were 1,132,513 attendances. The expenditure for providing these services was $16,481,518. Revenue collected from the services was $4,121,943. Thus, the subsidy came to $12,359,575 — about $10.90 per visit.

As part of the Ministry's program to encourage the development of a strong private sector and to help dentists set up their own clinics, government community dental clinics were leased out as private clinics. Since the scheme was launched in October 1984, 11 clinics have been leased to dentists.

Within the Training and Health Education department of the Ministry of Health there is the Dental Health Education Unit, which is responsible for dental health promotion and education. It has a full-time staff of two dentists and six dental nurses. The Dental Health Education Steering Committee sets the policy and direction for dental health education in Singapore.

At present, dental care is by and large provided on the basis of "fee for service." The public service, statutory boards, and other enlightened organizations do provide their employees with an annual subsidy for dental treatment. Others pay out of their own pockets.

Very recently, an insurance company offered to some selected dentists a capitation insurance scheme, while another organization is studying the feasibility of introducing a franchise scheme.

Singaporeans may pay their bills through the Medisave scheme, implemented in April 1984. Under the scheme, every Central Provident Fund contributor has 6% of his or her monthly salary income credited to his or her Medisave account. The Medisave savings can be used to pay hospitalization bills incurred by the contributor, his or her parents, grandparents, spouse, and children in both government and private hospitals. Because most dental treatment does not require hospitalization, the Medisave scheme has not benefitted people who need dental care.

Dentists

The registration of dentists in Singapore began in 1924 with the enactment of the Dentists' Registration Ordinance of the Straits Settlements. The practice of dentistry today is governed by the Dentist Act, Chapter 76, in the 1985 edition in the Statutes of the Republic of Singapore.

The Dentist Act provides for the establishment of the Dental Board, which oversees the following functions: (1) registration of dentists; (2) issue of the Annual Practicing Certificate, which authorizes a dentist to practice dentistry during the year for which it is issued; and (3) control over the professional conduct of dentists. The Dental Board has an Investigation Committee that advises the board on whether a disciplinary inquiry should be held on a complaint against a dentist.

There were 688 dentists on the Dentists' Register in December 1988; 593 were First Division dentists and 95 others were dentists without formal dental qualifications but were registered in 1950 and dental therapists registered after passing the Dental Board Examination. The dentist-to-population ratio is 1:3,847.

The distribution of First Division dentists was as follows: 128 (21.6%) were in government service; 27 (4.5%) were university affiliated; and 438, including 16 dentists not working (73.9%), were in private practice. Men and women comprised 64.2% and 35.8%, respectively; 91.9% were Chinese, 0.3% Malays, 6.0% Indians/Pakistanis/Sri Lankans, and 2.5% were of other ethnic origin. Breaking down the group by age, 37.3% were below 30, 30.8% were between 30 and 39, 19.2% were between 40 and 49, 7.8% were between 50 and 59, and 4.9% were above 60 years of age. The mean age was 36.5 years and the median age was 34.1 years.

Thus, the dentist population in Singapore is generally young, and the attrition rate will be low for the near future because only 12.7% of graduate dentists are above 50 years.

In 1987, there were 131 specialists of all categories compared to 523 nonspecialists (including 97 nongraduate dentists). Thus, there were about 25 specialists per 100 nonspecialists. This was high in comparison to other countries.

The incidence of dental diseases as reflected by the DMFT index of 12-year-old children is relatively low — 2.5 in 1984. Fluoridation of drinking water started in 1958, and successful preventive and excellent education programs have reduced the incidence of dental diseases. These, coupled with a small increase in population, will not be likely to stimulate high demand for much routine dental service. Patient shortage is therefore a problem that must be viewed with concern.

Training

Dental undergraduates are trained in the Faculty of Dentistry of the National University of Singapore. It is the only dental school in the country. The course takes 4 years and the current enrollment is 34 students. The faculty celebrated its diamond jubilee in September 1989. It is housed in a splendid building that has a total built-up area of approximately 6,000 square meters. It offers facilities for clinical service, for teaching of undergraduates and postgraduate students, and for dental research.

The Training Department of the Dental Division of the Ministry of Health trains dental auxiliaries, dental technicians, and assistant dental nurses to meet the needs of the Ministry of Health.

Postgraduate dental education had its beginning in 1949. At that time, the LDS (Licentiate in Dental Surgery) was replaced by the BDS (Bachelor of Dental Surgery), and a higher academic qualification, the MDS (Master of Dental Surgery), was introduced. The School of Postgraduate Dental Studies was formally established in 1970 with the following objectives: *(1)* to provide specialist training in dentistry and courses leading to postgraduate qualifications in dentistry; *(2)* to promote continuing dental education; and *(3)* to develop research in dentistry. The MDS degree is awarded by the school and is available to dentists who possess recognized dental qualifications and fulfill the entrance requirements laid down by the Board of Postgraduate Dental Studies. Government dentists are sponsored for training in local and overseas universities and centers for postgraduate courses under the Health Manpower Development Plan and other scholarship schemes. International experts or consultants are also invited to Singapore to lecture and conduct courses.

Professional organization

The Singapore Dental Association is the only national professional organization of dentistry. It was inaugurated in 1966 after breaking from the Malayan Dental Association. More than 90% of the graduate dentists are members of the Singapore Dental Association. Membership consists of five categories: ordinary membership, associate membership, corresponding membership, life membership, and honorary membership.

Various committees and subcommittees plan and carry out the association's activities. The more important ones are the Ethics and Dental Practice Committee; Dental Health, Education, and Research Committee; Editorial Board; Assist Young Graduates Committee; Dental Insurance Committee; Dental Fees Committee; Library Committee; and Task Force Committee.

The Singapore Dental Association is an affiliated member of the Fédération Dentaire Internationale and the Asian Pacific Regional Organization. Thus, it actively participates in international and regional activities. It will be hosting the 78th FDI Annual World Dental Congress in September 1990.

Whereas the association devotes much of its resources to continuing dental education for its members, its subsidiary, the Singapore Dental Health Foundation, undertakes dental health education for the public.

Summary

There is no apparent shortage of dentists in Singapore. The dentists are quite evenly distributed throughout the country. However, there is need for more trained dental technicians and chairside assistants. Good training facilities exist for all types of dental personnel.

Singapore is an urbanized and densely populated city with no vast and sparsely populated countryside. Therefore, accessibility to dental care service is easy. Also, the cost is within the reach of most people.

With the fluoridation of drinking water and vigorous and comprehensive dental preventive programs implemented by the Ministry of Health and the Singapore

Dental Association, the awareness of dental health is on the rise. The oral health status of Singaporeans is comparable to the best in the world.

Future prospects

It is our national aspiration to make Singapore a center of excellence for health care, providing quality dental care that is readily available and affordable to everyone. Sophisticated, current technology is added to the existing infrastructure. A National Dental Center providing all types of treatment is being planned to be established within the compound of the Singapore General Hospital.

Encouragement and assistance are given to expand the private sector, which complements the public sector in achieving our aspiration of becoming a center of excellence for dental care. The irony of this is that it brings about problems faced by other developed nations.

In the ensuing years, a few issues will warrant urgent attention.

Workforce. The number of graduates should be gradually reduced to that commensurate with the demand for services in order to prevent an oversupply of dentists. Even today there is already a perceived oversupply of dentists because in the private sector some young dentists are known to be underworked.

Training. Facilities for training undergraduates are good. However, local postgraduate training programs can be strengthened to obviate the need to spend a large sum of money to attend courses overseas. There should be formal, structured training for dental technicians and chairside assistants. The courses could be managed by a polytechnic so that on completion of study, a diploma or certificate is awarded. This will enhance their professional standing, social status, and income. The present shortage of these personnel should then be relieved because more people would then want to take up these occupations. Everyone knows good dental care depends on the service of a professional team — dentist, technician, and chairside assistant.

Certification/accreditation of continuing education courses. The importance of constant upgrading of knowledge and skills is obvious. No one can hope to provide the best service while remaining stagnant. A continuing dental education coordinating committee comprising representatives from the Ministry of Health, the National University of Singapore, and the Singapore Dental Association has been formed to establish such a committee. There is much more to be done.

Dental insurance. A scheme of third-party financing for dental services is desirable. The profession as a whole is still examining and studying the concept, mechanism, implications, and other ramifications. We believe that insurance companies should work with the Singapore Dental Association to develop a scheme or schemes beneficial to all concerned.

Fee schedule. In the interest of the profession, the Singapore Dental Association is considering providing guidelines on fees. Forums on this have been conducted and feedback received. The implementation of a fee schedule will have impact on the insurance scheme.

Medisave. The Medisave scheme was mentioned earlier. It is hoped that its use can soon be extended to oral surgical patients who need no hospitalization and to expensive nonsurgical dental treatment.

Professional audit. The Singapore Dental Association is doing its best in policing its members with regard to ethics and standards of practice, and the dental board is dealing with complaints against dentists. A formal body charged with the duties of auditing professional standards would be useful to ensure minimum standards are maintained.

Dental care for the handicapped and the elderly. As life expectancy increases, the handicapped and the elderly are being neglected. Their plight has not been fully appreciated. The Ministry of Community Development has taken steps to provide essential dental service to some of them and it is hoped that the program will eventually cover all of them.

Study/research of social factors on dental diseases. It is hoped a well-designed study can be done in the near future so that the results will help provide the basis for policy making and direction for future dental care planning and implementation.

Conclusion

The future is very challenging and there are many imponderables. Farsightedness and careful monitoring are needed to ensure that policy planning and implementation are maximally coordinated, to provide a dental service that is efficient and cost effective and with which both the providers and consumers are satisfied.

Chapter 14

Dentistry in the United Kingdom

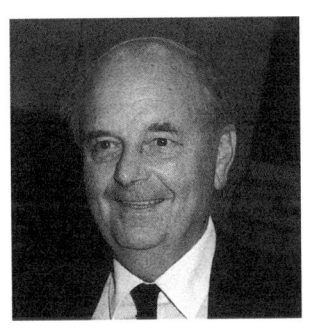

John W. McLean
London, England

Abstract

The provision of dental care under the National Health Service in the United Kingdom has, in many practitioners' views, reached a crisis point. The problem of funding an open-ended health service is becoming greater each year, and the escalating high technology, both in medicine and dentistry, has overwhelmed the state's ability to pay for it. The fundamental question that all governments now face is whether national resources can continue to fund the Health Service at the highest level of science and technology without sacrificing education, industrial training, and other vital areas needed to prepare Britain for the competitive world of the future European common market. It is the privilege of both the public and government to make these choices, and this paper suggests that a fundamental change in attitude to the welfare state is needed.

The original concept of Lord Beveridge in his classic reports on social security during 1942 to 1946 was that if the state provided a safety net for the underprivileged, chronically sick, or aging populace, then a new era would dawn in which demand for state aid would fall as people became more prosperous. Unfortunately, history has proved this illusory. It hardly needs stating that even the most prosperous Western countries are continuously engaged in a great debate on how to pay for their health and social services.

As each generation of doctors and scientists becomes more innovative, the escalation of high technology in medicine has overwhelmed the state's ability to pay for it, leaving in its wake a trail of frustrated clinicians and researchers all demanding priority for their pet projects.

In the United Kingdom, commissions have sat and come and gone, the great debate continues, and even dentistry has had its share of Royal Commissions, Dentists' Acts, and reports on unnecessary treatment. To catalogue these events would serve little purpose in this discussion, since it would certainly not shed much light on whether dental health has improved in the United Kingdom or whether there have been major advances in treatment patterns.

Essentially, the National Health Service in Britain operates like a central command economy, and dentists work on a fixed, itemized scale of fees. In the early days of the Health Service, the fees were generous, but as the Tattersall Committee of the British Dental Association reported in October 1964, such a system "puts a premium on speed and takes no account of quality. Standards tend to fall and the profession becomes preoccupied with 'turnover' and generally more commercially than professionally-minded. Since quantity is the main criterion, the less scrupulous are tempted to indulge in over-prescription and other dubious practices."

It is hardly surprising that incomes for some dentists rocketed in the early 1960s and the government stepped in. Fees were reduced time and again until today the dental profession in Britain has drifted into a low-fee, high-production service that has undermined both the morale and integrity of the young graduate. In my opinion, it is no longer possible to produce high-quality dentistry under the present NHS regulations, and yet no one wants to acknowledge this in public.

Even if the profession moved into third-party payment, it is unlikely that these problems will be solved. As Bernard Shaw so succinctly remarked, "No profession has a monopoly of ethics." Private practice is just as open to abuse as a state service, the only difference being that private practice does allow the dedicated practitioner to flourish.

High-quality dentistry depends on the services of dedicated, learned, and skilled people. If a country cannot secure this, then no amount of change in administration or policy will solve the problem in dental health.

The current clash between the British Medical Association and the Department of Health over the reorganization of the Health Service highlights this problem. Politics does not produce good medicine. If the professions are continuously downgraded by government and the media, then I predict a growing shortage of suitable recruits into both medicine and dentistry. The impact of this shortage on the public will not be sudden, but its implications have not yet been recognized by those in charge of the future of our profession.

The decline of dental caries in children is well documented,[1] and the impact of fluoridation programs and particularly the use of fluoride toothpaste, together with improved diet and dental health education, has had a major role to play in achieving this. However, despite this reduction we have not yet conquered dental caries and are still awaiting firm epidemiological evidence that the disease has not moved into later life.

The Department of Health in the United Kingdom has acknowledged the problem of continuing payment for dentistry on the basis of a fee per item of service and is now introducing capitation schemes to encourage total health care. This experiment is being watched with great interest but may only succeed in the treatment of the adolescent population. The ravages of periodontal disease, root caries, and attrition in the older population will still need addressing and at the present time involves high technology in dentistry.

A strong case can be made that if the state wishes to provide comprehensive dental care, it should institute a salaried service, equip surgeries and laboratories, and compete with private practice. This has not come about because the cost to the state would prove unacceptable.

Under the present regulations we now have a private practice system in which the fees are controlled by the state at a level they reluctantly accept but is totally divorced from the reality of what high-quality dentistry costs. To compound this practice the public is expected to contribute a major share of the cost and is led to believe that it is entitled to a sophisticated and comprehensive dental service. Fortunately, the British Dental Association is now coming to grips with these problems and has started to recognize bona fide private and dental health care plans. A glimmer of light does shine forth and it is possible that we shall see dentistry in the United Kingdom move forward into a truly preventive service.

The methods of payment and delivery of care must be left to gradual evolution in the light of experience. Neither the private nor state sectors have a monopoly on wisdom.

In Britain there are strong indications of an expansion of private health care, but it need not be at the expense of a state-run health service, as many people think. Unless we are prepared to act sensibly and recognize that both sectors have a role to play and can be mutually beneficial, then the less privileged will not receive the improved care that we all desire. The better-off must still be allowed to pay for excellence, since without this freedom a central command economy in health will become permanently established.

Financial constraints then tend to dispense mediocrity to all. Imaginative private practitioners should work in union with the dedicated hospital practitioners or researchers. This is the formula for improving health care.

Because of the decline in the rate of dental caries, workforce requirements in the United Kingdom have had to be reduced. The Royal Dental Hospital has merged with Guy's Hospital, and The University College Dental School is also scheduled for closure. Other closures are contemplated and it is likely that at least one more school will fall victim to the cuts.

However, despite the fall in dental caries, it is too early to assess future requirements for the adult population. Periodontal disease, root caries, and tooth wear all require extensive treatment in the older population, and it is interesting to note that major advances in treatment patterns during the last 35 years have been in new materials, techniques, and equipment, not in drug therapy.

Extensive work by Bertram Cohen and his colleagues at the Royal College of Surgeons of England resulted in the production of a caries vaccine. Professor Cohen's successor, Newell Johnson, has yet to see this vaccination program put into practice. We are still awaiting a cure for periodontal disease, perhaps our most formidable hurdle. The dental diseases of an aging population may present as great a challenge in the 21st century as caries has in the past. The replacement of diseased or worn tooth enamel with artificial materials will become an even higher priority than in the past, requiring great sophistication in our scientific and technical approach. This can only be achieved by harnessing the results of biological and material science research to an imaginative graduate and postgraduate training program. The contribution made in the United Kingdom to biomaterials research has greatly contributed to these objectives.

British research

Achieving permanent adhesion of materials to tooth structure in the hostile oral environment is particularly difficult. Any adhesive material has to compete with moisture at the tooth interface. Dentin is permeated by aqueous fluids transported from the pulp, and there is both loosely and tightly bound water in the surface of enamel. In the oral situation organic adhesives are either insufficiently polar to compete with water for the surface of dental tissue or, if highly polar, the bond they form is hydrolytically unstable.

Polycarboxylate cements

Smith[2] gave the first public report on the polycarboxylates to the British Dental Association's annual conference in Birmingham in 1967. His work in the United Kingdom presented the first solution to attaching dental materials to wet tooth structure. The use of polyacrylic acids ushered in a new era of molecular bonding to tooth structure.

Because of their multiplicity of carboxyl groups that form hydrogen bonds, these new cements could displace or even incorporate water into the cement. The bonds formed were of a permanent nature and not easily broken because these cements are dynamic materials and continue to ion exchange at tooth interfaces.

In addition, the nature of the polymer structure makes the polycarboxylate cements biologically compatible materials: diffusion of polyacid, with its train of associated H^+ ions down the dentinal tubules, is unlikely because of its high molecular weight and chain entanglement.

The significance of this research led to further investigations into alternative cements that could form long-term molecular bonds with tooth structure.

Glass ionomer cements

The development of the glass ionomer cements at the Laboratory of The Government Chemist by Wilson and Kent[3] resulted in the production of the first truly adhesive restorative material. Another barrier to adhesion besides water contamination is the dynamic nature of tooth material. Because enamel is an ion exchanger and dentin is a living material that is subject to change, it is rather like trying to bond to shifting sand. Under such conditions the adhesive bond must have a dynamic character, too. It will be broken as the substrate changes, and must be capable of being re-formed. Once broken, covalent chemical bonds cannot be re-formed. Dentinal adhesives based on phosphonate esters may fail because of this very point. By contrast, the ionic and polar bonds that attach the glass ionomer cement to the substrate can be reestablished, which, together with the multiplicity of the adhesive bonds, may account for this cement's unique property of being permanently adhesive under oral conditions. In addition, the glass ionomer cements have thermal expansions similar to tooth structure.

The glass ionomer cements are now used extensively as liners and bases onto which composite resins may be attached using the acid-etch technique.[4] Glass ionomer cements make excellent dentin substitutes, and their use as core build-up materials is expanding. The translucent nature of these cements has also enabled the restoration of Class V erosion lesions without cavity preparation, and they have the added bonus of leaching fluoride and exerting some anticariogenic effect.

Cermet cements

The abrasion resistance of the glass ionomer cements has been significantly improved with the introduction of the cermet cements by McLean and Gasser.[5] These cements, unlike simple mixtures of alloy particles or metal fibers, contain glass-metal powders sintered to high density that can be made to react with polyacids to form a cement. The set cement can be burnished, and in the case of the silver-cermets the sintered metal powder has a lubricating effect on the surface[6] and probably lowers the coefficient of friction.[5]

The silver cermet cements are used principally for core buildup, as bases for amalgam restorations, and in restoring early carious lesions via the tunnel approach. The glass ionomer cements may also be used in fissures and will probably replace amalgam alloys for this purpose. The treatment of early caries with glass ionomer cements has been used in the United Kingdom since the early 1970s, and it is predicted that their worldwide use as anticariogenic restoratives will make a significant contribution to public health in the next decade.

Alumina ceramics

The first high-strength aluminous porcelains were produced in the United Kingdom in 1964, and the principle of using high-strength ceramic cores for full porcelain veneer crowns became established.[7] More recently, new products have appeared in other countries, including Germany, France, and the United States. Nonshrink ceramic cores and slip cast alumina ceramics are all attracting great interest. The future of high-strength ceramics is promising because the all-ceramic restoration is generally recognized as the most esthetic of all our full veneer crowns.

Long-term resistance to static fatigue has also been studied in the United Kingdom and particular attention paid to reducing crack formation by bonding to thin metal foils such as platinum.[8,9] Thin porcelain laminate veneers are proving successful mechanically because of the reduction of crack propagation by resin bonding. The importance of protecting the flawed surfaces of ceramics is now being appreciated because long-term resistance to breakage probably depends more on this factor than raising mechanical strengths.

Glass ceramics

McCulloch[10] produced the first castable glass-ceramic material in the United Kingdom in 1966. More recently, newer types of mica glass ceramics have been marketed and used in the construction of veneer crowns, laminate veneers, and inlays. Outstanding esthetics can be obtained with these new materials by using them as reinforcing cores veneered with an aluminous porcelain. Experiments continue, to determine whether the strength and resistance to static fatigue of glass ceramics is adequate in high-stress–bearing areas. As yet these materials are not suitable for use as bridge connectors in fixed prosthodontics.

Composite resins

The most significant UK contributions made in the field of composite resins have originated from the British manufacturers. The development of visible light curing initiators based on alpha diketone-amine systems by Imperial Chemical Industries has received worldwide attention and represents a major advance in curing resin veneers to enamel surfaces. The work has, of course, been complemented by Buonocore's[11] original development in the United States of the acid-etch technique, an event of the greatest significance in dentistry.

The first major chemical development in resin chemistry was made in 1938 by the Amalgamated Dental Company, London, working with De Trey, Zürich, to develop alternative materials to silver amalgam alloys. The first epoxy resin, which used metal chloride catalysts, proved unsuitable for dentistry. Few people realize that this major breakthrough in industrial and household adhesives was a dental invention.

Future developments

The last two decades have been outstanding for the development of adhesive materials in dentistry. This work will gather pace and we shall see a new generation of glass ionomer and related cements (polyelectrolytes) challenging the current composite resins and amalgam alloys. Current scientific evidence indicates the adhesive materials such as acid-etched composite resins and glass ionomers can support and strengthen teeth, particularly the undermined cusp. We may use adhesive and anticariogenic materials such as the glass ionomers as dentin substitutes and composite resin to give occlusal support. The laminate restoration will come to the fore. For the more extensive restoration, laboratory-cured composite resin inlays are gaining popularity, and with all the advantages of using laboratory processing to secure high density and maximum monomer conversion, improved clinical performance may be expected.

Computer machining of ceramics is being looked at, and the ability to produce modified silicate biomaterials with mixed organic/inorganic functionality, possessing unique combinations of properties that would be unobtainable with either polymers or conventional ceramics, is now possible.[12] A sound understanding of microbiology and biochemistry may enable the future students to use sophisticated techniques to grow new human enamel in vivo from recombinant DNA synthesized protein. The treatment of the early carious lesion using the internal occlusal fossa or "tunnel" approach may be facilitated by using chemical solutions for dissolving caries. Other solutions may become available for remineralizing enamel.

Controlled drug release from biomaterials is another area of great potential. The use of chemotherapy to treat periodontal diseases may well represent the biggest change of all, in that organisms involved may be targeted by specific antibiotics. Small hollow fibers containing antibiotics may be placed around the neck of the tooth at the base of the pocket and then the area covered with a periodontal dressing. The antibiotics are slowly released and sterilize the area. The enormous value of this method of treatment is that only about one thousandth of the dosage is required of the antibiotic compared to that taken by mouth.

The future for dentistry cannot be covered without recognition of the outstanding work of Brånemark on osseointegration and the necessity of using materials with uncontaminated pure oxide surfaces to stimulate osteoblastic activity. It is likely that successful integration of implants depends upon oxygen screening at the implant interface, and this may also account for the bioactivity of the glass ionomer cements.

Orthognathic surgery, together with orthodontic correction, will continue to make great progress. The appreciation in the 1970s of the vertical dimension of facial growth led to the full range of spatial correction of facial anomalies that has become routine practice throughout the world today. Specialization in dentistry will increase to complement these advances, but it may be necessary for the public to reassess its priorities in order to pay for it. Health and education will have to assume the same attractive role as the pursuit of leisure and consumer goods. It is the privilege of not only governments but also the public to decide the issues. The future for dentistry remains very promising and we await further developments in its science and technology. However, it is easy to indulge in speculative research but more difficult to turn it into the reality of the marketplace.

References

1. Downer MC: Changing patterns of disease in the Western world. in Guggenheim, B. (ed), Cariology Today, Int. Congr. Zurich, 1983, pp 1–12.
2. Smith DC: A new dental cement. *Br Dent J* 1968; 125:381–384.
3. Wilson AD and Kent BE: The glass ionomer cement: A new translucent dental filling material. *J Appl Chem Biotechnol* 1971;21:313.
4. McLean JW, Powis DR, Prosser HJ, and Wilson AD: The use of glass-ionomer cements in bonding composite resins to dentine. *Br Dent J* 1985;158:410–414.
5. McLean JW and Gasser O: Glass-cermet cements. *Quintessenz Int* 1985;18:517–529.
6. McKinney JE, Antonucci JM and Rupp NW: Wear and micro-hardness of a metal-filled ionomer cement. *J Dent Res* 1986;64(Special Issue):344 (IADR abstr. 1577).
7. McLean JW and Hughes TH: The reinforcement of dental porcelain with ceramic oxides. *Br Dent J* 1965; 118:251–267.
8. Sced IR, McLean JW and Hotz P: The strengthening of aluminous porcelain with bonded platinum foil. *J Dent Res* 1977;36:1067–1069.
9. Piddock V, Marquis PM and Wilson HJ: The role of the platinum matrix in porcelain jacket crowns. *Br Dent J* 1984;157:275–280.
10. McCulloch WJ: Advances in dental ceramics. *Br Dent J* 1968;125:361–365.
11. Buonocore MG: A simple method of increasing the adhesion of acrylic filling materials to enamel surfaces. *J Dent Res* 1955;34:849–853.
12. Jones DW: The future of biomaterials. *J Can Dent Assoc* 1988;54:163–173.

Chapter 15

Development of Dental Care in Hong Kong

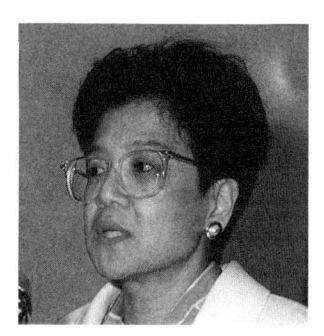

Wong Tin Chun
Hong Kong

Abstract

Dental undergraduate education started in 1980 in Hong Kong with an annual intake of 76 students; the first locally qualified dentists graduated from the Faculty of Dentistry of the University of Hong Kong in 1985. There has been a noticeable increase in the number of dentists trained abroad as well as the number of locally trained dental graduates. A low dental awareness in the population, coupled with the very successful water fluoridation program and Government School Dental Service catering to children between 6 to 12 years, has contributed to an underutilization of dental services.

Historical background

Hong Kong was acquired by Great Britain from China in 1842 under the Treaty of Nanking. In 1898, under the Convention of Peking, the New Territories, which makes up the major land mass of Hong Kong, was leased to Great Britain for a period of 99 years. Ninety-eight percent of the population of Hong Kong is Chinese, of Southern Chinese extraction, and predominantly Cantonese speaking. The population today is 5.6 million and has increased to this figure mainly because of the continuous influx of people over the border from mainland China, especially during periods of political unrest. Immigration, both legal and illegal, is continuing today. The social culture of the Hong Kong population is Chinese, although Western culture has had a great impact on most of Hong Kong society as a result of British influence and the realization of Hong Kong as a financial and trade center.

The treatment of dental diseases can be found in the records of the ancient civilizations of China. Emperor Huang Ti is recorded as having studied dental diseases in 2698 BC. He described oral inflammatory conditions, diseases of the oral soft tissues, and dental caries, which he believed to be caused by "toothworms." The primitive dental practitioners were "toothworm removers," tooth extractors, tooth cleaners, and tooth fitters. Dental practitioners were very much a part of life and would set up their stands in the streets of towns and villages. Tooth fitters or false teeth vendors are still in existence and can be seen plying their trade on the pavements of a busy marketplace in Hong Kong and within the famous walled city of Kowloon, a past haunt of Hong Kong's criminal underground, now to be demolished to make way for a park.

In the late 19th century, Hong Kong quickly grew as a busy trading center. The first modern-day dentists to practice in Hong Kong were the British and Americans who brought Western dentistry to Hong Kong to serve the needs of both the local and foreign population. Drs Poate and Noble, both University of Pennsylvania alumni, established their practices in Hong Kong during this period. Dr Noble also took an interest in the medical affairs of Hong Kong and was one of the founding fathers of the University of Hong Kong. Records show that the first Chinese man to travel to the United States to study for a dental degree was Dr Moon Hung Chaun. He was a member of the Class of 1899 at the University of Pennsylvania and he set up his own practice in Hong Kong in 1901.

The first Dentistry Ordinance was passed in 1914 and the first Dental Register appeared in 1916 with 22 names in the register, 8 of which were of formally trained dental surgeons. The Dental Board, which formed the earliest regulatory body, first met in 1934. By 1940 the number of fully qualified dental surgeons increased to 23. With legislation established, the Dental Council of Hong Kong came into existence in 1959 and it continues to play a large role in the regulation of the profession today. All practicing dentists from then onward were registered, with all additions to the register being controlled by the Dental Council.

Development of dental care provisions

With the increase in trade and commerce in Hong Kong, the population grew in proportion and gave rise to a greater demand for more dental care providers.

The Hong Kong government provides a dental service to civil servants, their dependents, and pensioners. A limited service is provided for prison inmates, and certain dental services are provided in government hospitals. There is no government dental service provided to the local population except for emergency care. In order to overcome the workforce shortage, the Hong Kong government initiated a scholarship scheme in 1954 whereby recipients were sent to certain overseas dental schools and in return they had to agree to a period of service with the government.

The general public therefore had to

rely on graduates of overseas dental schools who pursued their dental training on their own initiative and returned to Hong Kong to add to the number of trained dental surgeons practicing. Graduates of certain universities, mainly from the United Kingdom, the Commonwealth, and the United States were, and still are, granted the right of automatic registration with the Dental Council of Hong Kong under the Dentists' Registration Ordinance. For graduates of other universities, a statutory examination conducted by the Dental Council of Hong Kong is necessary for registration.

The number of registered dentists was still low up to the 1970s. In 1974, a White Paper was accepted by the Legislative Council, Hong Kong's law-making body, on the development of medical and health services in Hong Kong. Two important proposals accepted by the government were to change the dental scene in Hong Kong dramatically. One was the creation of the School Dental Care Service and the other was the establishment of a dental school in Hong Kong.

In response to the first proposal, a dental therapists' training school was set up in 1970 enrolling students on a 3-year training program. Dental therapists are trained in the Tang Shiu Kin Dental Therapists' Training School housed in the MacLehose Dental Center. Dental therapists provide dental care to schoolchildren under the Government School Dental Service, and they work under the supervision of professionally trained dental surgeons. To date, all primary schoolchildren, ie, all children between the ages of 6 to 12 years, receive dental care for a nominal annual fee. To ensure safety and to facilitate attendance, transportation is provided free to all primary schools in which children subscribing to this dental scheme are enrolled.

The second proposal, to establish a dental school, was based on the recommendation of the Medical Development Advisory Committee (MDAC). The MDAC also noted that there was no internationally accepted optimal ratio for the provision of dentists. An arbitrary ratio of one dentist to 6,000 population was set as the goal for the private sector. At the end of 1973, there were some 440 dentists practicing in Hong Kong, and it was then predicted that the stipulated ratio would be achieved by 1982, with approximately 450 dentists.

Construction of the dental school began in 1978 and the building was completed in 1980. Dental undergraduate teaching commenced at the University of Hong Kong in 1980, with an annual intake of 76 students, and the Prince Philip Dental Hospital was established in 1981. The first group of locally qualified dentists left the Faculty of Dentistry of the University of Hong Kong in February 1985.

The Prince Philip Dental Hospital is housed in an 11-story building and occupies some 33,000 square meters. There are 228 clinical positions, 161 of which are in open-plan clinics, 56 as individual surgeries, and 9 as special demonstration surgeries. There are five clinical departments: oral surgery and oral medicine, children's dentistry and orthodontics, conservative dentistry, periodontology and public health, and prosthetic dentistry, as well as supporting units such as pathology, hematology, related research laboratories, a library, and teaching areas. There is now also a school of speech science. The Department of Oral Surgery and Oral Medicine contains two operating theaters and facilities for sedation, relative analgesia, and general anesthesia, with fully monitored recovery areas. A large technical laboratory is available for teaching and production work. There is also an inpatient oral surgery unit with eight day beds. Twin operating theaters are also available at a nearby hospital.

The Hong Kong University dental students receive a dental education of the highest international standards. They are taught to fully utilize dental ancillary workers such as hygienists, technicians, and surgical assistants, all of whom are trained alongside the dental students.

Present situation

The number of dentists rose steadily up to 1973 and accelerated after 1978 (Fig 1). In 1975 there were 541 dentists in practice; in 1980 there were 638. In 1985 the number of registered dentists rose from 763 to 1,069. This surpassed the ratio of 1 to 6,000 population. Today, as of the end of July 1989, there are 1,437 dentists on the Register. Out of these, 1,343 are practicing in Hong Kong.

There are also 269 trained dental therapists offering dental care, under the government's School Dental Service, to a half million schoolchildren. The response rate is about 70%, indicating that about 350,000 schoolchildren are receiving dental care in Hong Kong.

A very important feature affecting oral health needs in Hong Kong is the very successful water fluoridation program started 29 years ago (Figs 2 to 4). This program has resulted in a dramatic decrease in dental caries in both children and adults.

Another factor affecting the workforce problem is the existence of unregistered (illegal) dental practitioners, who abound in Hong Kong. In the early 1980s it was believed that there were in the region of 1,000 illegal dental practitioners. They were made up of those who were not successful in the statutory examination of the Dental Council of Hong Kong or others who learned the trade through apprenticeship. They provided a cheap alternative to registered practitioners, though at considerable risk to the patient, who because of a lack of education, would not know any better.

The dental awareness of the population is generally low, although this is gradually improving. Priority for dental treatment is high only when pain is involved. Because a large portion of the population consists of recent immigrants from mainland China, dental education is low, if not nonexistent. Further, because there is no government public dental care system, this deficiency in dental education, combined with the cost, contributes to a relatively low demand for dental care compared to other Western countries.

An alternate source of dental treatment results from an allegiance to the motherland, combined with the lack of education and economic constraints, that drives many members of the local population to make the short journey to Shenzhen, a town over the border in mainland China, to seek dental treatment

The problem

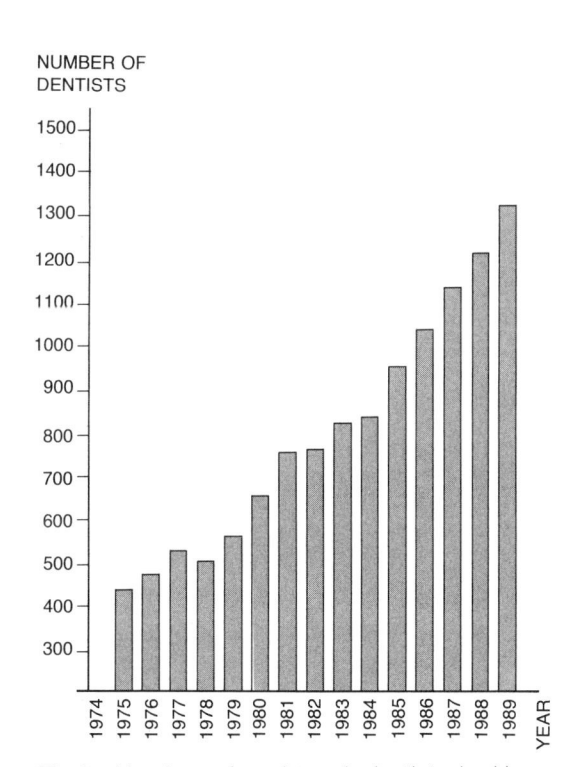

NUMBER OF DENTISTS

Fig 1 Number of registered dentists in Hong Kong, 1975 to 1989.

	1960	1980	1987
Mean no. Decayed/Missing/ Filled teeth per child	3.57	0.89	0.62
	Reduction 82.6%		
Percentage of children without dental caries	10.5%	60%	68.1%

Fig 2 Comparison of dental caries status for permanent teeth of children aged 6 to 11 years since implementation of water fluoridation in 1960.

	1960	1987
Decayed/Missing/ Filled Teeth	4.6	1.7
	Reduction 63%	

Fig 3 Comparison of dental caries status in 15- to 19-year-olds.

	1968	1987
Decayed/Missing/ Filled Teeth	11.3	7.3
	Reduction 35.4%	

Fig 4 Comparison of dental caries status in 35- to 44-year-olds.

there. As a result, many clinics have sprung up in Shenzhen that cater to the health needs of some of the Hong Kong population.

The problem

A review of the dental workforce situation carried out in 1979 suggested that the arbitrary dentist-to-population ratio of 1:6,000 would be achieved earlier than originally anticipated by the MDAC, and the target data were advanced to 1988 from the early 1990s. Much concern was voiced by the dental profession as to whether the supply of dentists was commensurate with the demand for treatment in the private sector. The dental faculty also echoed this concern and, with the approval of the university, reduced its entry from 76 to 60 dental undergraduates per year.

The government accepted the need for a thorough review of the dental workforce situation and decided to set up a Dentists' Subcommittee to study the matter. It commissioned a number of investigations, the

153

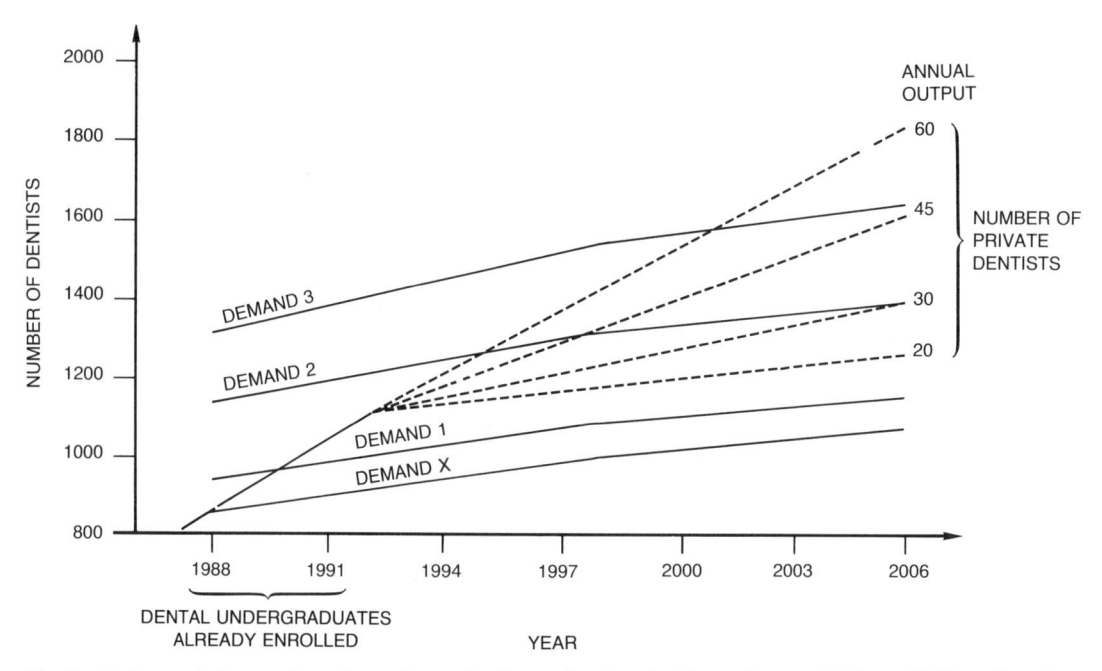

Fig 5 Estimated demand and number of private dentists in Hong Kong, 1988 to 2006, taking into account retirement.

most relevant of which is the Practice Profile Survey conducted jointly by the Hong Kong Dental Association and the faculty of dentistry.

The general pattern of major dental disease that emerged from the epidemiological studies is of a relatively low experience of dental caries in young adults. The older age groups show the greatest requirements for replacing extracted teeth. Loss of permanent teeth has not been shown to be a major oral health problem for most people below the age of 45. Dental calculus is widely found in the Hong Kong population and there are relatively few people who have clinically healthy gums. However, only a small proportion of the population go on to develop serious periodontal problems with advancing age. A small proportion of people demonstrate more serious oral conditions like dentofacial abnormalities, oral neoplasia, etc.

Incidentally, it has been established that between 10% and 20% of the population of Hong Kong are hepatitis B carriers. The figure for those tested HIV-positive is 148, of whom 24 have developed the full-blown syndrome and 14 have died. There is 10,000 to 100,000 times more hepatitis B virus than HIV per milliliter of blood; therefore, there is a much higher chance of contracting hepatitis than AIDS from blood and saliva. Hence, a considerable risk exists among unregistered dentists, whose standards of clinical hygiene tend to be well below acceptable standards.

The Dentists' Practice Profile Survey carried out in 1988 utilized a survey technique recently developed by the World Health Organization. The results indicated that private dentists considered that 67.5% of their available working time was devoted to productive work. In other words, one third of a private practitioner's day is spent idly. The figure for government dentists was 96%.

Annually there are 60 dental graduates from the University of Hong Kong. Figures for dentists being trained abroad and who will return to Hong Kong to practice are not accessible. There are about 100 aspiring to registration by examination annually. The number of dentists who may emigrate in the future is unknown, but the number of oral health personnel has become an issue in many countries, and thus opportunities to emigrate to developed countries are limited. Losses from the register due to retirement or death can roughly be estimated, but these figures are low because, with the current number of young graduates, the average age of practicing dentists is expected to fall.

The government has now accepted that an arbitrary dentist-to-population ratio can no longer be acceptable for planning a workforce. A workforce projection formula described in a joint FDI/WHO Working Group publication, *Health Through Oral Health: Guidelines for Planning and Monitoring for Oral Health Care* (Quintessence, 1989), was used to calculate the likely need for dentists up to the year 2006 (Fig 5). It was concluded, on the basis of this projection carried out in 1988, that there would soon be an oversupply of dentists if the present output of dentists remains unchanged, which it would until 1992 because of the 4.5 years of the BDS curriculum. This is the current situation.

Future development

It has been noted in a number of countries that economics presents a barrier to the seeking of oral health care, and there is no reason why this is not true in Hong Kong. In a community where the bulk of dental care is provided in the private sector, this is particularly true, especially because there are few schemes for underwriting the costs of dental treatment in Hong Kong. Even in the substantially free dental service provided by the Hong Kong government to civil servants and their dependents, the participation rate is only about 40%.

The demand for dental care and dental undergraduate admissions have a direct effect upon the workforce situation. If the demand changes and the number of students is reduced, the saturation point would be postponed for some time.

Demand levels rely on attitudinal changes in a society. Attitudinal changes take time, considerable effort, and commitment. Any workforce planning system must attempt to take into consideration future changes in demand.

The government has responded by the official permanent appointment of a dental subcommittee with wide terms of reference to constantly monitor and review the demand and provision of oral health care services to the population and to make recommendations to the government.

The demand for dental care can be improved through education and possible subsidy of dental care by the government. Much is dependent on the role of the government. Marketing can be pursued by the profession but must be done without detriment to the quality of service to the community.

The Hong Kong Dental Association is actively involved in the provision of dental education to the public and is making a high priority of marketing dentistry. With dental education, the demand for dental care will be coupled by a demand for excellence. A bright future for the profession is certainly there, but it cannot be achieved without struggle and possible hardship. Dentists not only must work inside their clinics but must be actively involved in the community, through the association, to bring dentistry to the public on a personal level.

Further reading

Davies WIR: The Development of Dentistry in Hong Kong.

Hong Kong Dental Association: Dentists' Practice Profile Survey 1988.

Dentists' Subcommittee 1988 Report. Medical Development Advisory Committee, The Hong Kong Government.

Chapter 16

Stomatology in Yugoslavia in the 21st Century

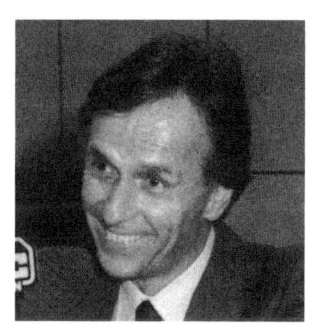

Matjaz Rode
Ljubljana, Yugoslavia

Abstract

In Yugoslavia there is no harmonized program for medical care since each of the republics has organized its own concept.

Because oral health not only involves dental or periodontal health, but also is an important part of the overall health of humans, we in Yugoslavia want to achieve two goals in stomatology within the 21st century:
- *to promote preventive oral measures instead of repair and rehabilitation,*
- *to move away from odontology and to reorient toward oral medicine.*

In the future we will continue to place emphasis on a number of population groups, which, however, have to be redefined. Besides dental care for children, we will also be organizing dispensaries for a number of risk groups. Preventive stomatological measures will be in the foreground for all citizen groups.

We will use the expression "Yugoslav stomatology" symbolically, because there is no harmonized program for medical (or dental) care in Yugoslavia. In Yugoslavia the organization and realization of such medical care is very heterogeneous.

Great economical and other differences between the republics of Yugoslavia demand different concepts in medical care and, in fact, a different concept has been devised locally in each case. Much of the discussion that follows will concern the republic of Slovenia.

Each republic has its own health ministry, the federal ministry is only responsible for global health strategy. This also applies to the field of dental care, which represents only part of the overall health strategy.

In Yugoslavia, dental care is almost exclusively organized as a public health service. There are only a few privately engaged dentists.

Dentists work in dental care dispensaries for treating children and adults; these are not lodged separately from the medical dispensaries in the health care

Table 1 Ratio of dentists to population and geographic distribution of dental positions[1]

Ratio of dentists to population		Towns (%)	Villages (%)
Yugoslavia	1:2,358	31.9	68.1
Slovenia	1:1,821	25.8	74.2
Bosnia and Herzegovina	1:3,143	26.7	73.3

facilities. These dispensaries represent the "front line" of dental care. The second line is made up of dental specialists, some of whom work in the health care facilities, while others are engaged in the university clinics. The third line is composed of stomatological faculties.

We already noted that between some parts of Yugoslavia there are great differences in the way in which dental care is organized. Table 1 serves to illustrate this.

The difference in distribution of dentists among the population is one of the reasons why in Yugoslavia a well-organized scheme of dental care is difficult to realize. However, for the whole of Yugoslavia the law applies that all citizens have the right to visit a dentist. Children, students, and a number of other groups can receive dental care (including orthodontics, periodontal surgery, and oral surgery) free of charge. Even for prosthodontics they pay almost nothing. Adults, however, have to contribute, particularly for prosthodontics.

In Slovenia, dental care has reached a good status. In general, dental treatment facilities are nationally available and accessible.

Organized preventive dentistry is slowly establishing itself. Laws and ministerial decrees govern the care provided. It is becoming increasingly clear that it will be possible to provide systematic dental care for defined population groups. Dental clinics can be found in almost all primary schools, and an increasing number can also be found in factories.

Perspectives

Oral health not only involves healthy teeth and periodontium, it is an important part of the person's overall health. This is because a person's physical, mental, and social well-being is, to a great extent, closely related to the health of the oral cavity. That is also the reason why in Yugoslavia we wish to achieve two goals in particular within the global philosophy of stomatology:

1. To promote preventive measures rather than repair and rehabilitation
2. To move away from dentistry and toward oral medicine stomatology

In the future, the emphasis of our work will be related to a number of population groups, which will, however, have to be redefined. *Conditio sine qua non* will be epidemiological data that will have to be available continuously so that dental strategies can be developed. At this point some information has already been gathered (Tables 2 to 4).

Table 2 Dental health per person — mean values for Yugoslavia[1]

Age	% Persons with caries	D	M	F	DFM
6 (primary teeth)	93.7	6.1	0.5	0.7	7.3
6 (permanent teeth)	39.7	0.7	0.0	0.1	0.8
12	98.7	3.8	0.5	1.8	6.1
35 to 44	100.0	3.1	10.2	4.7	18.0
65 +	100.0	1.7	25.5	0.9	28.0

Table 3 Healthy segments for some age groups — mean values for Yugoslavia[1]

Age	CPITN 0–1
35 to 44	0.25
65 +	0.02

Table 4 Current and projected age distribution (mean values) in Yugoslavia

Age	1981 (%)	2000 (%)
0 to 14	24.4	22.9
15 to 64	66.5	65.7
65 +	9.1	11.4

On the basis of this information we must organize stomatological (not only dental) care in such a way that improvements are made in the oral health of defined groups, and that this care can be monitored for effectiveness. The aims of such steps are oriented toward epidemiologically supported national indicators of oral health; the global health indicators as specified by the World Health Organization and the Fédération Dentaire Internationale are almost always identical with ours in Yugoslavia.

The specifications of such aims must also be based on the national and regional priorities derived from the demographic situation (particularly in Slovenia), the epidemiologically determined care requirements, the organization and effectiveness of the stomatological care system, and financial possibilities. In Slovenia, too, we will be paying particular attention to a number of target groups.

Children/students

For this group we will be perfecting a program of dental care that is already quite well established and includes the following measures:

1. Talking with pregnant women about motivation, oral hygiene during pregnancy, nutrition, and fluorides
2. Clinically examining and registering all 3-year-old children (providing therapy, control, and information when necessary)
3. Providing regular checkups (twice per

Table 5 DMF reduction from 1979 to 1988 for pupils in Ljubljana

School year	Child's age	DMF per pupil	D per head
1979/80	7	2.2	1.5
1987/88	7	1.2 (−43.6%)	0.4
1979/80	12	9.3	3.9
1987/88	12	6.2	0.8

year) up to the age of 6 years, with fluoride application and conservative therapy

4. Providing regular checkups at primary schools, where good results have been seen (Table 5)

Stomatologically, much has been done in Slovenian schools to improve children's motivation. Even in kindergarten, children are given help by dental and school personnel to practice proper toothbrushing and fluoride application. Additionally, in nearly all primary schools an annual competition called "Everything for beautiful teeth" has been organized for all classes. Here the school dentist performs random tests in each class using disclosing tablets; the results of these tests are published on posters for all to see. At the end of the school year we organize a festive promotion of the results of the best classes in Slovenia and we take this opportunity to distribute toothpaste, toothbrushes, and badges.

For older students we already have organized dispensaries for dental care.

Adults

Adults, too, should discover, not grudgingly, but with enthusiasm and positive information, that there is probably no area within the field of health care in which prophylactic behavior has been more successful than in oral health. That is why it is our aim for the 21st century to make available preventively oriented dispensaries for the oral medical care of adults. We will start in large factories and businesses to try to establish stomatological dispensaries within the framework of industrial medicine outpatient departments. Some outpatient departments of this type are already in operation in Slovenia and have proved themselves completely. Colleagues working in such factory outpatient departments have achieved extremely good results with a high care percentage (Table 6).

The main arguments for and advantages of such outpatient departments are:

1. Easy accessibility to dental care
2. Decreased absence from work (many millions of work days per year are lost because of toothaches)
3. Organized serial examinations and recalls
4. Early disease diagnosis
5. Collaboration with specialists for industrial medicine
6. The use of mass media (radio, posters, magazines, etc) to provide information, motivation, and oral hygiene instructions within the workplace[2]

The greatest disadvantage is financing, because the workers must pay for this service out of their own incomes.

Table 6 Results of preventively oriented stomatological care in a factory outpatient department in Slovenia

Age	DMF	D	M	F	F/(D+F)
33–44	18.1	0.7	3.8	13.6	95.3

Preventively oriented dispensaries will be organized for other adult groups as well.

On television, radio, and in many magazines we have opportunities to promote regular information about oral hygiene, oral diseases, oral health, etc. This all runs under the control of the Slovenian doctors' association so that the information is well coordinated.

Senior citizens

In Yugoslavia, particularly in Slovenia, the proportion of the senior citizen population is increasing, and it has been calculated that by the beginning of the 21st century approximately 20% of the citizens will be over 60 years old. In Yugoslavia-Slovenia we must also recognize that this growing proportion of the older population is also increasingly interested in their dental care. Aging may be a physiological process; however, it is a process accompanied by increasing morbidity. With increasing age the oral mucosa is subject to specific changes. During clinical examinations of the oral cavity of elderly people, besides the number of teeth, caries, periodontal disease, mobility and loss of teeth, and the degree of rehabilitation and quality, it is also possible to observe changes in the mucous membrane that make it possible to diagnose some diseases in their early stages. The oral health problems experienced by the elderly are gingival recession, xerostomia, abrasion and mobility, anodontia, denture stomatopathy, temporomandibular pain syndromes, and oral precancerous conditions, among others.

In order to coordinate an organized gerostomatological medical care system, it is necessary to establish a new standard of dental care for senior citizens.[3] Such a system must include dental care for the aged both in nursing homes and in private homes. Here, too, it is necessary to formulate priorities derived from the epidemiological necessities and requirements of old persons. However, although extensive information on the oral health of the youth population is available, this information on the older population is limited.

Our pilot study conducted with 200 aged persons of both sexes showed that in Slovenia approximately 20% are edentulous by the time they reach the age of 60, and of these, 30% have not been given dentures at all. Approximately 60% have carious lesions that have been cared for. We found white blemishes in the oral mucosa of 28% of the study group. We found denture stomatitis in 24% of the cases. Lingua fissurata was found in 26%. Dispensary care for the older population concentrate on the following:

1. Rehabilitation of the mouth
2. Hygiene awareness as well as im-

Table 7 Oral, neck, and head cancers in Slovenia during 1985

Cancer site	Men	Women
Lips	30	8
Tongue	46	8
Gingivae	6	0
Basis oris	25	2
Partes aiae oris	14	6
Pharynx, larynx, nasus esophagus	282	33

Table 8 Incidence of cancer per 100,000 population during 1985

Cancer site		Age			
	x	60–64	65–69	70–74	75–79
Lips					
Men	3.1	16.3	4.7	30.8	12.6
Women	0.8	–	–	7.5	13.9
Tongue					
Men	4.9	19.5	9.4	34.6	6.3
Women	0.8	4.2	3.1	–	–
Basis oris					
Men	3.7	16.3	14.2	11.5	23.6
Women	0.2	–	3.1	–	3.4

proved ability to perform individual oral hygiene measures
3. An individual care regimen for patients with physical, mental, or social handicaps
4. Special attention to the interdisciplinary collaboration between stomatology and gerontology

In organizing these services, we will try to (1) define a partly existing dispensary system for gerostomatology to provide facilities for early diagnosis of precancerous lesions and tumors, and (2) greatly increase the life span of patients' existing dentures with the help of free serial examinations, an information program, and motivational techniques.

Risk groups

Some of the population groups that require special dental care and attention are the so-called risk groups. Slovenia has already prepared a special program for the dental care of hemophiliacs, diabetics, and oncologic patients.

Special attention is being given to the dental care of the oncologic patients for two reasons:

1. Every dentist must be able to diagnose cancer and precancerous conditions in the oral cavity in their earliest stages.
2. The dentist must be able to mitigate the oral side effects of radiotherapy and chemotherapy.

In Slovenia, too, the cases of oral, neck, and head cancers are increasing, representing 9% of all new cancer cases each year (Tables 7 and 8).[4]

These two tables alone provide information that shows cancer in the mouth area is a serious danger. For this reason a scheme for semi-annual serial examinations is being implemented for the elderly. The highest priority in early diagnostics must be the recognition of precancerous conditions. Because the areas involved are easily viewable and accessible, experienced dentists have no problem making early diagnoses of precancerous conditions and other tumors in the oral cavity.

Together with oncologists, we are experimenting with a program we hope will mitigate the side effects of radiotherapy and chemotherapy for tumors in the mouth.[4] Our attention is focused on post-radiation caries, and xerostomia. For all our patients we are using fluoride pastes and mouthrinses. We are also preparing information on correct oral hygiene and are repairing caries-affected teeth with glass ionomer cements.

References

1. Vrbic V, Vulovic V, Rajic Z, et al: Oral health in SFR Yugoslavia. *Zobozdrav Vestn* 1988;43:3–11.
2. Schou L: Oral health promotion at worksites. *Int Dent J* 1989;39:122–129.
3. Künzel W, Sicha V: Anforderungen an die perspektivische Entwicklung der gerostomatologischen Betreuung. *Stomatol DDR* 1989;39:3–8.
4. Kogoj-Rode M, Rode M: Changes in the bacterial oral flora of patients treated with irradiation. *Zobozdrav Vestn* 1982;37:165–168.

Chapter 17

Dentistry in the 21st Century: Switzerland

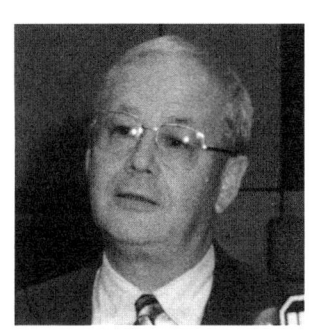

Peter Schärer
Zürich, Switzerland

Abstract

Because of the reduction in caries and periodontal disease, the goal of "optimal oral health" of the total population is achievable. A large increase in the number of prophylaxis auxiliaries and a reduction in the number of general dentists are thereby desirable. Specialization will increase because of higher demands for optimal restorative dentistry by a healthier patient population. Recent developments in Switzerland indicate that these changes are going to happen in the future.

Any outlook on the future of the dental profession for the next 20 years will always be an evaluation of future dental needs of the overall population and the services that our profession can provide. While in previous periods patient needs were rather large in relation to the number of practicing dentists, this situation seems now to be changing rapidly.

Through the enormous efforts in preventive dentistry, as provided in Switzerland from early childhood on, caries incidence has markedly decreased among children and young adults, and an increasing percentage of the total population will need less restorative treatment in the future. This trend, observed worldwide and expressed in World Health Organization reports[1] as goals for the future, is to a large extent already observable in Switzerland.

The goals in Switzerland with regard to "Oral Health CH 2000"[2] go even further than WHO. The Swiss concept of "Oral Health CH 2000" attempts to keep young adults free of dentinal caries to age 16, with a maximum of four occlusal fissure restorations at the age of 20. Every attempt will be undertaken to keep caries incidence at this low level and to minimize dental repairs through old age (Fig 1).

Such an optimistic goal can only be achieved by a principal change in dental service for the total population. With similar goals also outlined in regard to gingivitis and periodontitis (Fig 2), goals for preventive dentistry will include increasing the number of dental auxiliaries, providing preventive services, and reducing the number of restorative dentists (Fig 3).

While the number of dentists should only minimally increase (1989, 3,250 practices; 2000, 3,650 practices) or (preferably) decrease, the number of dental hygienists (1989, 1,000; 2000, 1,500) and especially of trained auxiliaries providing preventive services ("prophylaxis assistants") will markedly change:

- Prophylaxis instructors (teaching oral hygiene in schools, hospitals, etc): 1989: 1,200; 2000: 3,000 to 4,000
- Prophylaxis assistants (providing preventive measures under a dentist's supervision): 1989: 500; 2000: 3,000

With such a concept, the Swiss dental profession in the near future would have to accomplish two things: train and integrate on a very large scale new preventive auxiliaries into dentistry, and change the curriculum of dentistry, to teach students how to work with such a prophylaxis-oriented team.

Politically, the efforts of Swiss dentists to enlarge the number of prophylaxis auxiliaries and to integrate them into dental practices has met very little resistance from communities and public health officers. The possibility of reducing dental expenses is too appealing to be ignored by government officials. Resistance so far has come from some local dental societies and hygienist organizations that are not yet ready to change their primarily restorative-oriented attitudes.

Any change in the dental curriculum will not be as extensive as some academics fear. Basically, dental training will remain the same as long as the dentist will be responsible for the restorative aspects of the profession.[3] However, because the need for such work will decline in the future, a large reduction in the number of dentists with a modified curriculum will be the solution to the problem.

While orthodontics and maxillofacial surgery will be only slightly affected by recent developments, general dentistry, prosthodontics, and periodontics will need fewer dentists. Optimal dental services in the future could be rendered if: *(1)* 50% of the dental offices would be "prophylaxis offices," with the dentist acting primarily as head diagnostician and manager of a prophylaxis-oriented team; *(2)* 25% would specialize in restorative dentistry; and *(3)* the remaining 25% continued to provide conventional dental services to a smaller number of patients. Such a concept would provide optimal prevention and oral health and better restorative dentistry to those patients who still need it.

The effects of these changes on the income of dentists, dental technicians, and dental manufacturers cannot be predicted, but I would foresee a reduction of about 50%.

By comparing the average workload of a dentist in Switzerland in 1984[4] to that

Prevention of oral disease—caries prevention		
Etiology:		
bacterial plaque		
nutrition		
host susceptibility		

WHO-Goal for Europe in the year 2000:

5–6 yrs	50% caries free
12 yrs	DMFT ≤3
18 yrs	85% full dentition (28 teeth)
35–44 yrs	50% less toothless than 1981
65 yrs and older	25% less toothless than 1981

Methods, caries reduction in %, and duration of application:

Fluorides: Systemic and local		
— drinking water	50–65	lifelong
— tablets	25–80	birth–16 yrs
— salt fluoridation	60	lifelong
Fluorides: local		
— professional	30–40	1–2 ×/year
— individual mouthrinses; fluoridated	20–50	during school years
toothpaste	20–30	lifelong
Sealants:		
— occlusal	40–99	6/7 yrs and 12/13 yrs
low caries risk foods and beverages		
— quantity and frequency	?	lifelong
Oral hygiene		
— toothbrushing	?	lifelong
— interproximal oral hygiene	?	lifelong

Goals in Switzerland according to the concept "Oral Health CH 2000"

Children under 16 yrs
- the primary teeth except the fissures: caries free
- permanent teeth with max 3 fissure lesions, no approximal fillings
- bitewings without dental caries
- no additional caries in fissures

16 to 20 yrs
- no additional occlusal and approximal caries

20 yrs and older
Patients born 1960–1969 (20–30 yrs)
- no additional secondary caries on the max 4 fillings
- no crown and bridge work due to caries
- no devitalization due to caries
- no teeth lost due to caries

Patients born 1930–1959 (30–60 yrs)
- no additional caries
- no additional secondary caries
- no devitalization due to caries
- no teeth lost due to caries

Patients born before 1929 (over 60 yrs old)
- no additional caries in enamel areas
- a minimal amount of root caries

Fig 1 Comparison of WHO goals for Europe in the year 2000 and the goals of the Swiss "Oral Health CH 2000" in regard to caries prevention.

Control of periodontal disease

Etiology:
bacterial plaque
host susceptibility

WHO-Goal for Europe in the year 2000:

18 yrs	90% with min 3 healthy sextants (CPITN* = 0)
35 yrs–44 yrs	75% with min 3 healthy sextants (CPITN = 0)
65 yrs and older	max 10% have 1 or more sextants with CPITN ≥ 4

Methods:

individual	plaque removal, plaque disactivation, plaque disruption,
professional	subgingival plaque and calculus removal

Goals in Switzerland according to the concept "Oral Health CH 2000"

Children under 16 yrs
— max PBI-drgree 1–2 per papilla (total max 50)
— no probing depths > 3 mm

16 to 20 yrs old
— PBI max 20
— no probing depths > 3 mm

20 yrs and older
Patients born 1960–1969 (20–30 yrs old)
— PBI max 20
— no probing depths > 3 mm
— no attachment lost
— no gingival recession

Patients born 1930–1959 (30–60 yrs old)
— PBI max 20
— no probing depths > 3 mm
— no additional attachment lost
— no teeth lost due to periodontal disease

Patients born before 1929 (over 60 yrs old)
— no additional attachment lost
— no teeth lost due to periodontal disease

---

*CPITN (Wolf 1987): Community Periodontal Index of Treatment Needs
CPITN 0 = healthy: no hygiene measurements necessary
       1 = bleeding on touching: oral hygiene instruction
       2 = calculus: oral hygiene instruction with teeth cleaning and calculus scaling
       3 = shallow pockets: oral hygiene instruction, teeth cleaning, calculus scaling, and deep scaling
       4 = deep pockets: oral hygiene instruction, tooth cleaning, calculus scaling, deep scaling, and operative surgical therapy

Fig 2 Comparison of WHO goals for Europe in the year 2000 and the goals of the Swiss "Oral Health CH 2000" in regard to the prevention of gingivitis and periodontal disease.[1]

Dentistry in the 21st Century: Switzerland

Dental professions—description of profession

Dentists: (1989: 3250 offices; 2000: 3650 offices)
According to education, expenses of education, the expected knowledge and professional capability, the office structure, the office costs, and the social status, the dentist is primarily active as diagnostician and therapist, but he/she also offers a complete preventive treatment concept. In addition he/she is organizer, teamleader, and entrepreneur.

Dental hygienist: (1989:1000; 2000: 1500)
According to education, expenses of education, special knowledge, and professional interest and income, the dental hygienist is primarily a diagnostician and therapist for periodontal patients. She/he is responsible for maintenance and controls the other prophylaxis staff.

Prophylactic nurse: (1989: 1200; 2000: 3000–4000)
Specially trained people with preventive duties to instruct in schools and in institutions like hospitals and retirement homes.

Prophylactic assistants: (1989: 5000; 2000: 4000 half-day assistants)
Specially trained dental assistants with preventive duties, including maintenance under the control of dental hygienist and dentist.

Dental assistants: (1989: 5000; 2000: 5000)
Well-trained assistant for organization, preparation work, coordination, administration, and/or chairside assistance in the dental office. She/he guarantees an optimal office management.

Fig 3 Expected needs of dental professionals in the year 2000.[1]

Daily workload of a Swiss dentist in minutes. Confidence level 95% on the basis of 207 completed questionnaires in Fall 1984.

	U+K	MOTI	ZE	PARO	KONS	ENDO	KRBR	TEPR	TOPR	CHIR	PEDO	ORTH	NOT
mid ×	50	18	31	14	170	34	71	14	10	17	13	10	21
sh %	10.6	3.8	6.6	3.0	36.0	7.2	15.0	3.0	2.1	3.6	2.8	2.1	4.4
max	210	130	170	120	420	180	420	120	150	105	240	240	210
− VB	44	14	25	11	157	28	60	10	7	13	8	6	17
+ VB	55	22	36	18	182	3	81	17	14	20	16	15	25

U+K: Diagnosis and control; MOTI: motivation; ZE: calculus removal; PARO: periodontics; KONS: operative; ENDO: endodontics; KRBR: crown and bridge; TEPR: partial removable prosthodontics; TOPR: full dental prosthesis; CHIR: surgery; PEDO: pedodontics; ORTH: orthodontics; NOT: emergency treatment.

Fig 4a Daily workload of a Swiss dentist in 1984.[3]

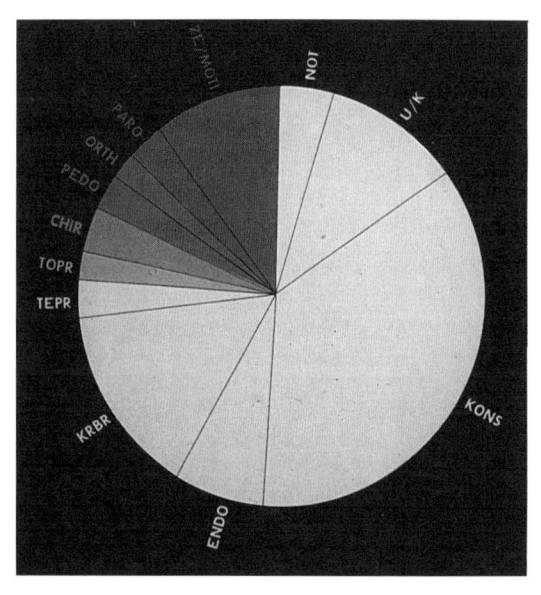

Fig 4b Total workload represents 100%.

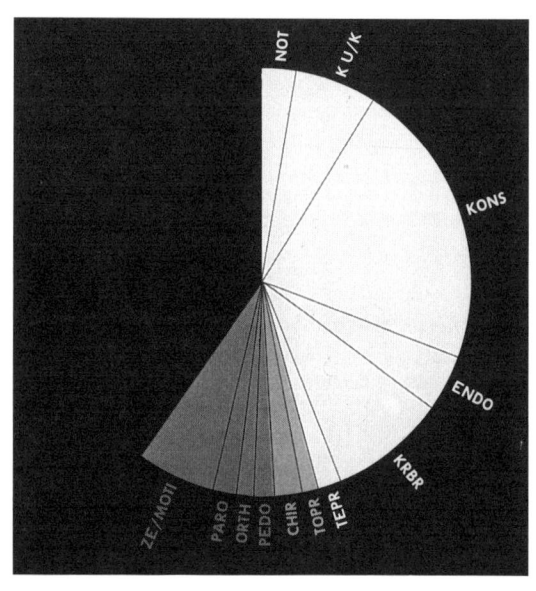

Fig 5 Daily workload of a Swiss dentist in the year 2000.[4]

predicted for the year 2000 (Figs 4a and b), one can see that a 40% reduction of caries and periodontal disease incidence will reduce the dental work considerably (Fig 5). If in the future prosthodontics and endodontics become specialized fields in Switzerland, the general dentist will keep around 25% of his or her present work. If the number of dentists should still increase in the future, this workload will be reduced even further. While there is a need in the future for more specialists in the various fields of dentistry, the general practitioners of the past might disappear. An estimated distribution in the future could be 20% fewer dentists overall as compared to 1989, with the remaining 80% comprising 30% dentists heading a prophylactic team, 25% specialists, and 25% general dentists.

Such a change in work will be the end of the general practitioner as known today. However, it would produce two positive results: *(1)* improvement of the oral health of the general population, and *(2)* improvement of the quality of restorative dentistry.

Developments in restorative dentistry

Reconstructive dentistry not only will experience a reduction in demand, but will be influenced by developments in the clinical and material sectors. The following recent developments are influencing restorative dentistry:

1. A marked reduction of caries and periodontal disease resulting from successful prophylactic measures during the last 20 years.
2. Increased patient demand for optimal esthetics, because a healthy, natural dentition will be "normal" for a large number of the population and a natural and healthy look will be popular.
3. The acceptance of dentin bonding, such as bonding to etched enamel, as an integral part of restorative dentistry.
4. Alternative treatment possibilities, such as porcelain inlays/onlays, laminate veneers, and adhesive restorations of the "Maryland bridge" type. If dentin bonding becomes a biologically accepted procedure, conventional luting cements, tooth preparation, and conventional crown-and-bridge materials must be reevaluated.
5. Implants, especially single-tooth implants, which will increasingly replace conventional fixed partial dentures as well as removable full and partial dentures
6. Changes with regard to optimal practice hygiene and management

These developments are going to increase the importance of graduate education and specialization.

References

1. *Alternative systems of oral dental care delivery. Report of a WHO Expert Committee.* Technical Report Series 750, World Health Organization, Geneva, 1987.
2. Lutz F, et al: Oral Health, CH 2000. *Schweiz Monatsschrft Zhhkde* 1989;8:928–939.
3. Ramfjord SP: Dentistry in the 21st century. *Quintessence Int* 1989;20:167–171.
4. Schärer P: Dental education at today's university. 100 Jahre Zahnärztegesellschaft Zürich: 153–160, Zahnärzte-Gesellschaft Zürich 1988.

Chapter 18

Dentistry:
A Profession in Transition*

Raymond P. White, Jr
Allan J. Formicola

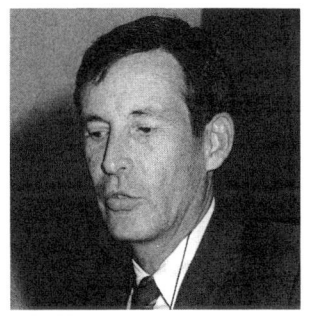

Raymond P. White, Jr
Chapel Hill,
North Carolina

Abstract

The United States enjoys a high standard of dental health care, an achievement that reflects well on our people and the dental profession. This high standard has been attained by a profession composed largely of general dentists oriented toward preventive health services and supported by dental specialists. Excellent schools of dentistry exist throughout the nation.

Although dentistry today is a profession held in high esteem by the public, underlying problems of great magnitude exist that prevent dentistry from being complacent about its accomplishments. Changing disease patterns, society's discomfort with the health care system, increasing overall health care costs, and a disinterest in careers in dentistry by college students are disrupting this system of care. This paper focuses first on important issues that are shaping academic dentistry and the dental care delivery system.

Issues shaping the dental care delivery system and dental education

Changing dental disease patterns

The epidemiology of the major dental diseases, dental caries and periodontal disease, has changed dramatically in the United States in the past two decades. As recently as 1971, screening for caries was felt to be a waste of resources because almost every child had the problem.[1] By the mid-1980s the situation was much altered. Klein et al,[2] reporting on the results of the Robert Wood Johnson Foundation – sponsored National Preventive Dentistry Demonstration Project, showed that much of today's youth is caries free. Other subsequent epidemiologic studies support these findings, and the expectation is that a high percentage of today's youth

---

* Modified from a paper prepared for the Future of the Health Professions Project funded by the PEW Charitable Trusts.

will move through their lifetime having very few problems with caries. Their need for dental restorations should drop considerably.[2-5] Attention on the promising increase in caries-free children — 13.3% in only one decade — has masked the scope of the problem remaining and the fact that the disease has only been brought under control, not eliminated. Other data suggest that the drop in caries rate is not being seen in the poor and that this small percentage of individuals with caries tends to have significant problems. No one is certain what combination of preventive and therapeutic measures will control caries in this less fortunate group.

A recent study by the National Institute of Dental Research of the working population can be interpreted to indicate that severe periodontal disease is diminishing, even though the more easily managed disease forms still persist. In the past, tooth loss from severe periodontal disease was initially seen in the population in the fourth decade of life. Extensive treatment could slow or arrest the progress of the disease but not eliminate it. Severe periodontal disease and the accompanying bone loss was the most important factor leading to tooth loss in the later decades of life. Although few are willing to predict the disappearance of periodontal disease and its sequelae, clearly tooth loss will not be prevalent in the future, as a result of earlier recognition, control, and treatment of periodontal disease. At present more than 45% of individuals over 65 years of age are edentulous in at least one jaw, requiring replacement of teeth with artificial dentures. If the incidence of dental disease is much less, the edentulous rate in the United States should dramatically decrease in future decades, and this would dictate a much different type of dental care for the elderly.[6]

The changes in disease patterns have influenced public attitudes and over the past decade have begun to change the character of dental practice. The American public who seek regular dental care today is less concerned about tooth loss from caries and periodontal disease, as well as the painful conditions that accompany acute episodes of these problems. With less caries and periodontal disease, the public's expectations for other aspects of good oral function are rising. McLain and Proffit[7] indicate that a significant percentage of the American population has malrelations of the jaws that are serious enough to warrant orthodontics and jaw surgery. Afflicted patients want this type of problem corrected. Patients expect to return to good oral function following trauma, and those that have ablative jaw surgery want jaw and facial tissue replaced both for function and esthetics. The prevalence of temporomandibular joint disorders seems to be increasing. Perhaps individuals have had such problems in the past, but today they are less willing to tolerate a disability that they now know can be alleviated.[8] Americans want the best from their health care system, and dental care is no exception to this expectation. More and more individuals have come to realize that good oral health and function are important to general well-being and psychosocial adjustment — all a part of the quality of life that is actively sought.

Dentists slowly are adjusting to the very

different demands being placed upon them as a result of the changing disease patterns and societal expectations. They must also be prepared to treat the growing numbers of older patients in their practices. Maintaining the natural dentition into old age will require the provision of care to patients who often will have medical limitations. At the same time, the dentist will need to satisfy a younger cohort with significantly different oral problems and expectations. Younger patients are concerned with prevention of dental disease, a desire for good occlusion, pain-free temporomandibular joint and jaw function, good lip function for speech, and facial skeletal harmony for a normal appearance.

The influence of research and technology

Rapidly changing technology, resulting from advances in the laboratory, continues to profoundly influence the delivery of dental care. Previously applied caries prevention strategies are credited with the clear trend toward a decreasing prevalence of this problem. The improvements are so significant that an entirely new strategy is suggested for the public health sector: targeting dental caries prevention only to those who are at high risk.[9] Information now emerging from research laboratories will improve the early diagnosis of periodontal disease.[10] Clinical tests for periodontal disease detection are becoming available to substantiate clinical findings. Tests that can be used in much the same way that serum chemistry determinations are used to monitor systemic diseases will dramatically change treatment of periodontal disease.

Expanding knowledge of biomaterials now allows new restorations to be bonded directly to the enamel and dentin of teeth.[11,12] Because carious lesions can be detected in the tooth quite early in their development, the disease process can be arrested and teeth can be restored without significant loss of structure. In a much different clinical approach than the fixed partial dentures of a decade ago, individual missing teeth may be replaced by bonding the replacement to adjacent abutment teeth.[13]

Because they have not benefitted from the decrease in caries and periodontal disease that is now apparent, many older Americans are edentulous or have multiple missing teeth. Partial and complete dentures are the conventional restorations for the missing teeth. Even in the best of circumstances prosthetic dentures cause a deterioration in bone and soft tissue over years of use. Now the lost bone and tissue in the jaws can be replaced with bone and bone substitutes, and implants made of biocompatible materials can be anchored in bone to support replacement teeth.[14]

A significant number of Americans have a malalignment of their jaws that creates functional and esthetic problems. By combining the expertise of the orthodontist, the oral and maxillofacial surgeon, and the restorative dentist with technology now available, jaws can be aligned properly, teeth straightened, and satisfactory oral function established.[15]

Because dental infections secondary to caries and periodontal disease were so painful and treatment under such circumstances was difficult, many adult Americans (as high as 20%) were fearful of dental treatment and avoided routine dental care. Current pain- and anxiety-control measures allow the dentist to treat these fearful individuals with medications that both reduce anxiety and provide anterograde amnesia, yet the patient is fully awake and has intact, protective respiratory reflexes.[16]

Though this list of recent advances is not comprehensive, these examples give some insight into the profound changes in dental practice resulting from advances in technology. The trend will continue because no one predicts anything but an expansion in our ability to generate new, useful information, applicable to patient care.

The need and demand for dental care

Society in America is heterogeneous, and our values and culture support individual choice. The health care system in the United States is reflective of this fact, making it difficult to predict the use of a particular health care service. Predicting the demands for dental care has been especially risky. Until very recently most dental care had been paid for by the individual from discretionary income, making the use of dental services extremely sensitive to the general economy. Although there are aspects of oral disease that if neglected can become life threatening, much of dental treatment can be postponed without immediate consequences. Further, the type of oral health care services a population seeks and receives appears to be related to a complex set of values intertwined with its view of health. The *need* for dental care and the *demand* for it by individuals can vary greatly, and recent history clearly demonstrates that it has.

Models to predict the need for dental care in the United States are based on the epidemiology of dental disease. As previously indicated, those surveys demonstrated that the incidence and prevalence of the two oral diseases responsible for the most loss of teeth appears to be changing favorably. Although the need for care of the two major oral health diseases on a population basis is changing, analysis of the implications of the changing nature of these two diseases on the demand for services is woefully inadequate. In the absence of such analysis wild speculation has resulted. The perception now exists among some that dental disease has been conquered and that the demand for services will drop precipitously. Other views argue against this perception. Recently Douglass[17] has attempted to explain these trends by examining them from an overall population perspective, by characterizing different age cohorts and then reviewing their potential dental problems throughout life. For example, he described those who fought in World War II as the "Iwo Jima generation," and current young adults as the "Atari generation." As groups, the Iwo Jima generation and the Atari generation have very different needs for dental care, based on disease patterns and behavioral attitudes. The Iwo Jima group did not fully experience the benefits of fluoride during tooth development, so their needs for restorative dentistry will be high throughout their lifetime. The need for restorative dental care for the Atari generation will be less for the group as a whole; however, a significant number of this group did not benefit from preventive measures and will require a high number of restorative services. Douglass further points out that attitudes about oral health care vary dramatically between generations. Whereas those in the Iwo Jima cohort and older came to expect tooth loss as an inevitable consequence of aging, younger cohorts find tooth loss unacceptable.

Douglass notes that changing attitudes will continue to fuel demand for dental services because the Iwo Jima cohort and those younger collectively will demand more care even though individuals in the youngest cohorts will need less care. Other than Douglass' analyses, few population studies exist on the determinants of the need for service and the demand for such services in the United States. Cohen[18] recently pointed out the need for such studies to include cultural and socioeconomic variables.

A complicating aspect of the demand for care goes beyond those predicted by epidemiologic studies of oral disease and is related to society's demand for sophisticated advances in the field. In the past, with no remedy available, individuals accepted grossly stained teeth, a result of tetracycline therapy to treat upper respiratory infection while teeth were forming. Today, dental restorations can reshape and recolor stained teeth through bonding directly to enamel, and afflicted individuals are demanding this treatment. Formerly, internal derangement of the temporomandibular joint was difficult to diagnose and satisfactory treatment was not possible. With computer assisted tomography and magnetic resonance imaging, however, appropriate diagnosis of internal joint disorders can be made, and open and closed arthroscopic surgical procedures can correct, repair, and replace joint structures. Afflicted patients demand this treatment to regain normal joint and jaw function. The development of a biologically compatible dental implant to anchor dentures for improved function has led to an escalating demand for this service.

Finally, no recognized professional standard exists in the United States to define acceptable basic or primary dental care. Such a question has largely gone unexplored in dentistry. In the absence of a professional definition, insurance plans appear to be shaping the standard. The private insurance carriers and industry clearly recognize the relationship between the demand for care, professional standards, and the incorporation of new sophisticated technologies into practice. Important policy questions remain to define what services constitute adequate dental care for the US population.

In summary, the need and demand for dental care require major thought from the dental profession. Epidemiologic data on changing disease trends, as well as the influence of cultural and societal perceptions, require more analysis to better predict the demand and need for care. Access to care for the lower income segment of the population requires more attention. More sophisticated technology will appear and biologic advances will continue. Their impact and effectiveness must be explored more systematically, particularly as they impact on society's demands for care.

The supply of the dental workforce

Dentistry in the United States remains a health profession of generalists who serve in a primary care role and provide the largest share of dental services to the public. These general dentists are supported by dental specialists, and working closely together, the two groups provide a very sophisticated level of oral health care. The great majority of general dentists are in solo practice. Dental specialists, on the other hand, often group together, with some specialists becoming subspecialized within their respective groups. Although there are some exceptions, the practice configurations in dentistry serve the public well, providing excellent geographic and generalist/specialist access.

By any measure, more dentists are available and geographically dispersed today to provide dental care than at any time in the past two decades.[19] The availability of dentists to treat the public is a direct result of federal and state initiatives to expand the number of graduates during the 1960s and 1970s. Such projections for a buildup in dental manpower were based on the anticipation of an expanding population and more third-party coverage for all Americans, either from government or private insurance. Private insurance has grown significantly over the past 20 years, but government coverage under medicaid is optional and very limited or nonexistent in most states.

There is no coverage for general dental services under medicare. New schools of dentistry continued to open, however, during the 1960s and the 1970s in anticipation of this broader access to care. Existing schools expanded their enrollments to a peak first-year class in 1978 of 6,301.[20] The number of civilian dentists has grown as a result from 75,000 in 1950 to 140,000 in 1987, and the dentist-to-population ratio changed from 49.8 to 57.8 per 100,000 as a result.[21]

Since 1978, a rapid decline in dental school enrollment has occurred, with the first-year class entering in the fall of 1988 consisting of only 4,196 students, a 33% decrease.[22] The American Association of Dental Schools projects that only 3,450 students will enter dental schools in 1993.[20] Women have enrolled in dental schools in greater numbers in the past decade, now comprising almost a third of dental students (31%).[22] The reasons for the rapid decline in enrollment are poorly understood, but many believe that dentistry's attractiveness as a profession to today's youth has waned as a result of the popular perception that dentists are no longer needed. The rapid buildup of graduates before 1980 and a poor economy in the early 1980s, which temporarily reduced the demand for services, created an atmosphere in the 1980s that there was no more room in the profession for new graduates. The high cost of education for dentistry also contributed to the problem. No one expects a rapid reversal of this trend toward lower enrollment, despite intensive recruiting for students by schools of dentistry. Not since 1939 will this country have educated so few new dentists. Some suggest that a shortage of general dentists will exist by the end of this century or early into the next century; others feel the lowered enrollment is a welcome adjustment. The drop in total enrollment from over 22,000 in the late 1970s to 17,000 today has already taken its toll on dental schools.[22] Five schools have closed and others are having difficulty maintaining a balanced program. Should several more schools close in the near future, there is a good likelihood that new schools will have to be built again in the year 2000.

The demand by the profession for individuals trained to be dental auxiliaries is now quite high, but dramatic drops in enrollment have occurred in these programs as well.[23] Traditionally, dental auxiliaries have been women, and women now have many other options for career paths. As a result of the lower birth rate of the 1960s and 1970s fewer individuals are in the age groups where dental and dental auxiliary students are recruited.[24] No significant change is expected before the turn of the century.

Dentistry has always been able to keep a balance between those practicing general dentistry (80% to 85% of practices) and dental specialists (15% to 20% of practices), a balance that has served the public well.[25] However, the rapid decline in dental school enrollment and the production of general dentists has not been followed by a similar decline in individuals studying to be dental specialists.[26] The public seeks care from the general dentists first, a relatively simple way for the public to gain access to all dental care. With a trend to a greater proportion of specialists, the question arises as to whether specialists in dentistry will become a primary entry point for caring for patients as it has become in medicine.

The appropriate training for general dentistry continues to be debated, with many leaders favoring expanded training over additional clinical years.[27] Issues of appropriate and mandatory continuing education and required recertification, and who should bear the costs of the process, continue to surface.

Today a consensus exists that there are adequate numbers of dentists to care for the American public but a severe lack of dental auxiliaries to assist them. But what about the future? Much depends on the configuration of dental practice in the future, and the assignment and allocation of tasks to dental auxiliaries, general dentists, and dental specialists. Major policy decisions must be made. However, the workforce issues in dentistry are confounded by the influence of changing technology, the shape of patient demands, demographics, and the financing of dental care. The complexity of the issues precludes a solution arrived at today being an adequate one more than 5 years later.

Financing dental care delivery

Almost all of dental practice is financed from fees charged to patients for services delivered. Most dental services are delivered in an ambulatory care setting. Overhead costs for the practice of general dentistry are high, in part because the dental office of a solo practitioner sits idle for a significant amount of time each week in comparison to facilities in a group practice. Also, the dentist must bear the cost of dental laboratory charges directly, and no adjustment is made if the patient or the third-party insurer does not pay. Overhead costs have increased significantly in the past two decades, often outstripping the solo dentist's ability to generate additional income from patient fees to cover the increases. Salaries for dental auxiliary personnel are rising rapidly, largely in response to the diminished availability of a dental auxiliary workforce. Costs for malpractice insurance have only recently begun to influence the overhead costs of running a dental practice. The problem of high malpractice premiums is significant for dental specialists who utilize conscious sedation and ambulatory anesthesia for pain and anxiety control, although the impact of rising costs for malpractice coverage are felt by every dental practitioner.

Increasingly, dentists are banding together in associations, and a few dentists are participating in managed care programs. However, dentistry still remains largely a profession of solo general dentists supported by dental specialists delivering services reimbursed on a fee-for-service basis. The shift to the ambulatory setting for medical services aligns the medical care sector with dentistry. However, health care expenditures and payments to physicians continue to rise as patients seek additional care. If more patients seek a wider array of dental services, expenditures for dental care also will rise. Over $32 billion was expended in the United States for dental care in 1987, representing 6.5% of the total health care expenditures of the nation.[28] Approximately 39% of the nation's dental care bill was paid by third-party insurers, with the bulk of the remainder being paid by the patient from discretionary income. In contrast with medical services, the federal government provides little support for dental services, less than 1% of the total.

Third-party coverage for dental services is a relatively recent phenomenon for the bulk of the US population. Dental insurance has been successful in emphasizing prevention and in using co-payments and deductibles to provide the widest scope of dental care possible with the financial resources available.[29] Clearly, private dental insurance has provided more patients access to dental care and made a wide scope of dental services available to these patients.

Significant changes are taking place in the United States in the financing of health care. In the face of attempts to decrease overall expenditures for health care, dental health insurance benefits continue to increase, covering an enlarging percentage of the working population. Those in the work force value their dental fringe benefits. It is difficult to predict, however, what choices will be made by individuals if they are forced to choose dental benefits from a "cafeteria" array of employee benefits. As long as Americans continue to value health services highly with dentistry among those services, patients will seek dental insurance plans from their employers and spend discretionary income for dental services. A severe economic downturn could eliminate discretionary income, or a radical change could occur in national health policy, both of which could affect the way dental care is financed.

The financing and delivery of comprehensive dental services is not assured for the future. Because so few federal funds go to finance dental care, dentistry is often forgotten as health policy is shaped. Some mechanisms must emerge to include a voice for the public who receive and the dentists who provide the over $30 billion in health care services annually. Similarly, a voice must emerge for the uncovered individuals who have no access to care at all.

The role of the dental school

The dental education system in the United States is small and it depends highly on the parent university and its medical center for continued existence. Few dental schools cover their full cost of providing clinical services. The system is under enormous stress as a result of the rapid expansion in the 1960s and 1970s and the precipitous contraction in the 1980s. Following the closure of five dental schools, only 55 dental schools remain in the nation. Many schools are under severe fiscal pressures because of dwindling resources superimposed on a traditionally inadequate financial base. The chronic situation has been made worse by the contraction of the number of students in the system: many private schools depend heavily on tuition revenue and many state systems allocate funds on numbers of students enrolled. Tuition costs borne by the students vary widely among the schools, with a high in the 1988–1989 year of $20,000. Instrument costs of $7,200, the national mean, add to the high cost of education.[30,31] Students finance dental education mainly through loan programs, and the high average indebtedness upon graduation continues to grow for each successive class of students. The high cost of education is a factor frequently cited now as a barrier for students to attend dental school, and financing education by loans is becoming a life-long burden. Little attention has been paid to the social implications of the heavy burden of the cost of an education to the student.

Dental schools could do more to increase their revenue from patient care. Currently only 14% of overall revenue comes from patient care, with only 3% of that revenue derived from faculty practice programs. The costs of operating dental clinics for predoctoral students is high. Dental students in a direct care role require an intense faculty teaching/supervision effort and a high faculty/student ratio. Such clinics, however, are a necessity because dental students in training must gain direct patient care experience before graduation and licensure. Schools reported losing over $40 million collectively in operating their clinics in 1987–1988, and some methods must be sought to use the clinic system more productively to reduce this deficit and meet the dual goal of education and revenue production.[30]

The role of the dental school in delivering dental services also needs to be reexamined.[32,33] To date, schools have only played a minor role in the overall delivery of dental care. As a rule the dental school sought patients only for teaching purposes. Individual schools have had outstanding programs of clinical research in targeted areas involving patients with specific problems. Patients are included in clinical research protocols and receive specialized dental care. For example, the University of North Carolina has had a consultation clinic for 15 years for patients with dentofacial deformities. Patients are seen in consultation by faculty and residents from multiple disciplines, the patient's problems are summarized, and a plan of treatment is suggested. Services to treat the problem are delivered both in the patient's home community and at the academic center in Chapel Hill. According to W.R. Proffitt (personal cummunication), the clinical data base accompanying the program includes records from 2,200 patients, with over 800 patients having been treated by both orthodontics and orthognathic surgery and followed for at least 1 year after completion of treatment.[34] The data generated serve as a major source of new knowledge in the field of treatment for dentofacial deformity.

In the past decade schools of dentistry have slowly expanded their role in care delivery through faculty practice plans and specialty clinics staffed by residents/graduate students. As demands for additional training for general practice have increased, individual schools have begun advanced general dentistry programs, which have expanded the institution's ability to provide general dental services. Dental schools have attempted to group dental students in different configurations, with supervising clinical faculty also delivering services.[34] Such models show promise for improved delivery of general dental services and educational experience, but no model has been adopted widely.

Schools of dentistry have not articulated well their role in the patient care delivery system or their possible contribution to developing systems of care to assist in covering those with limited access to care. Conflicts with local dentists and state and local dental societies are frequent. The challenge remains for all groups involved in patient care to work together to improve access for all to high-quality dental services.

Dentistry and the evolving health care system

Major concerns continue to be expressed by the public, industry, government, labor, and special interest groups about the health care system in the United States. Both dentistry and medicine will be influenced by the actions of these groups and by the major forces that impact on the economic future of the country. In this section, additional issues that clearly will influence the delivery of dental care and the education for dental health care are presented.

The changing knowledge base for science/technology and dental faculty

Scientific knowledge continues to expand at very rapid rates, and this knowledge base has and will continue to influence the technology surrounding the delivery of dental care. Academic dentistry has a small cadre of faculty who are contributing to the new knowledge in basic biomedical science. T.M. Valega, of the NIDR, notes that replacements for these faculty are being trained in the NIDR-sponsored dentist-scientist program, with an anticipated output of 25 faculty per year (personal communication, 1988). However, significant problems exist among clinical faculty who do not have the appropriate training to carry the new knowledge from the laboratory to clinical application. According to E.S. Solomon, over 900 full-time clinical faculty of a total complement of 3,000 full-time dental faculty are at the retirement age or will reach retirement age before 1995 (personal communication, 1988). Unfortunately, no funded program exists for training prospective clinical faculty for clinical research at a time when clinical research is becoming increasingly important and more sophisticated.

The impact of new knowledge and technology on health care must be observed under clinical conditions where there is less-than-perfect control of important variables. Research with patients is often confounded by effects unrelated to the clinical question being studied. The effects of interventions in dentistry are often small and undramatic. Evidence for or against the impact of different clinical interventions can often only be obtained indirectly, increasing further the complexity of the research design, analysis, and interpretation of data. The body of knowledge is evolving for improving methods for clinical research, design of experiments, and strengthening information obtained. Utilizing these skills takes training much different from that required for basic biomedical research. Clinician scholars need sophisticated, quantitative, and analytic research skills, and a program must be designed to provide these skills, along with clinical research experiences. Without such a program new knowledge will not be transmitted easily to the clinical setting, and the quality and the effectiveness of clinical services will suffer.

To improve the quality of clinical decisions, the clinician must be able to access the rapidly changing (and expanding) knowledge base and incorporate the information into a decision for an individual patient. The technology exists and will improve for managing information to assist the clinician in this process. However, the management of information from large data bases and the process of clinical decision making is not universally taught in dental schools or in continuing education programs. A concentrated effort is needed to enlarge the pool of academic dentists with the capability to design and interpret clinical studies and to manage large amounts of data.

The national economy and the financing of health care

Major changes in the productive capacity of industry have forced the developed nations to compete together in a world economy. It is rare for a consumer product to move from raw materials to a finished entity within one national boundary. Raw materials from one nation are fabricated into component parts in another, assembled in a third, and sold in an international market. The array of consumer goods and services available to those who can pay for them is astounding and beyond the comprehension of individuals born early in this century. Nevertheless, American industry must compete in this international market, where competition is intense. Any increase in production costs makes US industry less competitive. Health care costs of existing and retired workers are major costs for US industry, and the rapid escalation of expenditures for health care influence the competitive price of goods produced.[35]

The federal budget deficit is considerable and Congress is being forced to draconian measures to reduce the deficit. Health care expenditures and defense costs are escalating more rapidly than federal revenues. The states are beginning to report deficits as the 1980s close. The impact of these budget reductions and reduced expenditures for health care by government and industry are much discussed and include measures to ration the delivery of health care services. Government and industry have reached a consensus on the need to slow or even cap the expenditures for health care. The federal government must balance the budget and industry must cut its production costs to be competitive. However, the process for evolving such change is elusive. Dentistry will be affected by any changes in health policy and the overall health care systems. For example, because much of dental care is financed by discretionary income, increasing deductibles and copayments may require individuals to allocate their discretionary, after-tax income for medical care. Dental services are valued highly, but at least some individuals will be forced to abandon dental care in favor of medical services.

The United States spends a greater percentage of its gross national product on health care than any other industrialized nation.[28] Despite these expenditures, major gaps in financing health care exist, there is an uneven distribution of services provided, and large segments of the population have inadequate or no health care coverage at all.[36] The system in the United States leaves much discretion to the individual to select physicians and dentists to access all health care services. But often the individual does not have the knowledge to make an informed decision, one that would acquire the most appropriate health care at the least cost. The plurality of the US health care system has the major advantage of preserving the important doctor-patient relationship, but in this system a significant percentage of health care expenditures is allocated to administrative and overhead costs.

Any proposals implemented toward a national health policy and financing program will have a dramatic impact on dentistry whether dental services are included or not. The major problem for dentistry in discussing new national health policy and financing is that dentistry traditionally has had no voice in policy matters at a national level.

Changes in higher education and the health professions student

Dental schools exist as a part of a university community that has a major influence on society and on the future of the United States. Traditionally, American universities have provided a large segment of the US population with knowledge and information that has led individuals to a better quality of life and prepared them for the work force. The competitive pressures evolving from an international economy have led industry and government to turn more to the university as a source of new knowledge, which would provide US industry with a technological and competitive advantage in the marketplace. As a result, more pressure exists on the university to produce new knowledge through research and participate in the transfer of that knowledge to new products and services.

Most medical and some dental schools have had research as a major part of their mission for decades, and their research productivity has been considerable. As the university looks at each of its units to meet the challenge, all schools of dentistry will be expected to continue to improve the quality and quantity of their research effort without diminishing their education and patient care/service roles. All of this redirection must occur with constrained resources.[38] At present, American universities have a great backlog of needs for new facilities, renovation of existing facilities, and replacement of major items of equipment. At best, medical and dental schools will only receive their share of the total resources flowing to universities, making replacement of facilities and equipment in dental schools a major obstacle to an expanded mission. The best institutions will have cooperative agreements with industry and will be able to compete for available research dollars from the federal government. Units of the university, however, including schools of dentistry with no track record of research productivity, will have a difficult time mounting a new research effort and/or finding bridging support for research programs in transition. One major problem for dental schools is the fact that dental faculty trained for biomedical and clinical research are not being produced in large numbers. For example, the NIDR dentist-scientist program to train dentists for a basic biomedical research anticipates only 25 individuals completing the program each year, and no funded program exists for training dentists for clinical research — hardly the basis for an expanded research effort within the university.

The pool of individuals in the United States interested in a career in the health professions, including dentistry, continues to diminish. The number of individuals in the age cohort who traditionally might enter dental school will continue to decrease until 1995, with only a small increase after that time. To compound the problem, fewer individuals in the potential pool of entering students are interested in the health professions, and the major issues facing the health professions in the future appear to discourage those who might consider a health career. Cultural shifts in the population of the United States also will continue, with a few states experiencing the ensuing problems of incorporating new groups into their populations. Black and Hispanic individuals already are underrepresented in dentistry at the present time, posing a major recruitment problem for dental schools. With an increasing proportion of minorities in the population, a major new effort is necessary to solve the problem of minority underrepresentation. The American Dental Association and the American Association of Dental Schools have begun recently to work together on a national recruitment program, known as the SELECT Program. Much more must be done, again within an environment of constrained resources.

Directions for the future

Expectations for oral health and dental services

Academic dentistry and those dentists largely involved in providing clinical services can meet the challenges and continue to provide high-quality dental care to the public, even though difficult issues must be faced in the next two decades. Americans will continue to place a high premium on good oral health. Good oral function will be expected, and preventive health behaviors will enable the bulk of the population to retain their teeth and a high level of oral function throughout most of their lifetime. Americans will continue to be willing to spend discretionary income for dental services, further evidence that oral health is valued highly. Dental disease patterns will continue to change, requiring the dentist to provide different types of services to prevent and treat caries and periodontal disease. High-risk patients in younger cohorts will require much different treatment than their peers with no caries. Preventive dental services in the school systems will be targeted to those at greatest risk. Patients in older age groups will seek replacement restorations and expect missing teeth to be replaced with fixed restorations supported by implants anchored in bone and bone substitutes. Patients will expect good jaw function, including a temporomandibular joint with a full range of motion and a good occlusion. The 15% of the US population with handicapping malocclusion will have the problem corrected with orthodontics and orthognathic surgery.

Appropriateness of care will become an increasingly important issue. The dental profession will be required to show that alternative plans of treatment produce different outcomes. Few dental health status indices exist today, but these must be developed by the dental profession if it is to hold the public confidence. Patients, their employers, and third-party insurers will continue their focus on quality-of-care issues until the dental profession and individual dentists produce more data about the results of treatment. The transition to including appropriateness of care and quality assurance measures as part of clinical practice will be difficult, but once adopted they will become an integral part of providing care. Relicensure and recertification will be based on documented clinical performance. Less emphasis will be placed on initial licensure exams.

Throughout the United States, segments of the population will not have easy access to dental care, a smudge on an otherwise bright future for dentistry. Problems of providing these individuals with all health care services will be a major issue in the United States in the next two decades. Only a coalition of government and industry can solve these problems. In such forums dentistry has a very low profile, almost dictating that solutions for those not receiving dental care will be left untouched. The younger cohorts in these underserved groups will continue to benefit from improved preventive services. However, individuals with high levels of dental caries and periodontal disease will suffer, surrounded by the majority of the population who have forgotten that the severe sequelae exist.

Financing dental care

Dental care will continue to be financed by discretionary income and dental insurance. Because more dental services will be demanded by the public, expenditures for dental care will continue to rise. Changes in national health policy could deter spending for dentistry. For example, taxing employer contributions to dental health plans would reduce the dollars available for dental services. Shifts in federal policy to reduce the deficit will impact all health care spending; however, Americans make health services a high priority, want the best technology can provide, and will be willing to choose health care over other options.

National health policy will be debated widely, but it is difficult to see how a consensus can be reached. Many schemes will be tried for reducing expenditures for health care, and dentists will participate, though not in great numbers. To provide better access and reduce overhead costs, more general dentists will practice in small groups. The high indebtedness of recent graduates will force most of them to begin practice as employees, becoming partners or managing their own practice later in their careers. Women dentists will adopt more flexible career patterns than their male peers, but their productivity will be high.

Academic programs and the supply of dental manpower

Schools of dentistry will continue to play a critical role, educating dentists and dental auxiliaries, generating new knowledge, and providing specialized dental care. Enrollments in dental schools will continue to decrease, in spite of the best efforts at recruitment, because the number of individuals in the cohort who might enter dental school are decreasing and the health professions will be seen as less desirable as compared with other options. By the turn of the century there will be a consensus that not enough dentists are being trained to meet the needs of the US population. Rather than an increase occurring in the number of dentists being trained, dental auxiliaries will take on new roles, creating a career ladder and better employment prospects for these individuals. Educating general dentists and dental auxiliaries to provide increasingly sophisticated services will tax the ingenuity of the best dental educators, particularly when the new students must come from groups with a less intense science background and from minority groups not traditionally part of the health care system.

General dentists will continue to be the point of access for dental care. The roles of specialists and general dentists will be debated. Because solving complex dental problems requires multidisciplinary treatment, dentists will be forced to work together, each contributing special expertise.

Clinical dental faculty will continue to struggle to keep abreast of new knowledge and to efficiently transfer that knowledge to new dental students, but no longer will the dental school be required to graduate a dentist who can immediately deliver clinical services independently. At least 1 year of residency will be required for full licensure, that training being available in multiple settings with the faculty tied to academic centers. By necessity, academic centers will be coupled to community colleges, and the training of dental auxiliaries will take place in the same clinical settings as that of dental students and residents.

The delivery of dental services will continue to be profoundly influenced by a continuous infusion of new technology. Because the public will demand services that include new technology, keeping abreast of change will continue to be a significant problem for the general dentist or the specialist. To help solve this problem, regional clinical continuing education centers, staffed by the most appropriate faculty, will be developed and computer technology will be available to the dentist in the office for accessing large data bases of information to assist in clinical decision making. Academic institutions will forge partnerships with practicing dentists to assess new laboratory findings in clinical settings, a process accepted by patients.

Schools of dentistry will be under continued pressure to produce new knowledge through research. Faculty will be charged with addressing the major problems in their respective clinical fields. Individuals seeking clinical faculty appointments will have at least 2 years of research training before taking faculty positions, and many will have advanced degrees.

All full-time clinical faculty will be involved in delivering patient care, usually addressing problems of special patients. Faculty will be joined by residents and students in this effort. Clinical training for dental students will be conducted predominantly in the community. For patients with special problems referred to the dental school, multidisciplinary treatment will be the norm. From this effort specialized clinical centers will evolve, not only to provide patient care but to generate clinical data for research.

Predicting the future is clearly more hazardous than analyzing current trends. Because dentistry has been successful in the United States in preventing dental disease and providing services in a very complex health care system, continued accomplishment is almost assured. Many difficult issues must be faced, but the political will, knowledge base, and strategies are available for continued high achievement.

References

1. Lindahl RL, Young WO: *A guide to dental care for the early and periodic screening, diagnosis, and treatment program (EPSAT) under Medicaid*, American Society of Dentistry for Children and US Dept of Health, Education and Welfare, 1973, pp 11–13.
2. Klein SP, Bohannan NM, Bell RM, et al. *Am J Publ Health* 1985;75:382–391.
3. *National Survey of Oral Health in School Children 1986–87*. National Institute of Dental Research (Unpublished data).
4. Hughes JT, Rozier RG, Ramsey DL: *Natural History of Dental Diseases in North Carolina 1976–77*. Durham: North Carolina Academic Press, 1982.
5. Douglass CW, Gannon MD: The epidemiology of dental caries and its impact on the operative dentistry curriculum. *J Dent Educ* 1984;48:547–555.
6. Meskin LM, Brown LJ, Warren GB: Patterns of tooth loss and accumulated prosthetic treatment potential in US employed adults and seniors, 1985–86. *Gerodont* 1988;4:126–135.
7. McLain JB, Proffit WR: Oral health status in the United States: Prevalence of malocclusion. *J Dent Educ* 1985;49:386–396.
8. Rugh JD, Solberg WK: Oral health status in the United States: Temporomandibular disorders. *J Dent Educ* 1985;49:398–405.
9. Stamm JW, Disney JA, Graves RC, et al: The University of North Carolina caries risk assessment study. I: Rationale & content. *J Publ Health Dent* 1988;48:225–232.
10. Lamster I: Application of new methodology to the study of gingival crevicular fluid, in HM Myers (ed): *New Technologies in Dental Research*. Basel. Karger (in press).
11. Duncanson MG, Miranda FJ, Probst RT: Resin dentin bonding agents—rationale and results. *Quintessence Int* 1986;17:625–629.
12. Bowen RL, Cobb EN: A method for bonding to dentin and enamel. *JADA* 1983;107:734–736.
13. Thompson VP: Etched-metal resin-bonded prostheses. Report of the Council on Dental Materials, Instruments, Equipment. *JADA* 1987;115:95–98.
14. Albrektsson T, Zarb G, Worthington P, Eriksson AR: The long-term efficacy of currently used dental implants: A review and proposed criteria of success. *Int J Oral Maxillofac Implants* 1986;1:11–25.
15. White RP Jr, Proffit WR: Surgical orthodontics: A current perspective, Johnston LE Jr (ed): *New Vistas in Orthodontics*. Philadelphia, Lea and Febiger, 1985, pp 260–319.
16. Ochs MW, Tucker MR, White RP Jr: A comparison of amnesia in outpatients sedated with midazolam or diazepam alone or in combination with fentanyl during oral surgery. *JADA* 1986;113:894–897.
17. Douglass CW: Demographic point of a brighter future for dentistry. *Dent Econ* 1986;(Feb):8–12.
18. Cohen L: Societal expectations for oral health: Response of the dental care system. *J Publ Health Dent* 1988;48:83.
19. American Dental Association Bureau of Economic and Behavioral Research: *Distribution of Dentists in the United States*. Chicago, American Dental Association, 1987.
20. Solomon E: *AADS Manpower Project, Report No. 2*. Washington, DC, American Association of Dental Schools, Manpower Committee, Jan 1989.
21. Schwab P: *Medical and Dental Manpower Projections of the Health Resources and Services Administration*. Office of Data Analysis and Management, The Division of Medicine and Division of Associated and Dental Health Professions to the AADS Council of Deans, Nov 1988.
22. *Dean's Briefing Book, 1987–88 Academic year*. Washington, DC, American Association of Dental Schools.
23. *1988–89 Annual Report on Dental Education: Dental Auxiliary Report*. Chicago, American Dental Association, 1989.
24. Solomon LC, Wingard TL: The future demographic of higher education in the United States: Implications for the health professions. Future of the Health Professions Proceedings. Dallas, PEW Charitable Trusts, 1988.
25. *Advanced Dental Education: Recommendations for the 80s*. Washington, DC, American Association of Dental Schools, 1980, pp 15–16.
26. *The Relationship of Advanced Dental Education Programs and Declining Dental School Enrollments*. Symposium at the 30th Annual Council of Deans Meeting of the AADS, Nov 1988.
27. General practice residency and advanced general dentistry programs. *J Dent Educ* (special issue) 1983;47:359–413.
28. Levit KR, Freeland MS: National medical care spending. *Health Affairs* 1988;7:124–136.
29. Olsen ED: Dental insurance, a successful model facing new challenges. *J Dent Educ* 1984;48:591–595.
30. *1988–89 Annual Report on Dental Education, Financial Report, Suppl 6*. Chicago, American Dental Association, 1989.
31. *1988–89 Annual Report on Dental Education, Supplement 3: Dental School Tuition*. Chicago, American Dental Association, 1989.
32. Formicola AJ: Educational goals versus patient needs. Proceedings of the Third Conference on Comprehensive Care in Clinical Dental Education. *J Dent Educ* 1984;48:20–24.

33. Formicola AJ: "Service-first" philosophy. *J Dent Educ* 1988;52:509–512.
34. Cohen DW, Cormier PP, Cohen JL: *Educating the Dentist of the Future: The Pennsylvania Experiment.* Philadelphia, University of Pennsylvania Press, 1985.
35. Califano JA: A corporate Rx for America: Managing runaway health costs. *Issues in Science & Technology* 1986;(Spring):81–90.
36. Enthoven A, Kronick R: A consumer choice health plan for the 1990s. *New Engl J Med* 1989;320:19–37, 94–101.
37. Himmelstein DV, Wollhander S: A national health program for the United States. *New Engl J Med* 1989;102–108.
38. Hopper, et al: Future of the Health Professions Proceedings. Dallas, PEW Charitable Trusts, 1988.

Chapter 19

Dentistry in the 21st Century – A German View

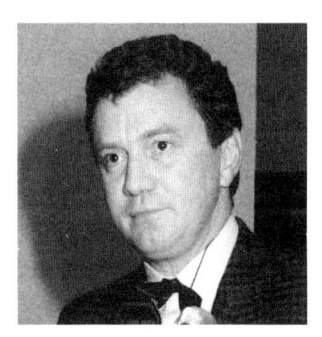

Heiner Weber
Tübingen,
Federal Republic
of Germany

Abstract

The perspectives on future dentistry cannot be based merely on technical and/or biotechnical considerations. Any kind of progress, no matter whether it is industrial or medical, involves a financial investment. Thus, further developments in dentistry will be strongly correlated with the social security situation in particular and/or with the economic situation of a country in general.

Furthermore, dentistry of the 21st century will depend on the dental health at that time. It can be anticipated that caries will decrease. However, tooth loss due to periodontal disease will become more prevalent as a result of a growing elderly population. Parallel to this development, the claims of our patients with regard to comfort and esthetics will increase, leading to sophisticated, complex rehabilitations that will include implants and prosthetic treatments.

The aspects of dentistry of the 21st century as addressed above can be reduced to questions of the amount and type of dental care possibly being needed at that time.

When the future of dentistry is to be discussed, the overall international aspects have to be differentiated from national concerns. Furthermore, if it is a European nation under consideration, confining the discussion to that country will be difficult and unrealistic. Thus, I will try to mix and interpret the international data with the data of my own country in order to give an objective, but personal, view. This view will basically include the amount and type of dentistry that will be needed in the future.

Amount of dental care

The amount of dental care needed is strongly correlated with the demographic development and with the dental health

Table 1 Age distribution of the West German population, 31 December 1984 and 31 December 2000

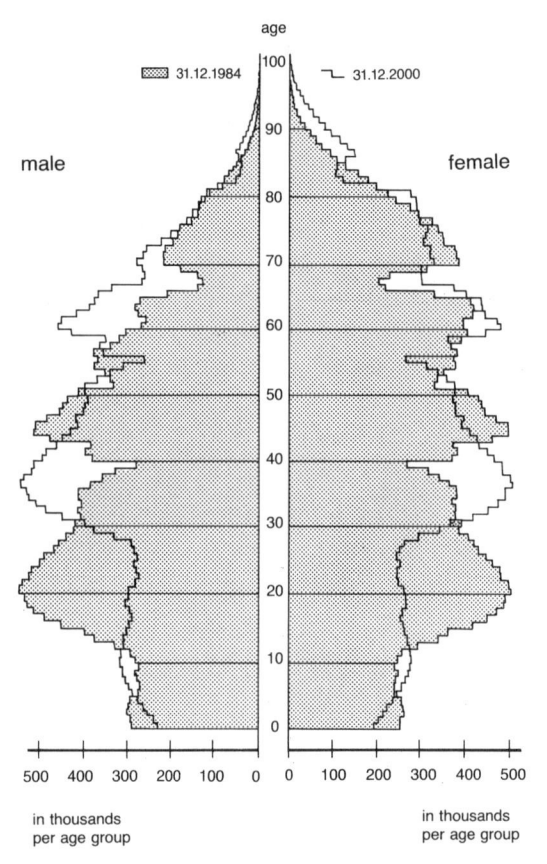

[Population pyramid chart showing age distribution for male and female, 31.12.1984 and 31.12.2000, in thousands per age group]

of our population. As far as the first parameter is concerned, all surveys indicate that at least West Germany will experience no growth or may even decrease in population (Tables 1 and 2). However, this will be offset by several facts that are specific to the West German situation:

1. The West German annual expenses for dental care are the highest of the industrial countries (Tables 3 and 4).

Table 2 West German population for the years 1970–2000

Age	1970 abs.*	%	1980 abs.*	%	1985 abs.*	%	1990 Model A abs.*	%	Model B abs.*	%	Model C abs.*	%	2000 Model A abs.*	%	Model B abs.*	%	Model C abs.*	%
< 20	17,423	29.6	15,929	26.9	12,898	22.8	10,990	20.0	10,955	19.5	10,903	19.4	10,479	20.1	10,682	19.7	10,540	19.3
20–60	29,119	50.0	30,503	53.9	31,586	55.8	32,010	58.3	32,438	57.9	32,480	57.9	29,182	56.0	29,587	54.6	29,676	54.3
> 60	11,720	20.1	11,656	20.4	12,158	21.5	11,894	21.7	12,652	22.6	12,747	22.7	12,479	23.9	13,962	25.7	14,387	26.4
> 75	2,586	4.4	3,484	**	4,072	7.2	4,031	**	4,408	7.9	4,483	7.9	3,454	**	4,219	7.8	4,506	8.3
Total	58,263	100.0	57,188	100.0	56,643	100.0	54,893	100.0	56,045	100.0	56,130	100.0	52,140	100.0	54,231	100.0	54,603	100.0

* absolute number of persons.
** data not available.

Table 3 European expenses for health care (including dental care) and for dental care (including prosthodontics) in 1982

	Expenses for dental care		Total expenses for health care		Expenses for dental care (% of health care)
	per person (in US$)	percent of gross national product	per person (in US$)	percent of gross national product	
Austria	35.46	0.39	644.40	7.37	5.32
Denmark	58.62	0.56	745.82	7.07	7.86
West Germany	104.76	0.98	872.65	8.71	12.60
Finland	41.80	0.40	692.83	6.71	6.03
France	75.35	0.70	931.20	9.30	7.57
Iceland	47.53	0.48	880.13	8.01	5.93
Netherlands	48.45	0.51	836.27	8.72	5.81
Norway	67.30	0.50	931.93	7.04	7.06
Sweden	101.70	0.87	1,168.50	10.03	8.68
Switzerland	112.00	0.72	1,157.30	7.40	9.74
Great Britain	22.36	0.26	510.25	5.88	4.38

Table 4 Expenses for dental care from 1970 to 1985. These data are based on the so-called socially insured patients (92% of our population); the expenses of the 8% of our population who are privately insured are not included here

	Type of treatment									
Year	operative/surgical		orthodontic		periodontal		miscellaneous		prosthetic	
	in Mill. DM	to prec. year	in Mill. DM	to prec. year	in Mill. DM	to prec. year	in Mill. DM	to prec. year	in Mill. DM	to prec. year
1970	1,708	–	–	–	–	–	–	–	828	–
1971	2,022	18.38	–	–	–	–	–	–	1,209	46.01
1972	2,250	11.28	–	–	–	–	–	–	1,524	26.05
1973	2,459	9.29	212	–	–	–	–	–	1,860	22.05
1974	2,810	14.27	589	177.83	–	–	–	–	2,086	12.15
1975	3,332	18.58	797	35.31	–	–	–	–	4,180	100.38
1976	3,377	1.35	920	15.43	–	–	–	–	5,312	27.08
1977	3,582	6.07	1,026	11.52	–	–	–	–	5,403	1.71
1978	3,806	6.25	1,162	13.26	–	–	–	–	5,755	6.51
1979	3,965	4.18	1,258	2.26	–	–	–	–	6,472	12.46
1980	4,160	4.92	1,357	7.87	–	–	–	–	7,351	13.58
1981	4,650	11.78	1,286	–5.23	–	–	–	–	8,110	10.33
1982	4,585	–1.40	1,274	–0.93	197	–	16	–	6,988	–13.83
1983	4,712	2.77	1,325	4.00	224	13.71	19	18.75	6,664	–4.64
1984	4,881	3.59	1,407	6.19	250	11.61	25	31.58	7,338	10.11
1985	4,938	1.17	1,429	1.56	259	3.60	30	20.00	7,666	4.47

Table 5 Social expenses for different dental treatments, in % (West Germany)

Type of treatment	Expenses			Number of cases		
	1977	1982	1985	1977	1982	1985
Operative/surgical	35.3	35.0	35.0	79.5	77.8	76.6
Periodontal	1.0	1.5	1.9	0.2	0.3	0.4
Prosthodontic	54.2	54.3	53.0	13.6	14.5	14.9
Orthodontic	9.5	9.1	9.9	6.6	7.3	8.0
Jaw fracture	0.0	0.1	0.2	0.1	0.1	0.1
Total	(100)	(100)	(100)	(100)	(100)	(100)

2. Half of our dental expenses are spent on prosthetic care (Table 5).
3. Our DMFT index does not reflect the position we ought to possess internationally (Tables 6a and 6b).

Thus, a decrease in the need for dental care is very unlikely in our country. Assuming that the average life-span for fixed and combined fixed/removable (telescoping/precision attachment) rehabilitations is in the order of 8 to 10 years, much extensive restorative work will have to be done in the coming decade and thereafter until, finally, these patients are edentulous. At the same time, our partially and completely edentulous patients will ask for greater esthetics and comfort in restorative treatment, even when they have to pay more money out of their own pockets. These circumstances will keep the need for and quality of dental therapy quite high. The increasing number of dentists (from 60/100,000 population in 1985 to 85–92/100,000 in 2000) might slightly enhance the effects described above.

Type of dental care

Discussing the future type of dentistry requires consideration of the different disciplines of our profession (as given in our country).

Preventive care (cleaning, prophylaxis, patient education)

Despite a well-organized social security system (including dental care), there is no nationwide, state-supported preventive program, and some statistics are disturbing: 10 million West German inhabitants did not buy a toothbrush within a 3-year period; 43% to 89% of all 3-year-old children and 72% to 93% of all 5-year-old children have caries. These statistics compel us to emphasize all activities that will help in lowering these figures and ultimately in meeting the dental goals of the World Health Organization given for the year 2000. Any private (patient-based) and/or professional improvement in this

Table 6a DMF indices of various countries

Country	Time interval	Age group	Index	Index beginning	end	Change in %
Australia	1954–80	12	DMFT	7.2	2.5	−65
Denmark	1973–80	15	DMFS	15.9	10.8	−32
England	1971–81	12	DMFS	9.3	4.3	−53
Ireland	1961–79	13–14	DMFT	8.0	4.4	−45
Netherlands	1966–80	12	DMFT	8.2	5.5	−33
New Zealand	1973–78	8–9	DMFT	3.3	2.0	−39
Norway	1955–79	15	DMFT	16.5	10.8	−35
Scotland	1970–80	12	DMFT	8.1	5.8	−28
Sweden	1973–78	15	DFS	27.7	13.7	−51
USA	1971–80	12	DMFS	6.4	4.2	−35
West Germany	1973–83	13–14	DMFF	8.8	10.8	+23
West Germany	1973–83	8–9	DMFT	3.3	2.3	−30

Table 6b DMFT index in West Germany in 1978 (number of patients: 14,491)

Age group	DMF	D	M	F
15 − 24	14.5	5.2	1.6	7.7
25 − 34	16.2	4.2	2.7	9.3
35 − 44	17.1	3.3	4.8	9.0
45 − 54	19.5	2.5	9.5	7.5
55 − 64	21.8	1.8	14.6	5.4
65 +	23.0	1.5	17.8	3.7

field will remarkably influence the amount and the type of dental care needed.

Operative care

Operative care will be influenced firstly and greatly by the efficiency of preventive care. As far as treatment is concerned, our patients will increasingly ask for restorative procedures that utilize tooth-colored, wear-resistant materials that necessitate minimal loss of tooth structure. This requires the development of appropriate materials such as improved resins or chemically bonding, wear-resistant luting agents.

Surgical care

The future of oral surgery will also depend greatly on the success of prevention. Bone regeneration and/or artificial

Table 7 Edentulism in Europe

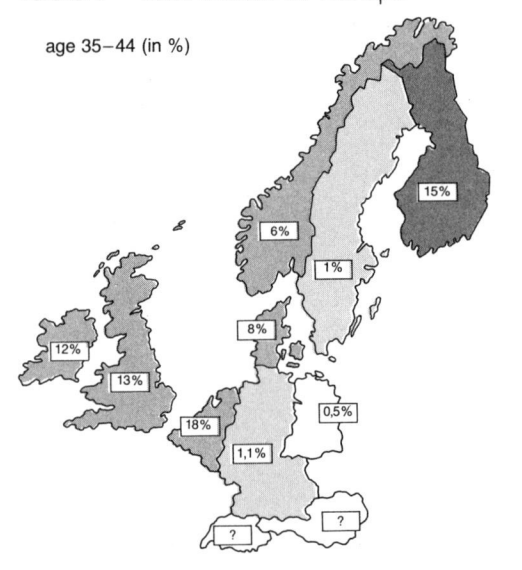

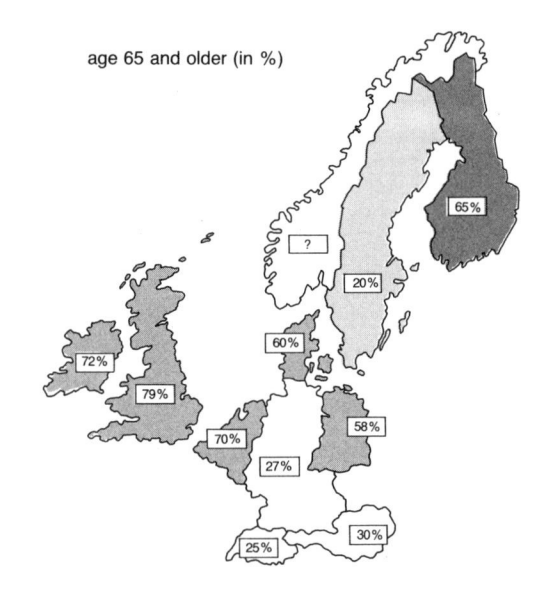

age 35–44 (in %): Finland 15%, Norway 6%, Sweden 1%, Denmark 8%, Ireland 12%, UK 13%, Netherlands 18%, Belgium 0.5%, Germany 1.1%, Austria ?, Italy ?

age 65 and older (in %): Finland 65%, Norway ?, Sweden 20%, Denmark 60%, Ireland 72%, UK 79%, Netherlands 70%, Belgium 58%, Germany 27%, Austria 25%, Italy 30%

replacement will be of outstanding importance. Maxillofacial surgery will be further challenged with regard to plastic surgery, especially microsurgical grafting.

Both oral surgery and maxillofacial surgery will be affected by the gradual and successful promotion of dental implant therapy. However, close cooperation between surgeons and prosthodontists will be mandatory in order to achieve the optimal results for our patients.

Periodontal care

Keeping in mind that periodontal disease is one of two major causes for tooth loss (caries, of course, being the other), it is amazing that only very little effort is directed in this field. However, statistics reveal that West Germany has a comparatively low percentage of edentulous patients in certain age groups (Table 7).

It can be stated that periodontal therapy must and will expand tremendously before and after the year 2000. Guided tissue regeneration will be the key for research and patient treatment.

Further insights into and success of dental implant therapy might have an impact on periodontics, too, inasmuch as the replacement of periodontally involved teeth by implants could yield a better result for so-called hopeless cases than extensive periodontal treatment.

Orthodontic care

Because orthodontic treatment is related to genuine malformation as well as to acquired diseases or poor oral habits, it is easy to conceive that prevention will again be influential. Major changes in the type of therapy cannot be foreseen at this point.

Prosthodontics

At least in West Germany, prosthodontic care will be of outstanding importance in the dental field for several reasons.

First, as indicated, many prosthetic restorations have been placed during the last 15 years; eventually, these rehabilitations will have to be removed, replaced, and/or modified. Also, West German patients ask for sophisticated prosthetic care with regard to esthetics and comfort. Another reason prosthodontics will be important is that in spite of all possible successes with prevention, there will be a continuous loss of teeth in older patients (50 years and older) as a result of periodontal diseases. This implies that more complex combined fixed/removable prosthetics can be expected for the future. Finally, as a result of the obvious successes of dental implant therapy, particularly with regard to the treatment of the edentulous mandible, more patients will ask for this type of treatment, which in turn will lead to an increase in extensive prosthetic rehabilitations (overdentures, fixed partial dentures).

The role of the prosthodontist with regard to implant therapy was well described by a consensus panel on the occasion of the Third Meeting of the International College of Prosthodontists held in Toronto in 1989. The consensus statement, a portion of which follows, was based on four questions given by Dr George Zarb, the fourth being related to the responsibility of the prosthodontist with regard to implant patients:

> The traditional role of the prosthodontist in the management of patients with implant stabilized prostheses, has been one of patient selection, treatment coordination, prosthesis fabrication, and its long term maintenance. This role should continue to be the preeminent one in patient treatment. However, consideration should be given to the placement of dental implants by prosthodontists trained in such techniques in graduate and postgraduate programs.

The state of the art of dental implants, as well as unanswered questions representing the basis for future research work and possible developments in this field, is well described by the Consensus Development Conference on Dental Implants (National Institutes of Health, Bethesda, Maryland, June 1988).

In general, future dental research work will derive from these areas that I have discussed (implantology, etc). While tooth loss due to caries will be reduced dramatically, tooth loss caused by periodontal disease will increase. Thus, more biological research will be directed toward the immunological aspects as well as to the healing/repair of periodontal defects. However, partial and complete edentulism will persist in spite of all of these efforts. The expected role of prosthodontics will scientifically be characterized by research activities dealing with the ease of manufacturing prostheses, including CAD/CAM, spark erosion, and/or sintering techniques. Furthermore, after a quite rapid growth of implant therapy, failures of implant/prosthetic treatments will have to be scrutinized, probably with emphasis on the impact of biomechanics.

Summary

In the industrial countries, practical and scientific dentistry of the 21st century will mainly be characterized by the prevention and therapy of periodontal disease (caries prevention will be managed on an individual, private basis) and by the treatment of partially and completely edentulous patients by increasingly utilizing implants. The technical possibilities of today will be limited by economic factors.

Further reading

Albrektsson T, Zarb G, Worthington P, Eriksson AR: The long-term efficacy of currently used dental implants: A review and proposed criteria of success. *Int J Oral Maxillofac Implants* 1986;1:11–25.

Brånemark P-J: Tissue-Integrated Prostheses: Osseointegration in Clinical Dentistry. Chicago: *Quintessence Publ Co,* 1985.

D'hoedt B, Schulte W: A comparative study of results with various endosseous implant systems. *Int J Oral Maxillofac Implants* 1989;2:95–105.

Gottlow J, Nyman S, Karring T, Rylander H: New attachment following surgical treatment of human periodontal disease. *J Clin Periodontol* 1986;13:604.

Gottlow J, Karring T, Nyman, S: Guided tissue regeneration following the use of Gore-Tex: *J Dent Res* 1987 (abstract).

Rekow D: Computer-aided design and manufacturing in dentistry: A review of the state of the art. *J Prosth Dent* 1987;4:512.

Rizzo A: Proceedings of the consensus development conference on dental implants. NIH, Bethesda, Maryland, June 1988. *J of Dent Educ* 1988; (special issue) Vol 52, No 12.

Sachverständigenrat für die Konzertierte Aktion im Gesundheitswesen: Jahresgutachten 1987 – Medizinische und ökonomische Orientierung – Vorschläge für die Konzertierte Aktion im Gesundheitswesen, Nomos Verlagsgesellschaft, Baden-Baden.

Schlagenhauf U, Rosendahl R, Netuschil L: Vergleich klinischer und mikrobiologischer Parameter zur Bestimmung des aktuellen Kariesrisikos. *Oralprophylaxe* 1989;11:70–73.

Setz J, Krämer A, Benzing U, Weber H: Complete dentures fixed on dental implants: Chewing patterns and implant stress. *Int J Oral Maxillofac Implants* 1989;2:107–111.

Spiekermann H: Implantatprothetik. in Voss R, Meiners H (eds): Fortschritte der Zahnärztlichen Prothetik und Werkstoffkunde. Band 3, Hanser, München, 1987.

Weber H: Technologie und Fortschritt in der zahnärztlichen Prothetik und Werkstoffkunde. *Deutsche Zahnärztliche Zeitschrift* 1989;44:572.

Weber H: Neue Technologien in der zahnärztlichen Prothetik. *Deutsche Zahnärztliche Zeitschrift* 1989; 44:817.

Weber H: Standortbestimmung der zahnärztlichen Prothetik. *Quintessenz* 1986;37:457.

Weber H, Schmelzle, R: Prothetische Rehabilitation von osteoplastisch rekonstruierten Defektpatienten mit Hilfe von implantatgetragenem Zahnersatz. *Z Zahnärztl Implantol* 1986; II: Sonderheft, 61.

Weber H, Schmelzle R, Schwenzer N: Optimierung von Rehabilitationsergebnissen bei kiefer- und gesichtschirurgisch versorgten Patienten durch implantologisch-prothetische Massnahmen. *Z Zahnärztl Implantol* 1988;IV:182.

Chapter 20

Dentistry in the 21st Century, with Emphasis on Operative Dentistry

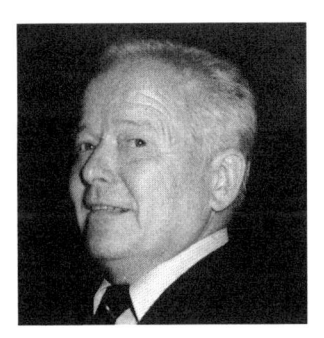

Ivar A. Mjör
Haslum, Norway

Abstract

Prognoses for the future are extrapolations based on experiences and recorded data from the past. They are hampered by the fact that new and unexpected changes cannot be included. A number of factors will affect the future of dentistry and dental health care, eg, the incidence, prevalence, and severity of dental diseases, the effect of preventive programs, advances in clinical techniques and materials, population development, attitudes towards dentistry, and the dental manpower situation.

Dentistry in industrialized countries faces a reduction in treatment needs. At present, the most marked effects are noted in the young population but gerodontology will be important in the future. Dentistry in developing countries must focus on the reduction of the need for dental treatment rather than on the "drill and fill" philosophy that has characterized operative dentistry in the main part of the 20th century.

Introduction

Being asked to look into the future is in some ways the same as seeking answers from a fortune-teller who looks into a crystal ball. Basing predictions on experience, data, and developments during the last decades add various dimensions to the predictions, and such extrapolations are indeed necessary in order to plan for the future. However, it is important to keep in mind that such prognoses are essentially educated guesses. Any unexpected or new situation cannot be included in the assessments. Thus, a major limitation in predictions is the fact that the future is unknown — a feature common to the fortune-teller and the scientist.

Dentistry in Scandinavia

About 50 years ago the concept of "drill and fill" replaced the "blood and vulcan-

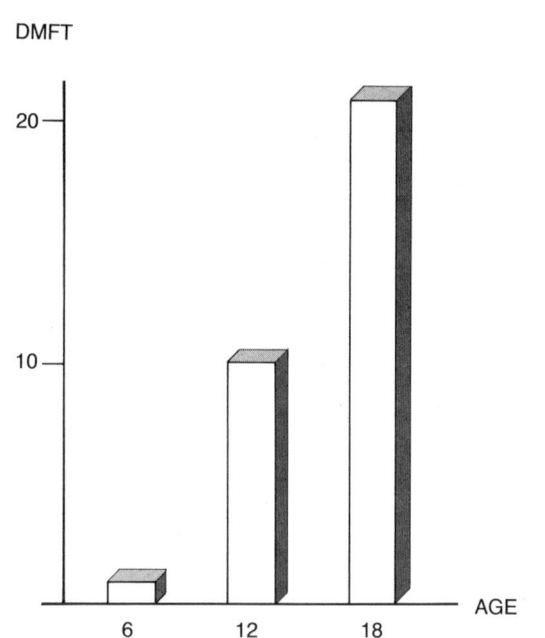

Fig 1 Bar graphs showing the DMFT values in permanent teeth at 6, 12, and 18 years of age in the 1950s and 1960s in a country with a high prevalence of dental caries (data from Norwegian Public Dental Health Service statistics).

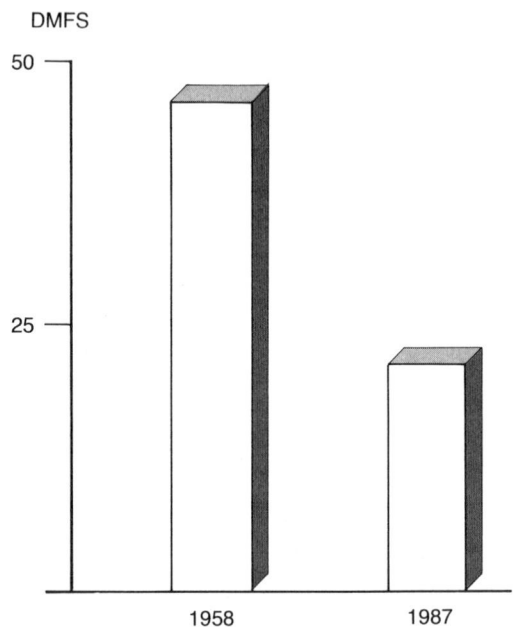

Fig 2 Bar graphs showing the DMFS values of 18- to 20-year-old Norwegian recruits in 1958 and in 1987.

ite" type of dentistry in the Scandinavian countries. Attempts were made to handle an overwhelming incidence of caries by removing the diseased tissue and inserting restorations. The situation in Norway was a typical example (Fig 1). Provided the workforce resources were present, the operative treatment resulted in a large number of restorations. For persons aged 18 to 20 years, the DMFS rate approached 50 on an average (Fig 2).

As time passed, it became apparent that dental caries could not be effectively defeated by inserting restorations, despite the fact that a seemingly effective school dental health delivery system was in operation providing free treatment to all primary schoolchildren. It turned out that re-placement and re-replacement of restorations became the major workload in operative dentistry (Table 1).[1–3] Despite the intensive restorative dental care in most industrialized countries, tooth failures occurred at a rate that led Lutz and coworkers[4] to describe the first restoration as the start of "the countdown" for the involved tooth. Dentistry was fighting a losing battle.

In the course of the last 30 years a reduction of more than 50% in caries has been recorded (Fig 2). This is impressive, and it is undoubtedly due to the general use of fluorides, especially those topically applied, including toothpaste, but also through the use of fluoride tablets. The well-developed school dental health system was particularly suitable for the systematic approach to such preventive programs.

The reduction in caries may be even more significant than the numbers indicate, because the restorations are generally smaller in size, which is not recorded by the DMF index. "Extension for prevention" is no longer a relevant principle, and it should be replaced by "maintenance for prevention." Thus, the deep-rooted principles of cavity preparation according to Black,[5] taught and emphasized in dental schools all over the world during the last 80 years, are not really applicable anymore. In fact, the reduced risk of caries and the possibilities for remineralization, combined with the properties of the modern restorative materials, call for an entirely different approach to operative dentistry. The changes that have occurred in the population's need for treatment have often not been followed up by modifications in the teaching programs, either in the undergraduate curriculum or in continuing dental education courses.

The altered caries situation in Scandinavia over a 30-year period as outlined above has had a marked effect on the workforce situation. About 25 years ago plans were made to open a third dental school in Norway. Finland opened two new dental schools during the last decade, and Iceland rebuilt its dental school and increased the number of students.

Table 1 Percentage distribution of restorations placed in an adult population (from Mjör[1])

Material	Primary caries	Replacements
Amalgam	29	71
Tooth-colored	21	79

Sweden had four dental schools and Denmark two. Half of these were opened during the last quarter of a century. It was estimated that on an average, one out of every 1,000 Scandinavians had to be a dentist if the population's dental needs were to be met.

Today (September 1989), one dental school in Sweden does not accept students for undergraduate training. Cutbacks in the intake of students have occurred in Finland and Norway, and despite a marked reduction at the two schools in Denmark, tough negotiations are presently going on to maintain both schools. The plans for a third dental school in Norway were abandoned. On the contrary, a slight reduction in admissions at the existing two schools stemmed the oversupply of dentists experienced in other countries, especially Denmark. Iceland has not experienced problems caused by an increase in the workforce, but the same caries reduction as in the other Scandinavian countries has not yet been noted.

Another change that affects the present and future of dentistry in Scandinavia and other industrialized countries is the gradual increase in the elderly population (Fig 3). An increasing number of these individuals have maintained their teeth,

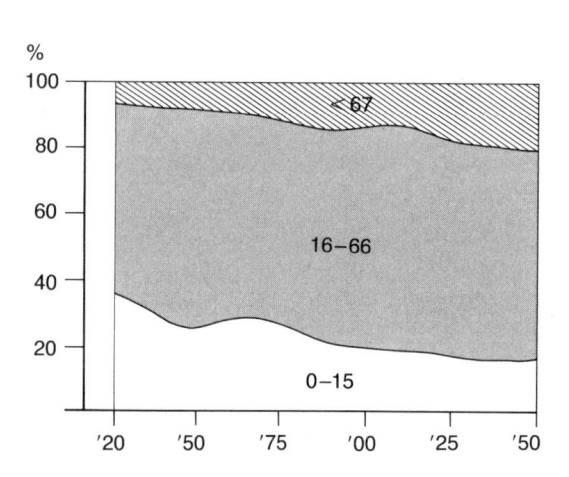

Fig 3 Graph showing the population development of the age groups 0 to 15, 16 to 66, and over 67 years old in Norway from 1920 to 2050 (data from Statistical Yearbook of Norway[10]).

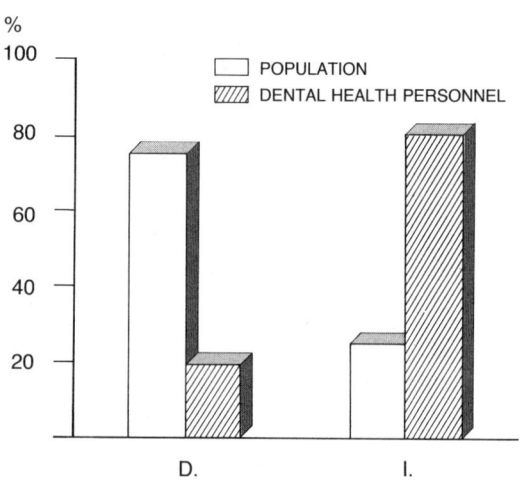

Fig 4 The percentage distribution of oral health personnel and of the population in developing (D) and industrialized (I) countries (data from WHO, 1987).

and they often present different and more complex challenges in conservative dentistry than adolescents. These people will require additional manpower, including different types of dental specialists, compared to previous decades. In general, they are "dentally" minded, maintain a good standard of living, and have the economic resources to preserve their dentition.

Global aspects

Extreme variations exist on a worldwide basis regarding the prevalence of dental diseases, the workforce situation, and treatment delivery systems. The skewed distribution of the dental manpower between industrialized and developing countries (Fig 4), where 80% of world oral health personnel care for 25% of the total population, is only one example of the distressing differences that prevail. Some industrialized countries have a history of dental disease prevalence and dental workforce resources similar to that in Scandinavia. In several developing countries, organized dentistry is unknown. All intermediate shades of dentistry are found on the global basis. Thus, the future of dentistry is not based on a well-defined entity; it will, therefore, be a conglomerate of extremes in disease patterns, dental awareness, and treatment delivery systems. Undoubtedly, dentistry in the 21st century will be as diverse as it is today on a worldwide basis. However, in a defined, limited geographical area, marked changes may occur.

The future

It is accepted that the development of primary caries may be reduced or prevented by lowering the intake of refined carbohydrates, optimizing oral hygiene, and utilizing fluoride supplements, the latter being by far the most important. Topical fluoride treatment also enhances remineralization of initial lesions and assists in the arrest of active caries. Although some disagreement exists as to the appropriate time for operative intervention in caries treatment, a tendency toward "treat to prevent" persists.[6] The decline in caries is expected to progress, although at a slower rate after the initially marked reduction has occurred. The World Health Organization goal of a DMFT rate of 3.0 in 12-year-old children by the year 2000 has already been reached in many areas. However, individuals are still found who do not benefit from the caries reduction at large. These risk groups must be targeted in the future. Preventive measures in addition to fluorides must also be sought to reduce caries, eg, chemical action on plaque and vaccines. In some parts of the world, caries is increasing. It appears as if dental caries is a price to be paid for economic development, at least temporarily.

A number of clinical surveys over the last 50 years has shown that the diagnosis of secondary (recurrent) caries is the main reason for replacement of restorations. However, meager evidence is available for a critical evaluation of secondary caries development, progression, prevention, and possible potentials for repair/remineralization. In fact, the clinical diagnosis of secondary caries is not a well-defined entity.[7] If the answer to at least some of these basic problems associated with secondary caries is solved in the future, operative dentistry in the 21st century will be different from what it is today.

The preventive measures as we know them today have focused on primary caries in children. The dentition of the adult and elderly population of the 1990s and for the first decades in the next century will have large numbers of restorations that need maintenance. The demand for conventional operative dentistry will, therefore, persist well into the next half of the 21st century, although the prevalence of secondary caries may decline.[8] Risk groups at all ages with a high caries rate will also exist. A gradual adjustment of the workforce needs is essential in order to adjust the number of professionals to the actual situation at any time, a task that is difficult because of the large number of variables.

Operative dentistry as it has been practiced in Scandinavia and in other industrialized countries has in some respects not lived up to its expectations, of "the countdown" theory by Lutz et al.[4] In fact, the history of operative dentistry has shown that caries cannot be permanently "treated away" by operative intervention. This observation is important for the countries where the caries rate is increasing and the need for restorative treatment is growing. The solution to these problems is not to be found in the operative approach to dental health care but through preventive programs, as demonstrated in Scandinavia during the last 50 years.

In the planning of dental treatment for populations with an increasing caries prevalence, it is important to learn from the mistakes made by others in the same situation. The answer is not to train more dentists but to put into effect preventive programs that lead to drastic improvements in the dental health. However, it is unlikely that this approach will be followed, for a variety of reasons; eg, the cost involved in preventive programs may be prohibitive, the gradual increase in personal incomes is unlikely to be spent on dental care, and the data valid for one part of the world may not be applicable or relevant for other parts. It can only be hoped that the "drill and fill" era will be shorter than that in Scandinavia and that effective dental preventive programs, based on relevant local data from dental research, will be developed. There is an urgent need for research data to assess the need for alternative, nonoperative treatments of dental caries. It is also feasible that a more permanent type of restorative dentistry will be developed than the one practiced up until today. Many factors will affect such a development. Two of these, the development of new materials and operative procedures, and assessments of the longevity of restorations, will be discussed below.

New materials and operative procedures

The increased awareness of the effect of the environment on health is affecting all parts of life, including dentistry. The biological reactions to dental materials, which are connected to material degradation and dissolution, have become an integral part of the assessment of the properties of dental materials. The search for inert materials in the absolute sense of the term or materials that have special beneficial properties has, therefore, become a main target for dental materials research. It will undoubtedly continue into the next century.

Among the materials that today are considered new candidates for routine use in conservative dentistry are ceramic materials, hydroxylapatite, and titanium, pure or alloyed. Their main advantage is that they are relatively inert and therefore biocompatible. The material cost is low; however, they have a decided disadvantage as far as cost is concerned in that they are based on indirect restorative techniques, ie, they have to be produced either by casting techniques or by computer technology such as CAD-CAM (computer-aided design – computer-aided manufacture).

The need for materials that are plastic for a suitable insertion time and set in situ will exist as long as restorations are needed. Today amalgam, composite resin materials, and glass ionomer cements are available for immediate restoration. It is doubtful whether amalgam will continue as the routine material into the next century, primarily because it is not esthetically satisfactory. Mercury used in dental practice also represents a potential risk for pollution of the environment. Furthermore, the mercury scare in the population may restrict its use. Composite resin materials have improved greatly during the last decade, but further improvements will be marginal because of inherent problems in their polymerization. They also contain a number of chemical reactants that may not be considered biologically acceptable. In addition, adhesion of resin-based materials to dentin remains a problem. Their use may therefore decrease rather than increase in the future. The main competitor to resin-based materials for esthetic restorations is expected to be a glass-ionomer type of material. These materials chemically bond to mineralized dental tissues and release fluoride. They are presently undergoing improvements, and they have come a long way during the 15 years they have been on the market. Their suitability for the treatment of root caries in gerodontology makes them essential for conservative dentistry in this growing part of the population.

Longevity of restorations

The long-term cost of operative dentistry is dependent on the initial cost and the longevity of the restorations. Today, restorative work with materials that are inserted in a plastic form is cheaper than those manufactured in a dental laboratory or by some CAD-CAM technique, primarily because of the time and specialized equipment involved. Glass ionomer cements are less expensive than amalgam and much less than composite resin materials. The cost of the materials used for indirect restoration also varies markedly, ie, gold alloys are more than 300 times more expensive than pure titanium per unit volume. However, the labor costs are more important than the material cost in most countries.

Once inserted, the relative price of a restoration is dependent on how long it lasts. Three quarters of the operative procedures performed for an adult population in an area with high caries prevalence and extensive restorative work may involve replacement of restorations (Table 1). Considerable information is available on the longevity of amalgam and composite resin restorations that fail, but only scanty information is available on restorations that do not need replacement. Many factors affect longevity of restorations: retention, the age of the patient, the size of the restoration, the tooth in question, the material, and the clinician's criteria for failure of a restoration. Operative dentistry has not been assessed accurately as far as cost/benefit is concerned, except for pit and fissure sealants as a preventive type of treatment, and for some other special types of treatment. Generally, sealing is not cost effective because it is impossible to predict which teeth will become carious.

The cost concern for dental treatment by the patients, health authorities, and insurance companies is expected to focus on the longevity of restorations in the future. It can be envisaged that private insurance companies especially, which play an increasing role in the financing of dental treatment in industrialized countries, will require a minimum longevity as guarantee for reimbursement of treatment costs in the future. The same applies to community dental health programs.

Concluding remarks

At present, about 75% of the world's population receive minimal dental treatment by only about 20% of the total dental health personnel available worldwide (Fig 4). The dental disease prevalence is increasing in these parts. The remainder of the world's population shows a decreasing need for restorative treatment, and they have 80% of the dental workforce at their disposal. This distorted distribution calls for an immediate change to prevent overtreatment[9] in industrial countries and to cover the the dental treatment needs in developing countries.

Assessments of the optimal training of the dental health personnel in the different parts of the world are urgently needed. However, changes in educational patterns, the design and establishment of appropriate training facilities for dental health personnel, the intake of students, and, most importantly, changes of the attitudes of practitioners are slow in any country. With a 5-year dental curriculum, as in many industrialized countries, decisions made today will have a minimum of 5 years to take effect. A longer planning period is needed in countries where training facilities must be built and where the economic priorities are tough.

A realistic assessment of dental treatment need and demand is essential for dental services to provide optimal oral health in the future. The number of variables in dental health care delivery systems are many, including altered disease patterns, new prophylactic achievements and alternative treatments, improved materials and techniques in operative dentistry, and the aging population. All these challenges call for ingenuity, inventiveness, and careful planning as guidelines for operative dentistry in the 21st century.

References

1. Mjör IA: Placement and replacement of restorations. *Oper Dent* 1981;6:49–54.
2. Qvist V, Thylstrup A, Mjör IA: Restorative treatment pattern and longevity of amalgam restorations in Denmark. *Acta Odontol Scand* 1986;44:343–349.
3. Qvist V, Thylstrup A, Mjör IA: Restorative treatment pattern and longevity of resin restorations in Denmark. *Acta Odontol Scand* 1986;44:351–356.
4. Lutz F, Krejci I, Mörmann W: Die Zahnfarbene Seitzahn-Restauration. *Phillip J Res;* 1987;127–137.
5. Black GV: *A Work on Operative Dentistry*, vol. 2. Chicago, Medico-Dental Publishing Co, 1908.
6. Thylstrup A, Qvist V: Is health promotion the main issue of preventive dentistry?, in Guggenheim B: *Cariology Today.* Basel, Karger, International Congress, Zürich 1983, pp 317–326.
7. Merrett MC, Elderton RJ: An in vitro study of restorative dental treatment decisions and secondary caries. *Br Dent J* 1984;157:128–133.
8. Hugoson A, Koch G, Bergendal T et al: Oral health of individuals aged 3–80 in Jönköping, Sweden in 1973 and 1983. *Swed Dent J* 1986;10:175–194.
9. Boyd MA, Richardson A: Frequency of amalgam replacement in general dental practice. *J Can Dent Assoc* 1985;10:763–766.
10. Statistical Yearbook of Norway, 107th issue. Oslo-Kongsvinger, Statistisk Sentralbyrå, 1988, p 48.

Chapter 21

The State of Dentistry in Italy

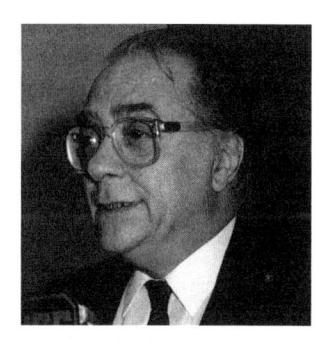

Mario Martignoni
Rome, Italy

Abstract

The author explains the state of Italian Odontology from an academic point of view. He also explains why Italy has chosen to create Schools of Odontology within the Faculty of Medicine and with the same programs as those of the European Common Market.

As for the predictable development of Italian odontology, the author thinks that it will have two directions: prevention and restoration. Both will be able to avail themselves of the use of computers according to the concept that prevention is the best therapy.

Particular attention is given to the future development of computerized robots and of electronic systems of analysis.

The author shows the results of an outstanding study, which, through magnetic nuclear resonance, gives the possibility of making a diagnosis and, at the same time, individualizes the anatomical biomechanical parameters used to analyze and correct occlusal function.

In 1912, a degree in medicine and surgery was required by law in order to practice dentistry. Later, the Specializing Schools in Odontology and Dental Prosthesis were instituted. According to the institutive law of 1912, odontology was considered "that section of general medicine that was particularly concerned with the health of the mouth." Therefore, odontology was acknowledged as a medical specialty along with otorhinolaryngology, radiology, ophthalmology, and clinical medicine. Regular university courses in odontology were offered by faculties of medicine and surgery. This meant that in order to practice odontology, a sole degree in medicine and surgery was adequate. Of course it was also necessary to pass the National Board in Medicine and Surgery. Individuals who wanted to expand their knowledge of odontology could enter a Specializing School of Odontology. At first, these schools had 2-year terms and at the end of the 2 years the title Specialist in Odontology was conferred.

Therefore, in Italy there were two possibilities of practicing dentistry: *(1)* as a physician practicing odontology, and *(2)* as a physician specialized in dentistry.

The first real change in this system was made 15 years ago when the organizations of public assistance required specialization in odontology in conjunction with the degree in medicine in order for an individual to practice dentistry. Almost contemporaneously, in order to conform with the European Common Market rules, the length of the university courses in specialization were extended to 3 years.

Finally, in 1980 a special law required that within a faculty of medicine the course of odontology and dental prosthesis be taught. The same program was adopted by all countries belonging to the European Common Market. Enrollment to these courses was restricted, and an entrance examination was required. Until this law was effected, no university faculty had ever had a limited number of students but, on the contrary, all students asking to enter had been accepted with the only requirement a high school degree.

Therefore, since 1980, the university faculties of medicine have had two programs: one in medicine and surgery, with a term of 6 years, in which individuals can enter simply by applying, and one in odontology and dental prosthesis, which requires an entrance examination and at the end of 5 years confers a degree in odontology.

The same law instituting the degree in odontology has established that in order to practice odontology in Italy one must be graduated in odontology. Therefore, those having a degree in medicine but no specialization could no longer practice odontology. Hence, in Italy there exist two professional figures: the "odontoiatra" (dentist) who is graduated in odontology and dental prosthesis, and the physician, graduated in medicine and specialized in dentistry. Again, both degrees are conferred by a faculty of medicine and surgery with the difference being the degree in odontology has a term of 5 years, whereas the degree in medicine has a term of 6 years to which an additional 3 years of specialization must be added.

At present in Italy there are 30 state universities, and every faculty of medicine has a course in odontology with a limited number of students (Table 1). These universities produced, up until 1984, 4,460 dentists.

At the present time all Italian universities can supply 932 new graduates in odontology and dental prosthesis every year. There are no specializing schools for the "odontoiatri" (having just the degree in odontology). On the contrary, there still exist 24 specializing schools in odontology for physicians (a course of 3 years) and they produce a total of 650 specialists per year. There are also six schools of specialization in orthodontics for physicians that produce 45 specialists every year in the following universities: Torino, Padova, Milano, Napoli (two schools), and Cagliari. Five schools of maxillofacial surgery also exist in these universities: Milano, Parma, Verona, and Napoli (two schools), with a total of 26 specialists every year.

Up until March of 1989, odontologists (graduated in odontology) and physicians specialized in dentistry could both practice odontology. During March and April of 1989, however, the Italian Constitutional Court (supreme legislative body) established that prohibiting graduates of medicine and surgery from practicing odontology was against the Constitution of the Italian Republic. Consequently, graduates in medicine could belong at the same time both to the category of doctors in medicine and to the category of odontologists. This decision has effectively returned Italy back to the year 1984 and has provoked strong reactions and controversies, especially within universities. This burning problem has been drawn to the attention of the European Parliament, from whom Italy awaits a definitive solution.

As far as odontology education in Italy is concerned, it is developing, and together with the economy of most industrialized countries, it must maintain the traditional values of a humanistic culture, which is characteristic of the Italian development. We must view the solution Italy has started to devise to the problem of adapting odontology education to the European Common Market within this perspective. As a matter of fact, Italy chose to institute schools in odontology with the faculty of medicine as a natural emanation of the traditional cultural values.

This solution is positive because it provides our dental students with the same biological knowledge as medical students, but it also generates unavoidable friction with some of the most traditional conservative values and with the privileges that they originate.

A similar situation occurred in the 1950s and 1960s. Contact with other European countries, particularly with the United States, became more frequent, and a group of young dentists (all physicians) improved their education in the United States, where they assimilated a different way of learning and more advanced technologies. They then brought

Table 1 Degree in odontology and dental prosthesis

Faculty of medicine	Number of students per year	Length of the course
Roma I (La Sapienza)	120	5 years
Roma II (Tor Vergata)	30	5 years
Roma (Catholic Univ.)	15	5 years
Milano	100	5 years
Napoli II	50	5 years
Napoli I	24	5 years
Padova	48	5 years
Torino	40	5 years
Palermo	40	5 years
Siena	40	5 years
Messina	32	5 years
Firenze	30	5 years
Bari	30	5 years
Bologna	30	5 years
Modena	27	5 years
Perugia	25	5 years
L'Aquila	25	5 years
Ancona	20	5 years
Chieti	20	5 years
Catania	20	5 years
Cagliari	20	5 years
Pavia	20	5 years
Brescia	20	5 years
Verona	20	5 years
Genova	20	5 years
Parma	20	5 years
Trieste	16	5 years
Ferrara	12	5 years
Sassari	10	5 years
Pisa	5	5 years

what they had learned to Italy, both on a university level and especially on a professional level. These cultural associations have strongly contributed to the diffusion of knowledge, technology, and different ways of facing odontology problems.

The number of young Italian dentists studying abroad (especially in the United States) has grown. In general, Italy has been experiencing, for the past several years, a real cultural and technological invasion from North American dentistry. This has generated what I would call the "Italian phenomenon," which consists of the creation of a new odontology class that joins the reliable traditional biological study and the new vanguard technologies, creating a strong professional group of the highest level.

This evolving phenomenon has in part taken place within traditional university institutions and in greater part in the professional field. It was led by professional associations whose development has been powerful and often uncontrolled. An excessive prudence and stasis of the institutions slowed down this evolution up to 1980, when after a long toil the modern schools in odontology were founded within the faculty of medicine.

What will the future hold?

It is always difficult to make predictions, but we can reasonably suppose that Italy, without betraying its cultural traditions, will range more and more with European nations overcoming rights and privileges that should no longer exist. That's what the help of the other members of the European Common Market will be determining.

As for public assistance and the social aspects of odontology, it is worthwhile to say that Italy is now completely revising the system, after it has proved to be a total failure. The change in the system is probably heading for an integration of public and private assistance. It is easy to foresee that greater attention will be paid to prevention in all sectors of odontology from public assistance and a growing use of private insurance assistance for diseases, affected not only by individuals but also by large firms and professional associations, so that it is possible to ensure a controllable standard in the quality of odontology assistance.

Odontologic research will follow two fundamental directions: prevention and restoration. Data compiled by the World Health Organization and found in the epidemiologic studies directed by Milano University (Vogel group) on two odontology diseases — caries and periodontal disease — are enough to show that prevention and hygiene education are nowadays the best therapies.

These longitudinal studies have also indicated the decline of surgical resective therapies, with the purpose of biological restoration of the loss of periodontal support due to disease. Therefore, we can forecast the use of simpler and less invasive means (for example, resorbable membranes) in order to obtain regeneration of the periodontal support and the alveolar bone. As for replacing teeth, research has already oriented toward materials that are biocompatible. This means orienting research and clinical practice in favor of restoration rather than reconstruction, using materials and techniques able to incorporate the new part into biological tissues. The restoration should be not only tolerated or even only accepted, but biologically integrated with vital tissues. Only in this way will we achieve a true restoration of the original.

This concept has been developed in prosthodontics by Martignoni's group and can be extended to all dental specialties. The application of the restoration concept has as its purpose the anatomical restoration of the marginal precision, anatomical contour, and biologically accepted texture characteristics, which together achieve the best biological fit.

Consequently, if the restoration is incorporated in the dentoperiodontal anatomy, it gives us the possibility to eliminate the possible iatrogenic damages that are almost unavoidable in most of our reconstructive cases so that they require an expansive program of maintenance. By the term maintenance I mean the hygienic measure directed to maintain the achieved result.

Regrettably, too often the maintenance program is only a therapy of the iatrogenic damage caused by imprecision, overcontour, and lack of surface texture at the moment of permanent cementation of the reconstruction. All these considerations bring us to the necessity to define or redefine the quality standard of prosthodontic therapy. Such standards should be the same in all the countries, and from this point of view it could be useful to range the quality of the dental practice as a guarantee of the health of every citizen and avoid overtreatment. It would be necessary to bring up to date such quality standards once they have been established, following the results of international research. The expected and already partially carried out use of computerized robots in restorative treatment, both to "read" the preparations and to achieve the master model without taking any kind of impression, will have much value to reach mechanical perfection and therefore a more complete elimination of iatrogenic factors of disease. We can also expect the complete elimination of the metal alloy casting procedure and its substitution with different methods in order to eliminate the volumetric variations.

Another field of certain development will be, without any doubt, maxillofacial surgery, especially considered as bioengineering corrective surgery, not only in the treatment of malformations but also for esthetic and functional restorations. We must look for a biomechanic permanent solution in this field, and with the principles already expressed, of the replacement of lost teeth using dental implants with the purpose of getting the formation of a relation between implant and biological tissue comparable to the natural dentoperiodontal relation.

Great contributions to maxillofacial surgery have been made in Italy by universities and by different specialized hospitals such as Verona, Roma, Milano, Torino, Napoli, Vicenza, and Parma.

Another field in which we are waiting for a development is that concerning the dysfunctional pathology of the stomatognathic system. Modern electronic systems and the use of magnetic nuclear resonance imaging have already made it possible to understand the neuromuscular mechanisms and most of the pathology of the system.

Particularly, I am firmly convinced that it is possible to develop, using magnetic resonance imaging, a complete analysis of the function of the stomatognathic system with the individualization of the personal anatomic parameters such as centric position, intercondylar distance, Bennett angle, Bennett side shift, protrusive pattern, overjet, and overbite, and also the possibility to establish the length of the maxillary anterior teeth.

We will also be able to transfer to our articulators those computerized data, and with this program, to analyze and to work out occlusal therapies with a predictable result. On this subject Roma University II (Tor Vergata) has been conducting a study for several years, with very encouraging results.

In conclusion, the predictable development of odontology in Italy will be oriented toward prevention and restoration, with the use of technologies more and more assisted by precision computerized instruments, so that it will be possible to obtain very high levels of precision and biomechanical results of full functional integration.

Chapter 22

The State of Dentistry in Poland and Predictions for the Future

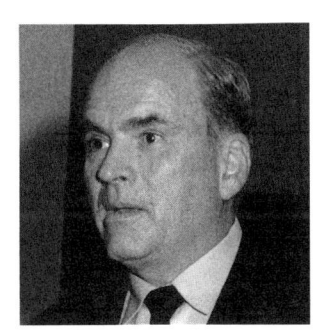

Wlodzimierz Józefowicz
Nawotki, Poland

Abstract

In Poland there are 18,000 dentists for 37 million people. More than 85% of Polish dentists are women. There are three sectors of health service: governmental, cooperative, and private. The governmental sector covers the whole country and provides free oral health service. The position of dental private and cooperative dental practices in the last few years has gradually increased, being the obvious result of political changes and insufficient government programs.

It may be predicted that in the future the reduction of dental caries will lead dentistry to oral medicine. Fewer dentists, better educated in medicine, will be needed. The actual barriers between dentistry and medicine will gradually be eliminated.

Poland is situated in the geographic center of Europe, with a population of about 37 million. Since the end of World War II, the country has been governed in a socialist way, which of course has greatly influenced the provision of health care, including oral health care. The present status of dentistry in Poland may reflect some of the advantages and disadvantages of the system as a whole.

Presently in Poland there are no adequate epidemiological data to illustrate the oral health status of the whole population. The published information usually concerns specific age groups, which are not sufficiently representative. In 1987 the National Oral Health Pathfinder Survey was conducted in Poland in close collaboration with the regional office of the World Health Organization for Europe in Copenhagen.[1] The objective of the survey was to establish a national epidemiological baseline for monitoring and evaluating oral disease trends, treatment needs, and workforce requirements. This survey was compared with the results from surveys conducted in other countries. The results of our survey were similar to those obtained in Yugoslavia and Hungary and better than those found in Greece, Malta, Morocco, Portugal, and Spain. The study also showed a great need for dental caries treatment and a need for tooth extraction in 7-year-old children that indicated the failure of preventive efforts.

Currently in Poland we are carrying out the International Collaborative Study of Oral Health Outcomes (ICS II). Participation in this study, organized by the World Health Organization, will bring us further knowledge about oral health care and will enable us to compare the results with those obtained from the previous study (ICS I)[2] and with the data from other countries.

In Poland there are three sectors of health service: governmental, cooperative, and private. In this respect the organization of health service differs from that in other socialist countries, where only a governmental sector operates.

The governmental sector covers the whole country and provides oral health services free of charge. Cooperative and private health services supplement the governmental health service. During the Stalinist years there were strong tendencies toward eliminating private practice and reducing cooperative practice, but such severe measures did not meet practical needs.

Dentists' earnings in private practice and in the cooperative sector are higher than the salaries in a governmental clinic, so they are obligated to work 35 hours weekly in governmental service; only then may they take work in one of the remaining two sectors. This obligation does not apply to retired dentists.

The governmental sector of dental care is organized in schools, in the workplace, and in the towns and villages. Cooperative dental services are usually organized in towns, and private practices are usually arranged at dentists' apartments. The position of private and cooperative dental practices in Poland in the last few years has gradually improved, which is an obvious result of political changes and the inadequacy of the governmental sector. This has had a great influence on the number and qualifications of candidates for dental education. When private practice was not so popular, the number of candidates for dental education was lower than for the medical education. Now, the opposite is observed.

Dental education in Poland comprises 17 years of study: 12 years in primary and secondary schools and 5 years in dental schools. Polish dentists can graduate from one of 10 dental schools. The schools are not independent but are subfaculties of faculties of medicine, with heads of these subfaculties being vice-deans of the medical faculties. The program of dental studies is more medically than technically oriented. For example, students are trained far less in laboratory prosthodontics than in clinical procedures; all fixed and removable dentures are fabricated by dental technicians.

Dentists in Poland may take up specialization in the following branches: oral surgery, maxillofacial surgery, periodontology, orthodontics, pediatric dentistry, prosthodontics, and conservative dentistry, as well as epidemiology, organization of health service, and social medicine.

The basic requirements for specialization in dentistry are equal to those in medicine.

Polish dentists can obtain a doctoral degree in medical sciences and may attain higher scientific positions in the same way as physicians. The close relationship between dentistry and medicine in Poland has gradually increased the prestige of dentists in Polish society. Some dentists have been chosen for such positions as rectors and prorectors of medical academies and deans of medical faculties.

A few years ago, dentists were assigned to the "first" group of employment, that is, the group whose working conditions make them eligible for retirement at the ages of 55 (women) and 60 (men). This privilege has led to a reduction in the number of practicing dentists. To compensate for this reduction, the number of students admitted to the subfaculties of stomatology has been increased, and the results of this action will be seen in the future years.

In Poland there are nearly 18,000 qualified dentists, more than 85% of whom are women. The reason that so many dentists are women is that in Poland most women must work, for financial reasons, and many want to work, for psychological and social reasons. They see dentistry as a suitable profession for women. (A similar situation is observed in medicine.) In an attempt to get more men into the profession, a requirement was made several years ago that medical school admissions be 50% men and 50% women, but this has since been rescinded because it violated the constitution. Also, men have a wider number of professions to choose from especially among technical professions; therefore, the number and quality of male candidates in dentistry and medicine is lower than that of female candidates. There are some disadvantages to the prevalence of women in the profession. Women retire earlier; they also take time off for giving birth to and raising children, and they are more concerned about home management. However, it is unwise to try to stem this natural predominance of women in dentistry through regulations.

The ratio of practicing dentists to the population is 1:2,300 and compared to other countries is rather high. In the public's opinion, the main cause of the inadequacy of the oral health service in Poland is the lack of dentists. This opinion is often supported by some administrators for whom increasing the number of dentists seems to be easier than making deeper changes in the system. The Polish Dental Association, however, has tried to show that dentists in public health service do not work effectively and that this is due to problems within the system such as improper provision of dental products, an insufficient number of auxiliary personnel, and a lack of correlation between the quality and effectiveness of work and income of dental personnel.

The provision of dental products is more than unsatisfactory. Planning and distribution, which requires a dentist to predict in detail what he or she will need in one or a few years (down to the kind, shape, size, and number of burs), cannot replace the normal free market in meeting the profession's needs for dental products. Similar situations may be observed in other socialist countries as well.

An insufficient number of dental auxiliary personnel is strictly related to their salaries. Dental technicians have some chance to earn a good salary in private practice, so their number is quite high. Conversely, the poorly paid dental hygienists and dental assistants often leave their positions for work in factories or other places that provide better incomes. At one time there were about 5,000 dental hygienists in Poland, but only about 1,000 of them have remained in the health service.

The bureaucratic management of the governmental health service does not allow for salary differentiation based on the quality and quantity of work done. Further, patient satisfaction or dissatisfaction has no influence on remuneration. In such a situation the dentist becomes dissatisfied, having a heavy and difficult workload, and so the patient may feel that he or she is unwanted in the dental surgery. An additional and important concern for the patient is that he or she cannot choose a dentist.

In Poland there is only one association that assembles dentists, the Polish Dental Association *(Polskie Towarzystwo Stomatologiczne* or PTS). The association has nearly 10,000 members. It comprises 24 local branches in the larger towns in Poland and 8 sections: maxillofacial surgery, periodontology, pediatric dentistry, conservative dentistry, orthodontics, prosthodontics, occupational dentistry, and radiology.

PTS collaborates with the Fédération Dentaire Internationale and with the World Health Organization. Particular sections of PTS work closely with other foreign and international societies of dental specialties. Poland has hosted some European and world dental conferences. PTS collaborates with the Polish Medical Association and with other societies for medical specialists. In 1990 the Medical Chamber will begin its work. An independent, self-governed, professional organization of Polish physicians and dentists, the Medical Chamber will be the continuation of a similar organization that existed in Poland before Stalinist times. The Medical Chamber will be responsible for the supervision of professional activities of physicians and dentists and will establish rules of ethics and dontology.

As can be seen from this discussion, dentistry is deeply dependent on the political, economic, and social situations of the given country. Some trends observed in Eastern Europe and on other continents may indicate elimination of totalitarianism as the way of governing, so most of the countries will be in a political situation that will enable the natural development of the dental profession.

It may be supposed that existing models of oral health services will undergo further changes. The first question is: How large a role will the governmental sector of the oral health service play after these modifications take place? In my opinion, prophylaxis is a crucial concern that should be addressed by the governmental services. However, dental and oral prophylaxis cannot be separated from the whole problem of preventive medicine. For example, the problem of water fluoridation cannot be treated without detailed analysis of possible methods of supply (air, water, food) in a given area. Physical exercises at schools may be another example. A large number of temporomandibular joint dysfunctions may indicate the need to include the training of masticatory muscles in our current physical education programs.

It may be supposed that dental practice will be organized into group practices, because the governmental service is expensive and ineffective and single private practitioners cannot handle their workloads. Dental health systems in other countries will be observed with regard to methods of payment for services and the proportions covered by government, insurance, and the patient.

Dentistry's evolution as an independent branch of medicine is a direct result of the treatment of dental caries. Most dentists spend a large portion of their time restoring teeth affected by disease. The restorative work had to be scientifically precise, but it also necessitated manual skill. From the practical point of view it was easier and cheaper to educate dentists separately from physicians, even though it was strange to divide the oral cavity from the whole human organism.

In the future, the basis for this division — ie, the need to train dental students to restore caries-affected tooth structure — will not exist. Theory and practice show that dental caries, like some other diseases, may be reduced or even eliminated. If this occurs, other oral health problems (oral diseases, neoplasms, anomalies, and traumas) will require treatment such as that being done by laryngologists and other medical specialists, and in this case dentists will require training similar to that received by physicians. A physician-specialist in oral medicine, for example, may specialize after 3 or 4 years of obligatory basic medical studies.

The barriers between dentistry and other areas of medicine should be removed as soon as possible. Of course, the change in the character of dentistry will mean fewer dentists will be required. This phenomenon has already begun in industrialized countries and will gradually spread throughout world.

Questions about the future role of auxiliary personnel remain, but obviously a medically oriented dental specialist will need continued support in procedures that are relatively easy but very time-consuming. Larger roles are foreseen for the dental hygienists rather than dental technicians.

The development of medicine, including dentistry, depends on progress in such sciences as chemistry, physics, biology, and psychology. It is highly probable that in the next few decades such progress will take place and will inspire further achievements in the medical field. I shall discuss only a few problems of this matter.

In the future, vaccinations may find application in dentistry, but I believe these will be used primarily in prophylaxis of the mucous membrane and periodontal diseases rather than dental caries. This does not mean that this method of prophylaxis might not be used on patients with a high dental caries risk factor. Dental phobia will be almost eradicated because of new developments in psychological, physical, and pharmacological methods of pain elimination. Many if not most surgical procedures will be performed with the use of the microscope, which will raise surgical precision to the levels currently enjoyed in the fields of ophthalmology and odontology.

Concurrent with the further development of implants will be reduced indications for the extraction of teeth. Each case of tooth extraction will be considered and documented in detail. Extraction due to an obvious lack of care by the patient may influence the cost of prosthetic rehabilitation. Similarly, a dentist will be held responsible for rushing to extract a tooth without trying conservative or surgical methods of treatment and adequate rehabilitation. New methods of surgically eliminating periapical abscesses and other pathological changes in this region, along with new pharmacological and biological treatments, will allow retention of those teeth that under current treatment limitations might only be extracted.

It is also probable that as civilization progresses some oral diseases will become more common and new diseases and abnormalities will be seen as a result of pollution and other changes in the environment. These might include allergies, neoplasms, mycosis, and as-yet-unknown viral diseases. In the future, dentists will have to be trained in the diagnosis and treatment of diseases affecting the mucous membrane, the soft tissues, and the bone rather than the teeth.

Summary

Poland actively takes part in the International Collaborative Studies and has carried out the National Oral Health Pathfinder Survey in partnership with WHO. The results showed that the state of oral health in Poland is worse than in the highly industrialized countries.

In Poland there are 18,000 dentists for 37 million people. More than 85% of Polish dentists are women. There are three sectors of health service: governmental, cooperative, and private. The governmental sector covers the whole country and provides free of charge oral health service. The position of dental private and cooperative practice in the last few years has gradually increased as a result of political changes and the inefficiency of the governmental sector. The public health service does not work effectively because of inadequate supplies of dental products, an insufficient number of auxiliary personnel, and the lack of correlation between the quality and effectiveness of work and the incomes of dental personnel.

It may be predicted that in the future the decreased incidence of dental caries will cause dentistry to evolve into oral medicine. Fewer dentists will be required but they will need a broader medical education. The actual barriers between dentistry and medicine will gradually be eliminated.

The governmental sector of the health service will be mainly responsible for the complex prophylaxis of all diseases, and group practices will predominate over clinics and private practices.

Scientific developments in dentistry may include vaccinations, elimination of dental phobia, the use of microsurgery, and a considerable reduction of the number of tooth extractions.

References

1. Möller IJ: *Oral Health in Poland,* POL/ORH 001. Copenhagen, World Health Organization, 1988, pp 3–5.

2. Arnljot HA, Barmes DE, Cohen LK, et al: *Oral Health Care Systems. An International Collaborative Study Coordinated by the World Health Organization.* London, Quintessence Publ Co, 1985, pp 125–126.

Chapter 23

Dentistry in the 21st Century: Germany

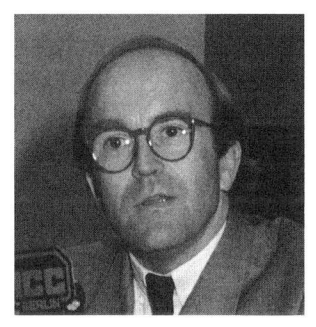

Frank Braun
Düsseldorf,
Federal Republic
of Germany

Abstract

All important political and economic events of the past and the present find expression in all spheres of life. These events leave their marks on the development of our profession as well. Therefore, I would like to cast a brief glance backward to establish a historical framework on which we can base our projections for the future.

I am convinced that history takes a course determined by humanity: it does not follow its innermost laws, as the philosophers of the Enlightenment and even Hegel and Marx assumed; it is not fate but our work that determines our future. We cannot with utmost certainty predict whether we will face good or bad times, but we should contribute our share to the best of our ability to ensure the good.

Are we — the privileged dentists enjoying practice in the free part of this world — not inclined to look at the world merely from our limited "dental horizon?"

The devastation caused by World War I exceeded even the most disastrous predictions of the greatest pessimists. Europe lost its world supremacy, and Germany suffered the greatest setback in her historical development with regard to her national, cultural, and traditional values. Also, in the field of medicine and dentistry she lost her former leading role permanently.

The most disastrous of all wars was followed by an equally disastrous treaty of peace that inherently bore the basis for the next world war. The year 1929 was the year marking the beginning of history's worst economic crisis, one to affect the entire world. This crisis had its roots in the United States, the nation that was to become the leading economic power of the future. The United States has remained that power ever since and will continue to do so in the next century, exerting an increasing influence on our profession, too.

As a consequence of World War II the two superpowers — the USSR and the United States — developed; later these two countries became adversaries and fought a "cold war." In the course of this development we witnessed the foundation of the two German states, the North Atlantic Treaty Organization, the Warsaw Pact, and the decolonization of Africa and Asia.

The two defeated nations of 1945, Japan and Germany, recovered their strength much faster and showed far more productivity than they would ever have been able to do during their former "glory."

This factor was also to determine the outstanding economic development of both countries during the postwar era in the field of dentistry, where Japanese and German dentists were to hold top positions both with regard to the international comparison of their income and that of other free professions. The overcompensation of particular professions will remain the consequence of a free enterprise economy, as its regulative forces always produce corrections: in both cases mentioned, incomes have long since peaked and their high levels will not be reached again.

A glance at the further developments in 20th century history reveals astounding scientific accomplishments: the development of nuclear technology for military and various peaceful purposes; the discovery of genetic technology with its promising and weighty possibilities; the computer — the "electronic brain," as it was originally called — which will mimic and surpass the human brain in the next century; the beginning of electronic data processing, a new science and experience in human life; and finally space technology.

In political developments we have witnessed the revival of religious wars, involving especially a militant Islam centered in Iran, the former classical empire and once the most reliable ally of the United States. The withdrawal of the United States from Iran was one of the gravest political mistakes in American world strategy. A further setback was the belief that the European Enlightenment could be transferred as the dominant cultural concept to continents colonized by the European states and later dominated by the United States. In most cases only a comparatively small portion of the upper class could be reached, and today many of these individuals have been exiled or executed.

This phase of regression affected the entire medical field with negative consequences for decades.

Global developments in the 21st century

Realizing past developments we must keep options open for future generations and avoid accumulating additional burdens.

The next century might perhaps prevent less than the last, for the issue will no longer be the creation of an infrastructure, the rehabilitation after two world wars. The key to the future will be consolidation and dissemination of what has been achieved. We are facing a development toward a more homogeneous world.

Freedom and democracy will set free an epidemic effect, and communism, dictatorships, and oppressive military governments will belong to the past. It is impossible to erect barriers against the ideas of freedom and human rights in the age of worldwide communication and satellite television. In the next century there will be a free European society, based on common peace negotiations, that will include all East European countries and enable Germans to establish their national unity in free self-determination together with their neighbors in East and West. Freedom and the rights of humankind will prevail; borders will lose their importance.

Along with the elimination of the causes for tension between East and West, armaments will lose their dominant role within Europe. Ecological social orders have become self-evident; the protection of the environment will be considered part of the human rights. Europe will finally have a functioning government elected by the European Parliament. It will have a common currency and pursue a common world policy.

Present world powers will be brought vigorously into balance with the rest of the world community. Besides the USSR and the United States, China and India will emerge, as well as a Pacific economic union with Japan as its nucleus. Europe will become an independent power with global responsibility based on its economic and cultural tradition.

An international, socially oriented economy will change the world toward more direct responsibility and prosperity for all its peoples. Armed conflicts will more and more be solved by diplomatic means and determined solely by the world powers.

Technical progress and environmental protection will no longer be conflicting issues. The impact of industry as a dominant force in society will have lessened considerably. The needs and conditions of industrial production will no longer determine the life of humans; on the contrary, production will be determined by the necessities of the life of humans.

Just as the protection of the environment will dominate in the next decades, the ethics of consumption will be the prevailing issue in the years that follow. The field of recreational activities — the purchase of goods and services connected with tourism, hobbies, sports, education, culture, media, and entertainment — will become one of the largest economic factors in the world.

The desire for so-called individuality will increasingly be realized via consumption. Leisure-time consumption, especially care and health of the body, will almost assume the character of an "ersatz religion." Our current work-oriented society, in which one works to live, will lose its fascination and be replaced by a society that celebrates life.

Also in the next century economic, social, and cultural aspects will largely depend on the quality of our educational system. In view of the dynamics of progress the curricula will continuously have to be adapted to scientific and technical progress, with ethical considerations taking priority — "Man is the measure of all things."

Primary school education will have to provide a solid foundation on which any further education can be continued, because the acceleration of progress and the structural changes caused by it demand a permanent actualization of those qualifications acquired during the time of training. In this context postgraduate medical education in our profession will gain a new, legally embodied importance. It will have to be accepted by medical practitioners that not only will the government check the continuity of postgraduate medical education, but also, the results of medical services will be measured according to state standards.

Demographic development in Germany

Projections concerning population growth have proved surprisingly correct in recent years. Statisticians believe that the tendency toward a decreasing European population versus an increasing Asian and South American population is irreversible. Consequently, estimates for Germany imply that in less than one generation age groups will have halved, with general life expectancy steadily increasing. If the present trend continues there will be twice as many people above the age of 60 as under 20 years in the year 2030. Not only would this necessitate decisive changes in our health and pension systems, it would also mean that the world would be seen from the perspectives of older rather than younger people. This decrease/stagnation in population can be observed in most industrial countries. In contrast, the population of the world is steadily increasing and in only 40 years' time a decrease is likely when prosperity and changes both in consciousness and attitudes will have attained a new balance.

Politicians in industrial nations are thus challenged to pursue a policy favorable to the family and open to the upbringing of children. On one hand the demographic development will have a considerable influence on the impact of individual ways of thinking, with regard to economic and political beliefs, while on the other hand the family will play an important role because it will continue to offer a haven from danger.

The future cannot be realized amid a loss of family and other social ties, because this loss estranges, destroying human beings even if they live in affluence. A solid network is needed as a basis. The state must remove obstructions and provide economic alleviations.

German social insurance

For more than 100 years Germany had a progressive system of international prototype quality of social insurance that represents the basis for the medical care of all citizens and at the same time is the foundation for the prosperity enjoyed by the medical professions in Germany.

The imperial decree enacted in 1883, substantially influenced by Bismarck, introduced the legal regulation of comprehensive compulsory insurance in Germany and may be considered the origin of our present-day health insurance law. With compulsory insurance it was intended that all citizens would be given a legal right to dental care.

At the same time one had in mind a social compensation between all groups of the population.

On the basis of the law on panel doctors, which was improved in the following decades, independent free practice is essentially ensured today. It is not a supervisory system that decides what is correct and useful but one that allows the individual dentist, as a member of a free profession on a high scientific and technical level, to treat according to the health requirements of the patient, who is free to choose him or her. Every citizen is insured but at a certain income level he or she may be exempted from the statutory illness funds and may enter the private health insurances.

Through sound competition among various illness funds and the commitment of the dental profession, the necessary "self-propulsion" for the further development of dentistry is well ensured.

In an autonomous system with an equally autonomous jurisdiction of the dental profession, the elected representatives of the professional body can agree on the extent of dental services and their financial rating in negotiations with the illness funds. Only if the dental profession fails to provide the dental care for the population does the state intervene. This is necessary to ensure the protection of the citizens; however, no such measures have been taken during the past four decades since the end of the war.

An individual system of social insurance similar to the German model would prove suitable for many countries in the 21st century.

The working principle of today and tomorrow must be: services in return for service. The aim is to remain in a system of comprehensive social security, the basis of which is founded in the individual responsibility of every citizen, also for those risks that can only be covered collectively.

Fédération Dentaire Internationale

It was no accident that just in 1900, at the beginning of the 20th century, the Fédération Dentaire Internationale was founded by Charles Godon. He had realized that terms like *knowledge, disease,* and *health* were not confined within the borders of individual countries. His work proved to be lasting; from small beginnings a powerful international organization has emerged that today includes more than 90 nations. Except for the International Red Cross, FDI is the oldest international medical association and today by far the largest professional organization.

In tracing back the history of the FDI, one realizes with amazement that the founders were skilled "politicians" for their profession. They all fought hard for the status and recognition of the dentist within the scope of the medical professions. In some countries dentistry existed somewhat independent of other health care areas; in others medical doctors also dealt with dentistry. They all thought of themselves as dentists but suffered from the dominant influence of the medical profession. These problems have almost entirely been solved in Europe, North America, and Japan but internationally they will remain into the 21st century.

Today the FDI represents more than 400,000 dentists worldwide, and the parliamentary solidarity of more than 90 member organizations is difficult indeed and will be more so in the future. Nevertheless, one can proudly emphasize that methods have been developed to manage the various problems of dentistry in the world nearly to the full extent (though not always exhaustively, due to financial reasons).

Unfortunately, many colleagues in their "intact dental ivory tower" have not yet embraced the idea of international cooperation, nor are they aware that their dental training has already become subject to international conditions. Besides the idea of international understanding, ie, of idealistic, cooperative ties, the advantages of international cooperation have to be transparent for the individual colleague. By sharing our experiences, we can better evaluate and thus improve our own systems. It is imperative for our profession that a large majority of colleagues support the idea of international cooperation, for in the final analysis, through their fees paid directly or indirectly to their national associations, they support this international cooperation.

Earlier I referred to historical events of this century as they have gained an overall importance to our basic perspectives. I tried to avoid a discussion narrowly focussing on our profession because in the future, as in the past, political and economic developments of individual countries will be reflected in the field of dentistry. In this context I would also like to highlight an increasing dependence of every country on its neighbor. Today nearly every political decision implies consequences affecting other countries, just as developments outside our own boundaries will have effects on our own national policies. Already today European law within the European Community may conflict with, or even break, national laws also in the field of dentistry. Thus, we can increasingly observe that political measures are no longer determined solely by the two world powers but that today, unlike in the past, developments in smaller countries affect dentistry worldwide, and this will be even more true in years to come. External influence will become multifarious and thus the demand for our professional policy must be a "great" policy, ie, one that accommodates expanded international perspectives.

Concerning the FDI, it is to be hoped that it will develop considerably yet remain politically independent for the benefit of all dentists. Its independence is certainly its strongest unifying force; the FDI should by no means yield to the destructive temptation of excluding countries on the basis of so-called political realities.

The solid future development of the FDI will imply:

1. Expansion and improvement of the Dental World Parliament

2. Improvement of international cooperation in research and education
3. Establishment of an international dental media center supporting public relations and education by means of a comprehensive dental world library and dental video library
4. Publication of a leading world dental journal
5. Organization of world congresses of the highest scientific standard in connection with coordination of dental trade fairs
6. Foundation of an international university serving the needs of international dentistry at the headquarters of the world organization

Creating a "world" dentist

The European Regional Organization of the FDI has been successful in creating a type of "European" dentist — a dentist trained at an internationally regulated and recognized university who can serve and be accepted throughout the European community. Since 1980 there has been mutual agreement by the 12 member states of the European Community recognizing dental diplomas issued within those countries. At the same time, a common dental educational training scheme was enacted. This was established 12 years ago and the national governments are now following with their policy.

Thus, it is not presumptuous to assume that in the 21st century it will be possible to create a "European" dentist, notwithstanding the fact that there are still enormous differences in the dental status in the various countries.

Looking at North America we cannot but notice that so far it has not been possible to create either a compulsory dental training scheme or mutual recognition of the diplomas issued by the individual states. Although some states do recognize diplomas from other states a European dentist is able to establish a practice in another European country more easily than an American dentist can in his or her own country. This is true despite the fact that the differences between the individual European countries concerning their dental training schemes are even greater than in the United States in addition to the further difficulties that arise out of language differences in Europe.

This harmonization in the recognition of national diplomas will be completed in the 21st century and the same trend will extend to Canada and parts of Central and South America. Nevertheless, a type of "American" dentist already exists as a result of the tremendous importance of American English as a world language. Just as Latin, and before that Greek, were the world's scientific languages, today English — specifically American English — has taken that function. Consider, for example, the unquestioning way in which many of us, as non-English, non-Canadians, and non-Americans, accepted the invitation to this international symposium, knowing that the presentations would be in English.

In the 21st century this process of Americanization will continue and the influence of the American dentist not only as a model in the field of research but also as a model for the Asian/Pacific area, and above all the Japanese dentist, will increase. Parallel to this process, the European dentist will develop independently but will not succeed in escaping the trend toward Americanization. The African and Asian dentist — especially the Chinese — will be necessary in an initial phase of development in these regions, only to be assimilated over time through improved education and steady adjustment.

In summary, I would like to answer the first question: If it will not be possible to create the "American" dentist with uniform educational and qualification standards in the United States, the "land of unlimited opportunities," until the end of this century, how much more difficult will it be for the world to reach a comparable standardization?

A "world" dentist will not yet exist in the 21st century. The European dentist will undergo an independent development because of stratified cultural traditions and a necessity to integrate the Eastern European countries; however, he or she will not be able to escape the Americanization of the profession. The American dentist will further consolidate his or her lead position because of language and scientific achievements in the United States.

Will the future development of dentistry depend only on the competence of the dentist?

Generally speaking, one can say that in industrial countries of similar cultural and economic levels a comparable standard of dental knowledge has evolved. However, the extent to which the practitioners of those countries actually put their knowledge to use can easily vary for each country. There are countries in the world where dentists are undoubtedly highly trained but where the masses do not benefit.

The facts reveal that the practice of dentistry not only depends on the qualifications of a country's dental professionals but is deeply rooted in the social structure of the individual countries. It will be one of the preeminent tasks of dentistry in the 21st century to eliminate this discrepancy, for society will no longer tolerate dual standards in medical care based on social class. The solution to this problem will determine whether dentistry will continue to exist as a free profession. Let us not ignore the fact that internationally an increasing polarization on the issue of the treatment of patients in free practice versus state institutions has evolved. By institutions, I refer to the practice of dentistry in state institutions or outpatient departments of both private and state-run health insurance systems.

I have already mentioned that the FDI represents more than 400,000 dentists, more than one third of whom do not work in free practice. For the 21st century I predict a further decrease of the institutional dentist as the process of democratization continues worldwide, and I expect an increasing resignation of socialism to commit itself to economic activities. Nevertheless, it will remain a special international task for the Americans and Central Europeans to see that the balance will not be shifted to the disadvantage of the free practice.

Dentistry in the 21st century

Dental departments at the universities will become recognized on a mutual basis by countries worldwide. Research and teaching will be generally separated, with research being pursued primarily by industry. The former ethical conceit of the European dentist with regard to the dental industry no longer exists; a close cooperation between the two will develop. The differentiation of the dental specializations as in the United States will not become a trend. In Europe orthodontics and oral surgery will remain mutually independent fields of specialization. A specialization in the field of maxillofacial surgery will require a medical degree. However, combination or group practices, already common in the United States, will increasingly develop in Europe, mainly because of economic considerations.

The present prestige in being a doctor will not be maintained in the 21st century, and the status of the dentist will probably differ only slightly from that of a professional technician or scientist holding a university degree.

The controlling function of the state, of the state-run health insurances, or the patients, will revolutionize the dentist-patient relationship for the worse. The following reasons will account for this: computer transparency, a skepticism and extreme political awareness of the patients, and changed legal positions with regard to dental services.

Statisticians rightly point out that there is an "overproduction" of university graduates in Europe, especially in our profession. Against this, politicians in the European Parliament argue that in the individual countries of the European Community ratio of dentists to patients varies between the countries from 1:1,000 to 1:9,000. A theoretical balance of figures will not occur in spite of a higher mobility of the European dentist, thus leading to a university graduates' proletariat, as can already be observed in Scandinavia. This trend will also affect the working and living conditions and the status of the dentist; another consequence will be an approximation of incomes with respect to dental auxiliary occupations, as is already the case for our northern neighbors. The decision to work past the age of retirement will be restricted by legal regulations. The achievements of technology and scientific findings will lead to further improvements in dentistry. The resulting rationalizations will affect the dentist less than the dental auxiliary occupations, but it is the dental technician whose profession will change dramatically. The manual portion of the technican's job will become relatively small, consisting of making corrections to machine-made computer products, and refining crowns to improve esthetics. In the next century more than half of the work of the dental technician will be replaced by computers.

The dental practice in the 21st century

The ergonomic accomplishments concerning the construction, planning, and design of dental practices have already theoretically reached a limit that can only be refined to a negligible degree. For the 21st century, however, dental managerial economics, ergonomics, organization, and the use of computers will be integrated into the dental training scheme.

Practices will be more uniform for ergonomic and financial reasons, more functional in their planning and design, with a view to atmosphere or adapted to popular styles, and run on a more efficient basis as a result of better training of auxiliaries. Also, the continuous training in emergency treatment will have become normal both for the dentist and the dental auxiliary. The special disposal of medical waste from dental offices will be subject to legal regulations.

Protection for the mouth, eyes, and head will dominate the attire of the dental team. Every practice will be connected to a data bank and a computer center, which will allow direct communication with colleagues of all medical branches and sick funds. This will facilitate the transmission of information regarding patient histories, the direct referral of patients, pharmacological and specialist agreements on high-risk and problematic patients, information on available dental supplies, and data exchanges between the dentist and his or her tax consultant and tax authorities. All accounting will be done exclusively by computer. Fiscal control will become easier, as will controls of quality and warranty by the private and state-run health insurances and the patients, respectively.

The computer will also be indispensable for regular patient examinations. In the case of malfeasance, fines will be charged to the patient's account. Even if it might seem a nightmare for us today, the storage of data in a computer will be regarded as a kind of safeguard.

Economic associations of dental practices will increasingly be found in the industrial nations.

Public health and conservative dentistry

The power of the sugar industry will be broken by the beginning of the 21st century. No producer will be able to exist economically if its product is directed against human health.

Political associations, as in the case of the countries of the Common Market, will in the 21st century enable fluoridation of drinking water in large parts of the world. Regulations concerning the sanitation of drinking water will allow a therapeutically sufficient fluoridation of the drinking water in EC countries as early as 1992.

The decisive change of the general consciousness with regard to more care and preservation, combined with the positive results of the worldwide dental campaigns for prophylaxis, will delight statisticians in the industrial nations. However, these factors, which will cause an enormous reduction of caries, will lead to a decrease in conservative treatment. Possible vaccines against caries will further this process. The field of endodontics as an expression of further development in dentistry will strongly increase. Amalgam will disappear from dental practices and be replaced by restorative materials that resemble the natural tooth substance, can form a compound, and can provide a perfect color match.

Inlays and onlays will be provided with the aid of computers. Gold, as the best dental material, will no longer be a choice material for restorative dentistry, will only be of antiquated nature, and will be replaced by low-priced plastics matching the natural color of the tooth and equalling gold in performance.

A new generation of transillumination instruments will have replaced the old X-ray machines.

Prosthodontics

Computers will be used increasingly in prosthodontics. Computer technology will allow a more perfect impression technique and the creation of crowns, bridgework, and plates with automatic jaw registration. Efficiency and quality will be improved. Esthetic perfection in dental technology, insofar as manual skill is concerned, will peak by the end of this century: in the 21st century the dentist or the dental technician will only execute the individualization of the computer-designed product. Computer-generated audiovisual information will be used both in general and specific ways for projecting treatment outcomes in prosthodontic cases.

There will be fewer developments in prosthetics in the industrial nations despite a longer life expectancy of their populations and an increase of geriatric treatment. We may, however, assume that in developing countries a large demand for basic prosthetic treatment will remain for decades.

Orthodontics

For this special field an increasing demand is also to be expected in the next century, even if hereditary anomalies in the maxillofacial region are eliminated through genetic interference. The increased demand for esthetic perfection will guarantee both the need and the success rate of orthodontic cases through improved cooperation on the part of the patients. In addition, the number of adult patients will grow. To the same degree, the quota of preorthodontic treatment for prosthetics, orthognathic surgery, and craniomandibular periodontology is already incorporated in the dental education.

Periodontology

Periodontology will have to be assigned a new importance in the 21st century as its essential influence on all the fields of dentistry will be recognized. The percentage of those patients who will lose their teeth to periodontal disease will become very small because these patients will have practiced better oral hygiene. In addition, further developments in artificial bone and tissue replacement materials will enlarge the therapeutic range of periodontal treatment. Genetic engineering may also play a role. A more conservative periodontal treatment will have replaced surgical alternatives.

Oral and maxillofacial surgery

The quality of dentistry reveals itself in the decrease of extractions observed in some European countries for many years. The last study by WHO also confirms this: in the Federal Republic of Germany only 1 person out of 100 aged 35 to 40 years is edentulous. In Denmark this rate is 8, in Ireland 12, in Finland and the Netherlands 17. This comparison is even more pronounced for the older generation. Whereas in Ireland, the United Kingdom, and the Netherlands 3 out of 4 people above the age of 65 are edentulous, only 1 out of 4 in Switzerland and FRG, and only 1 out of 5 in Sweden, have lost all their teeth.

In the industrial nations a further decrease in dental surgical treatment will occur in the 21st century. Unfortunately, this will remain the only form of dental treatment in many developing countries.

Parallel to the decrease of extractions, the number of tooth resections will rise in the industrial countries. Oral and maxillofacial surgery, minor and major endeavors, respectively, will essentially be distinguished by outpatient and inpatient treatments, with a medical degree required for the field of maxillofacial surgery.

Through further developments and innovations, mainly with regard to pharmacology, the spectrum of preprosthetic and orthognathic surgery will be expanded. These developments will include new artificial bone replacement materials, medicaments accelerating the process of healing, and medicaments for total control of inflammatory and allergic reactions in both bone and tissue. Along with further strides in implantology, which will reach its peak in the 21st century, the portion of problematic patients will decrease drastically in the future. Because of an increased life expectancy, the number of high-risk patients and disabled patients will rise considerably.

Through profound knowledge about the interaction of medicaments, which will to an increasing extent determine the life or death of patients, the risks of operations for trauma and cancer patients will be decidedly lowered.

An important demand with regard to dental education both for the present and the future will be that attention must be paid to early diagnosis of tumors and precancerous lesions as well as to oral manifestations of systemic diseases and infectious oral diseases and infections.

Neuralgic pains

In the 21st century the neurophysiology of the masticatory system will be clarified, will be part of the dental education, and will expand the range of dental treatments considerably.

Neuralgic pains in the region of the head, throat, neck, and temporomandibular joint will rise enormously, as will muscular functional disorders. As is common with these disease complexes, the psychological component often has an initiatory effect; thus, treatment will require psychotherapy as well as the removal of occlusal disturbances, which can be diagnosed with the help of the computer.

The development of the affluent society of industrial nations will imply the inclusion of psychotherapy as a necessary addition to the spectrum of dental treatment.

Whether dentistry will succeed in enlarging and transcending its limited scope by the integration of new medical fields, and thus evolve from dentistry to "dental medicine," will to a large degree determine the future of dentistry in the 21st century. Even if we witness enormous shifts within the various fields of dentistry such as a decrease in conservative, prosthetic, and surgical treatment versus an increase in orthodontic, periodontal, and endodontic treatment and implantology, the absolute demand for dental treatment in the industrial countries, with their growing numbers of dentists, will not rise significantly. This means that in the 21st century the "dental cake" will be sliced in smaller pieces unless the dental workload can somehow be increased.

Proper prophylaxis should not begin with the cleaning of the teeth but must start with the correct choice of food. The dentist not only has to become the responsible "custodian" of the oral environment but must also become a teacher of proper nutrition. The direct interdependencies between poor nutrition and disease are well established, and dietetics will become increasingly important in the next century.

In Europe, unfortunately, this obvious replenishment of the dental education and general enlargement of the medical spectrum has so far been neglected by the dental profession. The chance to develop concurrently with the growing field of masticatory neurophysiology will be regarded as a step into the field of oral medicine. If dentistry develops no further, it will cause an irrevisible setback, especially in light of the rapid developments in general medicine. A renewed gap between dentistry and general medicine would be a logical consequence that could not be compensated financially. It would be anachronistic to believe that the Hippocratic oath of this century could be transferred to the next millenium, yet it would mean a degradation of our dental profession to renounce it entirely in the 21st century.

This is why I am firmly convinced that the medical professions will only be able to successfully defend their social and political roles in the future if truthfulness will remain the maxim of their action or if they will again call to mind the ethical values of our profession.

I think it is completely legitimate for the medical profession to defend its rights in order to take an active part in the economic process, but in any labor and trade disputes our arguments have to be on a high level. The respect for our medical service and the credible presentation of our problems are the arms in our fight.

It remains fascinating and at the same time encouraging for the future that the ethical and moral maxims of Hippocrates, which could only develop on the basis of a democratic philosophy, have never entirely left our medical profession, especially in light of the political odyssey democracy has taken, at least in parts of our globe.

This is why the oath of Hippocrates and the pledge of doctors, initiated and accepted by the World Medicinal Association, is almost a "profession of faith." I am firmly convinced that the attraction of and satisfaction in our profession will remain as long as a free dentist in free practice in a free state is allowed to exist.

We have already transcended the peak of our individual freedom, because more knowledge will not give us more freedom but will make our ancient soul poorer, more anxious and lonely.

However, being an optimist, I will continue to believe in the future of our profession, though with essentially different perspectives: more uniform, less individual, and with less "highlights."

Further reading

Official Journal of the European Communities, L 233, Volume 21.

Liaison Committee for Dentistry in the EEC Countries (Study of Professional Qualifications and Fields of Activity of Dental Practitioners in the Nine Countries of the EEC).

Zahnärztlicher Verbindungsausschuß zur EG. Anlagen zur Untersuchung über die berufliche Qualifikation, die gegenseitige Anerkennung der Diplome und den Tätigkeitsbereich der Personen, die in den 9 Ländern der EG die Zahn-, Mund- und Kieferheilkunde ausüben.

Vergleichende Darstellung der Systeme der sozialen Sicherheit in den Mitgliedstaaten der Europäischen Gemeinschaft (1. 7. 82).

"System der zahnärztlichen Versorgung in der BRD" (Tiemann/Herber).

"Die Welt" (30. 7. 88), Axel Springer Verlag.

Publications by Dr Rolf Braun.

Chapter 24

Dentistry of Today and in the Future

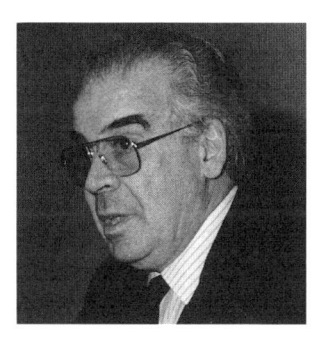

Roberto
Gonzales-Giralda
Tenerife, Canary Islands

The Chairman of IBM Corporation in 1943 actually said: "I think there is a world market of about five computers." World market! And Field Marshal Fock, a hero of World War I, said: "Aeroplanes are interesting toys but have no military value!" So it is difficult to predict the future.

About what is going on currently throughout the world, we have heard plenty, so I am not going in any way to try to add to that. We do have people who are actually looking into the future of dentistry, but the future of dentistry, for me at least, is brighter than what has been anticipated.

First of all let me remind you that the Fédération Dentaire Internationale, which is the worldwide organization of dentistry, comprises the national dental associations of 92 countries. It does not represent the governments, it does not represent public dental health, it does not represent dental education. We do hold within our congresses conferences of dental deans, conferences of chiefs and officers, but we do not represent them. We represent the private practice of dentistry.

Dentistry needs to know what lies in its future, and the only way to predict the future is to understand the present. Unfortunately, dentistry is failing to understand what is happening to the profession and what is happening around us.

Society, as we know, is changing, and dentistry itself is highly dynamic. We are caught between two different epochs of high turbulence because we are between the painful present and an uncertain future. Again, however, unless we understand the present we won't be able to predict the future. First of all we will have to analyze ourselves as dentists, and we have to be objective and try to do an exercise in prospection. That exercise in introspection will give us the picture of what we are doing, how we are moving, and where we are going.

We are actually in a society with completely new structures, new values, new concepts. And that society has, first of all, multiple options and also likes to have wider models of provision of services. There was a time when the provider went to service and the dental profession had the power of decision, but the power of decision is no longer with the dental profession, with whoever may be providing services. The power of decision today is with the consumer, and we try to go out to the consumer, try to give to the consumer what he or she wants.

For 200 years dentistry has been delivering services in the same way. Now we are at a point where, thanks to research, we will have the technology that we need. The only problem is that we are unable to provide the services being demanded from the dental profession.

Thus, we have the technology, we have the profession, but unfortunately we we do not know who is going to pay for the provision of these services.

We have been told in the preceding pages how in some countries, such as in Scandinavia, where the state provides dental health, the costs of such services are outrageous.

Let me remind you of something: In Vienna at the time of the FDI World Dental Congress, there was a country that was presenting as a model the school dental services of that particular country. What was the pride of some from that country was also the shame of others because it was very costly to the country. And at the end of the year, at the end of the program, there was no relation (costwise) between the input into the system and what was being provided.

Therefore, if we have the technology, if we have the dental workforce, we must develop different models for the provision of our services. We must be more imaginative, we must go out to the public, we must utilize marketing strategies, we must awaken the potential demand. And that will create a demand that we need and a brighter future for dentists.

There are a few things I would like to speak of because we really have to be proud of who we are. I am very proud of having been a practitioner. I am very proud of the FDI representing the general practice of dentistry. Dentistry has performed tremendously in improving the oral health of different nations, and of course dentistry, the organized profession, has helped governments provide better services for better health for their own people.

In 1985 the World Health Assembly in Geneva passed a resolution recognizing that governmental action by itself was not sufficient to really attain the goals of health for all by the year 2000. That was an official acknowledgment by government in the World Health Assembly that by themselves they were not able to attain that goal, and they called in the resolution for governments to go to the profession in their own countries to help them attain for the people what they were not attaining by themselves. WHO has made those goals their own, but it was actually the profession together with government through the WHO and the FDI.

The FDI will have to find an equilibrium between the promotion of oral health and the protection of the profession, because we do have some rights to be protected, too, in the same way that the public has rights to be protected.

And last, of course, the FDI is against the extrapolation of models. What may be good for one country may not be good for another. A model that is applicable in the Federal Republic of Germany cannot be applicable to other parts of the world where there are not the same socioeconomical conditions. Governments do have the right to provide their own people with the best that they have.

DISCUSSION

DENTISTRY IN THE 21st CENTURY
A GLOBAL PERSPECTIVE
BERLIN

SEPTEMBER 10, 1989

Simonsen

This symposium was organized in conjunction with the celebration of the 40th anniversary of the International Quintessence Publishing Group, and the 20th anniversary of *Quintessence International*. I would like to thank all of the speakers for taking time from their busy schedules to be with us today in this exciting symposium. We have heard some extremely interesting papers presented today. It has been stimulating to sit through many presentations from so many people, from different countries, cultures, and points of view.

The floor is now open not only to speakers but also to guests and anyone else who would care to ask questions. I would particularly like to encourage participation by our colleagues from the Berlin Dental Association who are present. I also see some people in the audience from other countries. I believe the President of the Zambia Dental Association is with us, Dr Caroline Mmembe. And so, please, don't be shy! Speak your mind and let us hear your opinions on some of the issues raised today. My role here is to keep out of the discussion as much as possible and let you have as much opportunity as possible to speak your minds.

Dr Löe, please start us out.

Harald Löe

It is about 10 hours since I had a chance to say something, and in the course of these 10 hours we have heard many thoughts, many challenges to our minds. There is one thought, however, that has not changed at all in my mind and that is based on the fact that when we had these tremendous changes of patterns of oral diseases that have occurred, nobody was able to predict them.

It says something about predictions. I do not think it is possible to predict too much beyond what you can foresee on an annual basis. But I want to impress upon you that what we saw came out of a scientific approach to dentistry. That it was an understanding of the underlying causes. There were technologies that were developed because of the scientific effort.

Further, I want to remember that today science is moving even faster and it is therefore even more difficult to predict. I spoke very superficially today about the new biology that is coming about. This is nothing less than genetic regulation of tissue responses, genetic regulation of diseases, and genetic regulation of defenses.

Today there is no question that the new technologies, for example, the monoclonal antibodies, provide tremendous opportunities for diagnosis. And that is going to be to the dentists what urine is to the urologist or blood is to the hematologist.

We are able to show the first scientific evidence of risk for caries, periodontal disease and even predict some of the outcomes. These technologies are opening an entirely new stage where research and practice are going to come together.

But, as we say in Norway: "You ain't seen nothing yet!"

So the old approach to caries vaccines are all abandoned and we are on to new approaches to developing technologies that would immunize patients in the future against caries and juvenile periodontitis or other types of periodontitis.

So I must remind you that science is changing very fast. The researchers are still in the driver's seat. There is also no question in my mind that never has the gap between science and practice been so small.

I know that China is going to do something very exciting in terms of prevention of oral diseases. It may come to almost a sacrifice of a whole generation. But they may have sidestepped the entire path that we have been through in restorative dentistry. And prevention is going to be the whole mark of approaches to developing countries. To see prevention at work in a population of a billion people would be something to behold. I won't be present, but some of you people will be, and it is going to be very exciting. Thank you.

Simonsen

Thank you very much, Dr Löe, for starting us out.

Degner

I am from Berlin and Mr Haase was kind enough to ask us to say something. We have heard that science and dental medicine are progressing. But I see a problem, and this problem is that the different states in Europe, and all over the world, may be too far apart. The different social systems will sometimes cut off the advances of dental medicine. The social problems in one country cannot be equated to those of another country. It will take time, maybe a long time, before we all can have dental medicine in one high standard as you ask here.

Leontiev

I would like to say some words in our discussion. When referring to the question of stomatology in the 21st century, three important factors must be taken into account:

First: The current status on development of treatment methods as well as prophylaxis depends on scientific progress.

Second: A careful choice of priorities is essential in determining individual stomatological discipline for the general public.

Third: On the structural, economical, and ideological aspects of the society, psychological awareness or readiness of society for new technologies, economical questions, and, of course, to priorities, is essential.

Thank you.

Simonsen

Thank you. I would like to ask you a question, Professor Leontiev: I understood from some of your graphs from your presentation this morning that you have, in the Soviet Union, dentists and stomatologists, and it was not clear to me what the difference is. Could you please clarify for the record how you define a stomatologist in the Soviet Union?

Leontiev

In our country, a stomatologist is a specialist with a high education. We have no dentists in our country.

Simonsen

No dentists?

Leontiev

No dentists. We have specialists with middle education in German called "Zahnarzt" or dentist. But he or she is of middle education. A stomatologist is a specialist with a higher education.

Simonsen

So a stomatologist has a higher education than what we would call a dentist. Thank you.

Professor Martignoni.

Martignoni

Thank you for permitting me to come to the discussion so I can clarify better what I could not in the first presentation.

Following what Braun and our colleagues from Russia told us in our discussions earlier, I can tell you about stomatologists, because I participate in the elaboration of what the difference is because we in Italy had the same problem at the beginning.

The title stomatologist is given to those who are physicians first and then took a second degree as a specialist in oral disease, or in stomatology. Stomatology means all mouth diseases whatsoever.

Now what is a so-called dentist? We in Italy call a dentist all the physicians that practice dentistry without any specialization in dentistry. That is what we call a dentist.

Simonsen

In the Soviet Union does the stomatologist have medical training?

Leontiev

Yes.

Simonsen

In addition to or before dental training?

Leontiev

A stomatologist completes training at the Stomatological Faculty of the Medical Institute. And the stomatologist has a 3-year complete education and a more than 2-year special stomatological education.

Simonsen

Thank you; that explained it. Professor Weber, you have a question?

Weber

I would like to try to get back to the purpose of why we are sitting here, which was carefully defined: we are supposed to give a somewhat — well, let's say — futuristic outlook or forecast perspective. That means we are supposed to collect data and we are not supposed to give well-defined concepts.

So what I would like to do is to compare some antagonistic statements here. One was made by Dr Löe, and the other one was made by Professor Leontiev. For me being a young, inexperienced scientist — certainly as compared to Dr Löe — I would say one statement made by our Russian colleagues seem to me a pragmatic statement.

When we talk about the 21st century the time is very, very limited. So for me a pragmatic solution in defining the problems and defining socially acceptable models seems to be the first step.

The other part Dr Löe was talking about is the futuristic part, and if I understood you correctly you were talking about diagnosis, helpful diagnosis. So first we have to establish the diagnosis by use of these extraordinary techniques you have been describing. And then, what about therapy? Once you have defined the risk patient, what about therapy as far as caries and periodontal disease are concerned?

So, in other words, for me it appears to be necessary for a step-by-step planning for the future. I would like to follow these ideas first without omitting the other scientific research work.

Simonsen

Dr Caroline Mmembe, President of the Zambia Dental Association. We are very happy to see you here in the audience. You had your hand raised?

Mmembe

Thank you very much, Mr Chairman, for allowing me these few minutes. I have been an observer of this unique meeting. It's been wonderful to see the 21st century through the eyes of all the distinguished people gathered here.

And one thing that has come out of it is the fact that, in fact, what we are working towards is the same in all countries, whether very developed or underdeveloped. And we are all agreed here, from what I can hear, that the future of dentistry lies in prevention. That much, at least, has not been disputed by anybody here and that is reassuring.

From what Dr Löe was saying it is clear that research is important and it is obvious also from the presentations that have been made that some countries are probably going to have more time to do research than others. Here I am looking especially at the African situation. The paper presented by Professor Reddy highlighted the wastefulness in the African continent.

Let me just concentrate your mind on Africa. I am sure you are all very aware of what Africa is. It is actually right in the center of the world. And it is represented by many diverse countries. If you start from the North you have countries which have a Mediterranean influence, so they have a bit of Europe. You have countries that are associated with the Middle East. You have countries farther south and you start looking at what you understand as Black Africa. Therefore, Africa presents a conglomeration of the ideas that have been proponded here and yet they are largely untapped.

I have been extremely interested in this Quintessence International World Symposium. There is a wealth of similar information that is largely untapped in Africa. I would like to suggest to Mr Haase that a similar symposium, just looking at what is in Africa, would have a lot of significance and probably would open more vistas for research, in the countries that can do research. Our problems are not unique. I do not think they are unique because, as I have already pointed out, we all know the problem; we know the answers. But, how do we go about improving the situation throughout the world?

With these few words I would like to thank you for your attention.

Simonsen

Thank you very much, Dr Mmembe. Professor George Zarb.

Zarb

I started dental school 30 years ago, and for the first two decades of my dental education, which I helped perpetuate because I have been an educator for a quarter of a century, most of what I learned, and most of what I taught, was based upon anecdote. It was glossy anecdotal stuff but anecdote nonetheless.

And in very recent years, as the result of the kind of work Dr Löe referred to, we are seeing entirely new vistas opening up in dentistry because already we are beginning to teach and apply things which have the strength and the compelling evidence of science to back them up.

I think if we do not recognize the tremendous impact that science has had on our field, we are going to go on perpetuating mythology and being nothing other than glorified carpet makers in the mouth.

But in reality we have a very profound professional and humanitarian obligation to go on attacking dental disease. Let us not take ourselves too seriously. We are talking about a series of infective processes, of which two are very definitively responsible for the ubiquitous periodontal disease and caries. Already they are on the way to cure.

Let us acknowledge the fact that probably we are the only health field which, within the next quarter of a century, will make ourselves obsolete.

I think we should be honest and open about realizing the possibility that dentistry is going to become a very, very minor part of the overall health service of the future.

Simonsen

Obsolete in 25 years?

Zarb

Think about it. Before you reject it just think about the possibility.

Simonsen

I am not rejecting it, George. I am simply the moderator. I would like to pick up a little straw here and there and try to stimulate some discussion. Professor Melsen.

Melsen

I think that we are sharpening the consciousness of the population so that now they want more. They want esthetic dentistry; there are age changes going on. And we all know that age in these days is something which the public has an extreme interest in. The consequences of aging are also in the dentition. And we have more teeth to care for than we ever had. We have fewer people but we have more teeth to care for. And this will mean some sophisticated treatment even if we can wipe out periodontal disease and caries.

I think that sometimes politicians come out with statements which are not representative of the population. I sit on a committee in the Dental Health Ministry and our Minister wants to cut back on orthodontics. He wants to cut back on orthodontics for cosmetic reasons because he says: "Oh well, if orthodontics doesn't help periodontal disease or prevent caries, why should we do it? Let's cut back." So he claims to represent the population when he says: "We can eliminate orthodontics for cosmetic reasons."

A survey was done on a representative part of the Danish population: 87% of the Danish population wanted orthodontics for cosmetic reasons.

You cannot cut back on the development that people want esthetic teeth also. And we have changes going on in our body. We have changes in our bones. We have less resistance to tooth migration. What was stable at a certain time may not be stablé later. And you will have to work your way up to another kind of stability. I think that is a job to be done there.

Zarb

I am not suggesting that it will be cut back; on the contrary, the more sophisticated our society becomes, and one could say that perhaps the triumph of Western science has been predicated on the fact that the individual's notion of health, of a higher standard, is paramount. And it is on the basis of this that different levels of sophistication of dentistry will always be needed. I welcome the notion that orthodontics should be needed by everybody. And we should make it available to everybody.

Today we are no longer embarrassed to admit that a lot of what we do in dentistry is of an esthetic nature. A few years ago it was not considered to be a reason for motivation. Plastic surgeons a few years ago were embarrassed to admit that they did certain things. Today a large percentage of the practice is those "certain things." So I am all for this. Please understand, I have no intention of throwing out the clinical baby with the bath water either. I would like us to be a little more honest to motivate people.

Melsen

I think it is very important to have the consumers being part of the decision-making process.

Simonsen

Is it the consumers? Dr Dugoni, how much of the increase in adult orthodontic care in the United States over the past few years is, do you think, attributable to a major advertising campaign that the American Association of Orthodontics initiated some years back? I remember seeing some advertisements that specifically were encouraging adults to seek orthodontic care.

Dugoni

Well, certainly the impact of public education programs influenced the number of adult patients seeking out orthodontic care. I think also the advancements in tooth movement, in the biology of tooth movement and in esthetic appliances, created a demand. But I don't know that we have any actual data to show how much the increase in adult orthodontics was influenced by marketing programs. But in my state of California, where we did do controlled studies of our marketing programs to influence the public in seeking dental care, we found that while the rest of the United States was getting less busy, the state of California was getting busier. The dentists were getting busier and that's because of a major public educational program.

If I may change the subject for a minute — one of the areas that I heard discussed was demographics — as we look at all countries, people are living longer. The effect of prevention is saving all of those dentitions. So we're having less edentulism and a larger population that's keeping their teeth. This has forced upon the dental schools in the United States, over the last decade, more comprehensive training in geriatric care, and therefore greater knowledge of medicine. Dental students are being trained to truly be physicians of the mouth. There is expanded education in pharmacology, more intense education about patients that are medically compromised, and so on.

That is an important aspect of the future practice of dentistry. As we take care of those older patients, their care will bring a closer alliance with medicine.

I am concerned that we will lose some of the autonomy that we have had in dentistry. In the United States we have a model of education that separates dental education from medical education. At the same time we have many adjunctive courses, many alliances with medicine, but we remain an autonomous profession. Although dollars have gone for dental research, so often the bulk of research dollars goes primarily to medicine, which has more appeal.

I am troubled because I want the dental profession to remain very strong as it competes with medicine for research dollars and for curriculum time. And so I get concerned; I want to be closer to medicine, but I don't want to be absorbed by medicine, or controlled by medicine.

Simonsen

Four or 5 people have raised their hands to speak. I am going to take you in the order that I saw your hands. Professor Weber.

Weber

George, I hope I got the message. First of all the good news: in 25 years from now Germany will be very happy to accept all the unemployed Canadian dentists!

Now, seriously, I know what you have been aiming at and I think there is no misunderstanding between the two of us. I have never intended to generate the impression that I would think that this basic research work could be omitted. Not at all. I would like to emphasize this again. For me there is no doubt about the fact that we do need this type of research work and that we do need the outcome, the hopefully positive outcome, for improving dental care. There is no doubt about that.

I would like to address three different topics here, which, in my opinion, have to be answered.

First, could you agree on the statement that there are individual levels of oral hygiene, individual "dental IQs," which will have a certain influence, in spite of all the prevention which might be introduced to our population?

Second, there are hereditary diseases, for instance, in terms of disease which have to be treated on an orthodontic basis — at least on an orthodontic basis, maybe even on a maxillofacial surgical basis, too. I am talking about tumor patients. And they will always be there, there is no doubt about that. At least, it is very likely that they remain there longer than the 21st century.

As far as your statement is concerned with regard to the unemployment rate, or time we need for having unemployed dentists, just look at the German DMF index which clearly shows that it's the only index in Europe which is still going up. And now I am being somewhat sarcastic when I say, this might be a reason for still increasing the number of our dental students while all the other European countries try to cut down on the student numbers. I don't mean this seriously of course.

It is a matter of fact that the DMF index is increasing. So what I am aiming at is that there is an obvious difference between the different countries. And this is what it is all about when you compare the different statements of the different speakers in this day. At least, there are, let's say, continental differences.

And finally, when you say that we might be the first profession which is digging its own grave, I think we should think about a new definition of dentistry. I think that we might have to change our professional goals in terms of diagnosis and treatment. But I cannot share the feeling that dentistry is dying. Somebody has to inform the people, somebody has to motivate people, and somebody has to do the basic treatments that will remain: removing calculus or doing some orthodontic treatment.

And I would like to ask the question to Dr Dugoni: Could you give me some idea as to what extent this orthodontic treatment being applied to adults is due to tooth loss? Is it just the question that the patient wakes up one morning and says: "I would like to have my tooth rearranged?" Or is it due to the fact that the teeth start to move? For me there is a tremendous difference.

Dugoni

I think the reasons for adult orthodontic treatment are diverse. For example, the patient may want to have better esthetics, or may want to have the orthodontic treatment they did not have as young people, now that they are adults. I think a great deal of it is related, of course, to lost teeth or teeth that have migrated, or to periodontal disease in which orthodontic treatment and comprehensive restorative dentistry become complementary to maintaining the dentition.

There is a multifaceted explanation as to why adult patients are seeking orthodontic care. It also relates back to the profession. If we look at the United States and the sophisticated level of the dental care rendered, we observe that dentists themselves are recommending more orthodontic care for their patients than they were in the past, just as they are recommending more periodontal treatment. Similarly, they are

Discussion

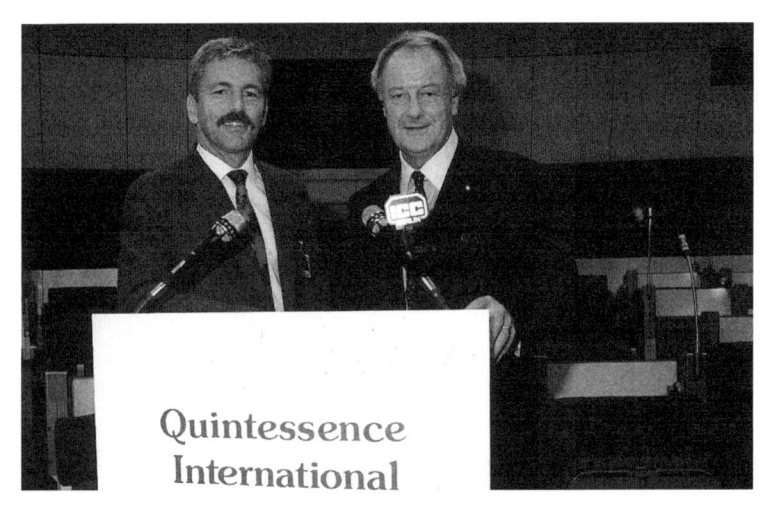

Mr H. W. Haase introduces Professor Richard Simonsen as Chairman of the Symposium.

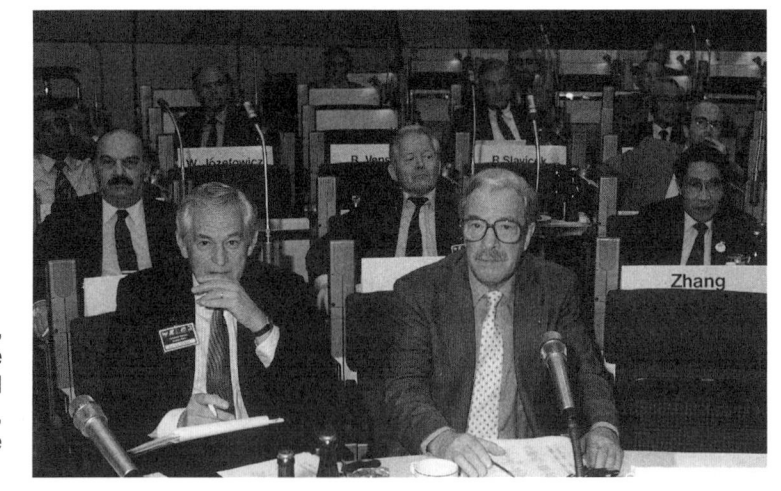

Professor Arthur Dugoni, Dean, University of the Pacific, San Francisco, and Dr. Harald Löe, Director, NIDR, seated in front of the other speakers and guests.

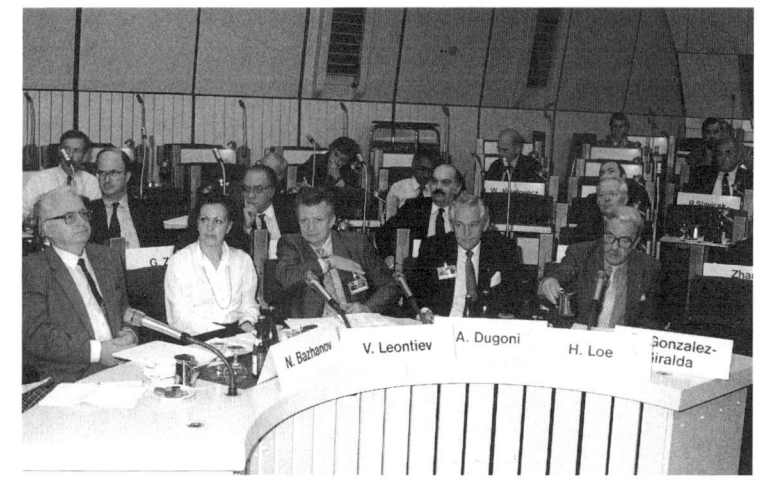

The delegation from the Soviet Union *(left)*, led by Professor Valery Leontiev, seated next to the delegation from the USA.

Discussion

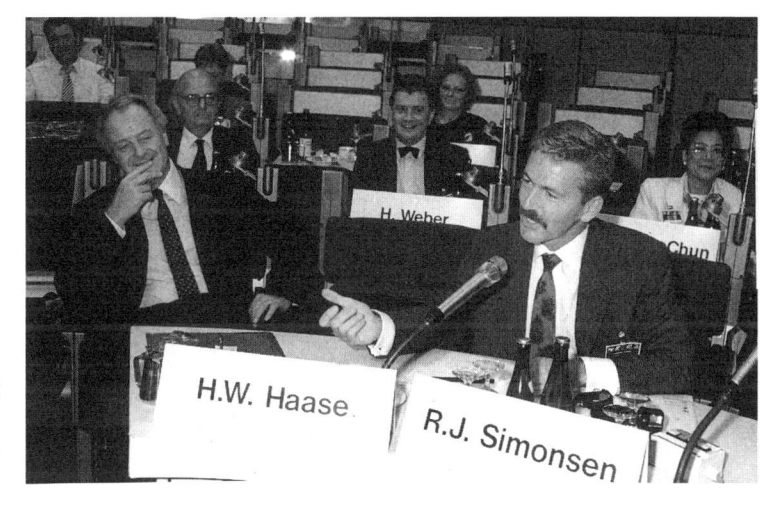

Professor Richard Simonsen shares a humorous moment with Mr H. W. Haase and, seated behind Mr Haase, Dr John McLean.

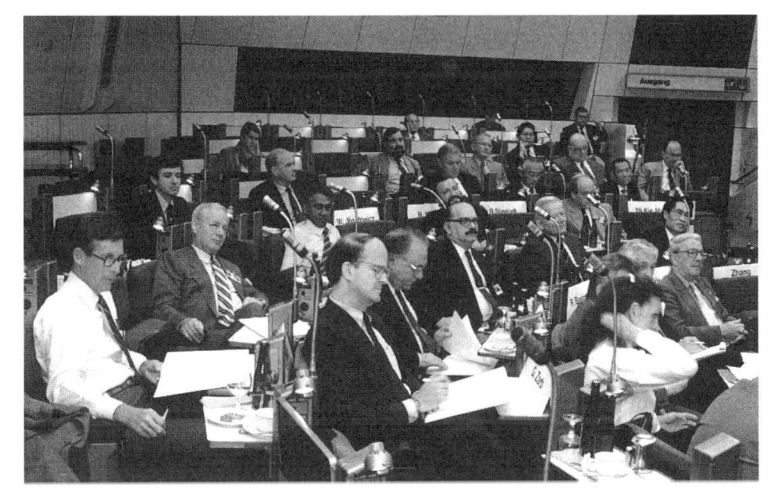

A portion of the audience and speakers. Foreground *(left)* Professor Raymond White (USA), *(center)* Professor George Zarb (Canada), and *(right)* Dr Larisa Panova (USSR)

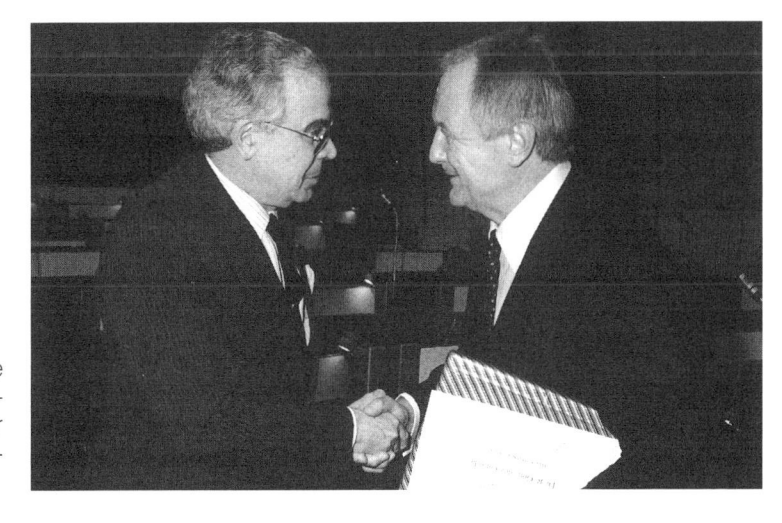

Mr H. W. Haase thanks the President of the FDI, Dr Roberto Gonzalez-Giralda, for his contribution to the Symposium.

doing more nutrition counselling, more cosmetic dentistry, and more implants. I think we have become scientifically more knowledgeable. We have a better educational foundation based on science, biology, and research. I think we have moved 50 years beyond that statement of dentists "working like tooth carpenters." We became a scientific profession when we identified the effects of research as an important component of our educational programs.

Simonsen

Professor Weber again.

Weber

Your question, Dr Simonsen, adressed to Dr Dugoni, implied that there will be a tremendous remaining amount of patients asking for orthodontic treatment. My question clarifies that once you have successfully fought against decay and periodontal disease, the amount of adult patients will decrease. This is the end of the equation. You said that there will be numerous patients — adult patients — asking for orthodontic treatment. And I think my question clarifies that you cut down on this number of patients as soon as you find solutions for caries and periodontal disease.

Simonsen

That depends on your assumption as to what the causes are for people seeking orthodontic care. I am not so sure that the reason you suggest is the correct one. I presume adult patients seek orthodontic care primarily because they wish to be better looking and we are living in an age of esthetics. Adults know that orthodontic treatment is not only for young people.

We can follow up later — but I have Professor Reddy next on my list to comment.

Reddy

Thank you, Mr Chairman. I just would like to shift the focus of the discussion a little bit because it seems that the bulk of the discussion concerns a part of the world that has a great deal of treatment. For example, I believe it is true that 80% of the world's dentists treat 20% of the world's population. The other 80% of the world's population have, in fact, very little treatment. So when we are talking about overtreatment in esthetic areas, we should keep this in perspective.

Dr Gonzales-Giralda earlier talked about the goals of the FDI and he spoke very strongly about preserving the right to private practice. I have no problem with that. But that particular system of health care may be inappropriate to certain developing countries.

So the ethical obligation for me from a developing country, and I think to Caroline Mmembe as well, is not to preserve private practice or health service or whatever the system is. It is to look at what is the best system, the most cost-effective system of utilizing some of those advances that Dr Löe talked about in delivering health care to a population that desperately needs it.

When we have hundreds and hundreds of orthodontic patients in South Africa we are not looking at their esthetic needs. We are looking primarily at what biological needs they have — how biological treatment can improve them if we give them orthodontic treatment.

So there are vast differences here. And considering that what I am talking about probably represents 75% to 80% of the population of the globe we should keep this discussion in perspective.

Simonsen

Thank you, Professor Reddy. Those were very appropriate comments since Caroline Mmembe is next on the list. It is my sincere hope that this discussion not focus entirely on the industrialized world, but also consider the very many needs of the developing nations. Dr Mmembe.

Mmembe

I would like to concur with what Professor Reddy has just said. But also to point out that we need to concentrate more on the moralistic aspects of dentistry. The sort of population we are serving in developing countries covers a cross section of the type of people that have been discussed here. We should never lose sight of the fact that the needs of different people must also be taken into account.

In other words: what Professor Melsen was saying also becomes important in our situation where there are some people who demand sophisticated dentistry. What often happens is that these people end up having to travel many thousands of miles, for example, to Germany, to get this type of treatment. So that cost factor also must be taken into account. Obviously, not everybody can do that.

Therefore, I just want to emphasize that although we know what we need, we must also be cognizant of the fact that we must be able to provide a sophisticated type of dentistry to the few people who demand it at some point.

Second, I want to highlight the point brought up about educating the public. In our situation in Zambia we have been, as an association, promoting dental care and increasing people's awareness of potential preventive and restorative treatment. The majority of the people have always felt that if they have a toothache they should just go and have the tooth extracted and that is the end of the story. We have started educating the people as to what they should be looking for in preventive care. That has created an excess of patients coming to the clinic to have their problems solved. Then we end up with too few dentists to solve their problems.

Education is important, but at the same time we need to marry the two sides of the problem that I am highlighting. We improve people's awareness and then we must be able to provide back-up service. That is equally important.

Lastly, I just wanted to point out another issue which, perhaps, you may not have thought about but which became clear to me during the presentations today. And that is the fact that for many countries, especially on the African continent, there are no dental schools. So in order to build up the dental segment of a population we have to send people to other countries for their education. Now, for example, out of the 12 indigenous dentists that we have in Zambia so far, 25% were trained in Russia. When they come back home, the basis, or the emphasis, of their training in Russia may be very different from the realities that they face when they come home. So that also has some bearing on the problems that we are experiencing. Thank you very much.

Simonsen

Professor White, you had your hand up some time ago.

White

Dr Mmembe made the more profound statement that's been made here today and that is: given a choice — and many people in the world do have a choice as a result of education, socioeconomic status, political status, and the like — given a choice, I can make the case that the public, the patients, people in society, are ahead of the dentists.

The people's definition of dentistry encompasses providing them with the kind or oral health that Dr Melsen mentioned and that the World Health Organization has adopted — an oral health that gives one well-being and allows maximum function in daily life.

I am continually amazed that, not only in the United States but in other parts of the world, patients are demanding sophisticated care that dentists haven't worked out. If you look at the older population in the United States, people who are my father's age, they do not accept that they are going to have dentures that slop around in their mouths and won't stay in place so that they can't eat.

If you look at the patients — and Dr Dugoni and I maybe need to compare our notes — but the orthodontic patients that I see for the most part are self-referred. They won't accept the fact that they can't function well because their teeth don't come together. They want to get orthodontic treatment because in their mind it improves their oral health and allows them to function better.

And I can give you examples all the way down the line. They want to come to the dentist and they all seek the most sophisticated procedures. Many times the dentists are not prepared to deal with a lot of these things that perhaps are controversial, or that we have not worked out yet. But they are willing to come and have these things done. Also, not only do they speak as individuals, they speak through their political entities, they speak through labor, they speak through management, and they demand dental services far in excess of anything that I would have anticipated. It is the attitude of the people that amazes me.

We don't see this big opportunity and we are unable to respond appropriately to what the patients are asking.

Simonsen

Dr Löe, you wanted to say something?

Löe

Yes. I want to comment on the topic of medicine and dentistry. You just heard Dr Dugoni walking this fine line between the concept of a physician of the mouth, without moving dentistry into the clinical fields of medicine. The separation of dentistry, or dental medicine, from the rest of medicine was an accident of history. It has turned out to be a benefit to dentistry and has turned out to be a benefit for populations.

There is no question in my mind that dentistry has evolved and developed in a much more beneficial way in its separate walk through history than it could have as a part of medicine. But another question is whether you are more interested in substance than in process. If you have a physician of the mouth, you have substance. If you want process you either include it in medicine or you don't. I would maintain, however, that dentistry — since 1840 when the formalization of the separation took place, at least in America when the first dental school was established, outside medicine — has been on its way back to medicine the whole time. We have incorporated more basic sciences into the dental curriculum to the point where at the University of Connecticut, where I served as Dean, we had exactly the same basic science curriculum for dental students as for the medical students. And some dental students even took the National Board examination for medicine.

Now that is very important because there is no reason why a physician of the mouth should have less basic science that a physician of the nose. So that, I think, should be very consistent in our approach.

And I can't get excited about whether we are calling ourselves stomatologists or physicians of the mouth or something else. The real issue is: what is the basis for dental students' education — what is in the curriculum for their education? I have said dentistry has increased the intellectual level of the profession all through history. And I think we are getting to a point where we are in a bona fide clinical discipline — of medicine — without being part of the medical school curriculum.

Another thing is, I have a reason to be proud of this development. I think the system works. And I, from the research point of view, must tell you that dental research is very much part of the main stream of medical research. We are no less capable than other clinical disciplines. Comparing ourselves with otolaryngology, orthopedic surgery, ophthalmology — we are competitive and comparable. There is no question in my mind that we are doing very well, even compared to some of the specialties in internal medicine. It should be made clear that we have reached a level of capability, scientifically and professionally, that gives us every reason to be proud of our profession.

The other thing I wanted to say is that the publishers in this environment — this environment of fast-moving science and a profession very hungry for new scientific information — have a very special responsibility.

I think that publishing companies are going to be very important for the next century. I don't believe that we are each going to have our own computer and then everything is solved. No. I think publishing houses are going to be very important. Probably more important than ever.

But there is a certain screening that has to take place in publishing houses, and there has to be a review, a rigid review of material prior to publication and dissemination so that the profession does not get confused. And I know this is done. But I think this is a very important function for any publication that is going to be read by both the initiated and the uninitiated, so to speak.

These symposia, then, serve a very important function, and I would like to compliment you, Mr Haase, for having brought all these people together. I am delighted to have been a part and I am proud to have been given an invitation to participate in the program.

So as far as I am concerned: the models that the FDI President spoke about, that each country will have its own model system and that we are not here to design one model system that is going to fit everybody, is wisdom — that is real wisdom to me. Whatever we are doing we are just continuing to adapt to changes and build a better and better profession.

Simonsen

Thank you, Dr Löe. Professor Frank Braun.

Braun

I listened today to some very remarkable reports. But let me be honest. Sometimes I feel we must remember that dentistry is not the center of the world. We should not forget that we are only a little stone in the garden of the world. Yes, we can discuss fine dentistry. And here I think it is very important that one speak of the future of dentistry, thinking of the industrialized countries and, of course, of the developing countries. Because there are two different kinds of future. And, of course, one has to come back to what Dr Zarb said. The absolute demand for dental treatment in the industrial countries will essentially not rise; one has to realize this. And even if there is a little part, in the orthodontic field, which can increase, this does not mean there is a general increase in demand and that the number of dentists should grow.

We are now able in Europe to close dental schools — in Holland and also now in Scandinavia — which I think is fantastic.

There is only real future of our profession if our society system — especially the East, the communist countries — will change, and we do hope so. And there is a fantastic situation happening in the last couple of years with perestroika and glasnost.

But society must change first. Then there will be a growing economic factor that will then, in the end, allow our little dental field to be developed. And so the change really very clearly depends on economic success in a country and in change in society.

Simonsen

Maybe we could change direction a little bit and try to see if there is anything that any speaker has said that anyone here totally disagrees with? — No? Well, I guess we have more consensus than I had hoped for, in terms of generating some stimulating point/counterpoint discussions. Professor Josefowicz. You are next.

Josefowicz

My colleague said that in communist countries we are changing and it is a fact. We are not satisfied with this system. We want to change many things. We noticed even from this discussion, which was very helpful and fruitful for us, many things have to be completely organized in another way — 180 degrees differently.

For example I, as a teacher, can't have private practice in my teaching office. But I can have private practice later, after my work. That means I want to get home as early as possible. Now, I do not have a practice, but most of my assistants do.

Students in Poland must pay for taking courses in the United States and other countries. But in my country we pay the students. And if students do not have to go to classes they are very happy. They are not interested in gaining more knowledge because there is no examination for the whole country, like in the United States, and also there is no competition. So the quality of work does not matter. It is nothing.

For example, if from my students somebody says: "You know you will have a course for implantation." They say: "Oh, we are very busy; we have a sport match," or "We want to watch television." In the United States they ask: "Will you pay me for attending? — No. — Oh well, we will go anyway. Because even without payment we learn something more."

And other problems: for example, we have only 15% males in dentistry. In the United States this is completely different. We have other problems: for example, patients don't pay for dentures or for drugs. This leads to them take advantage of the system and they demand 10, sometimes 20, dentures. Because if they don't have to pay they don't want to put up with some difficulties in the beginning. It is the same with prescription drugs. You can find a lot of prescription drugs in homes which are not used at all.

Also, in dentistry there is no relationship between quality and quantity of work. So we have noticed that the best medicine and dentistry is in countries where the social administration system is decided by society. In our country the Minister of Health was the man who decided. And, of course, there is centralization — the system where one person in the Ministry of Health decides everything. It is not good. There is no feedback between the needs of society, treatment, and organization.

So as a representative of the Polish Dental Association I am very glad to be here. We should do more for a new way of Polish dentistry. For example, if the child of a mother who works goes to a preschool, it costs society three times more than it would to pay this worker; it would be easier and less costly to give the money to the mother to stay at home.

But you see if the political system governs too much it is not good. For example, in the United States dental health care is essentially private. In Poland there is only the Government Health Service. This is not a good idea. We should have competition between private practice and governmental practice.

The government pays less than 5% of the fees for health service. This is not sufficient to have good dentistry. So people who want to find good dentistry with good materials and with good equipment are willing to pay private fees. It is not true that dentistry in Poland does not cost society, because society pays, in the form of flowers (which are very expensive), cognacs, vodka, and such things. It means society loses money. But the dentist has no money either — I cannot buy anything with vodka! So I drink it, of course!

But the President of FDI told us that there is not one way for each country and of course this is true. For example, the connection between medicine and dentistry in Poland has been viable for over 40 years — it works quite well and we are not afraid that we will in the future be a branch of medicine.

The title is another problem. The Polish stomatologist is also a dentist. We have the same identical degrees. For example, I am a doctor in medical sciences. And my degree was taken in the Faculty of Medicine.

Simonsen

Thank you. You mentioned that it was a disadvantage that 15% of dentists in Poland are men and the rest are women. I think there are some people here who would see that as a great advantage! How do you see that as a disadvantage?

Josefowicz

I think that it is a disadvantage because a lot of women have children and then they stop work. Also, when their children are young, most of the women are less active in society. Most men are active. So I think that 40% women in dentistry would be quite enough.

Simonsen

We had better leave this subject, I think!

Josefowicz

Let me just say that dentists in Poland were, and are still, paid at a very low salary, less than other workers. Workers sometimes have two times higher salary than dentists in official practice, that is, governmental workers. So men prefer to be technicians or other disciplines which are paid better. But now, because private practice is better, we have a lot of good candidates and also the number of men is higher. It is simply an economical problem.

Simonsen

Thank you. I'd like to get to one topic; maybe this will have to be the last topic — overtreatment. In these days of limited resources it seems tragic that there is overtreatment going on. Dr Ivar Mjör, unfortunately, had to leave before our discussion, and I know he would have been very vocal this afternoon, particularly on this topic where he is very knowledgeable and outspoken — I am therefore sorry that he had to leave. He left a note as a point of discussion: his question is, "Has the time come when a dentist should be paid for the fillings he or she does *not* make?" So Dr Mjör is wondering if the time has come to compensate dentists for keeping people healthy rather than treating sick people. Anybody care to comment on this? Yes, Dr Gonzales-Giralda.

Gonzales-Giralda

Thank you, Mr Chairman. May I just by reference refer back to a comment by Professor Jairam Reddy. By the way, Professor Reddy, we come from the same continent — you know my home country is the Canary Islands?

Perhaps you did not understand me, or I did not express myself as well as I should. Dr Löe, by the way, has said that he is in favor that each country will have to find its own model for the provision of dental care. Because I personally believe in the exercise in the practice of dentistry in freedom and in private practice. But we do not have anything at all against any other model. Each country will have to find its own model. This is for sure. I want that to be clarified.

Simonsen

Before you get on to the subject of overtreatment I just want to ask you one question, since you are talking about the FDI and the relationship to the dental associations — does the FDI willingly accept more than one dental association from a country? That is to say, if there is more than one dental association in the country?

Gonzales-Giralda

Yes it does. The only thing is that the application from a national dental association from a country that already has an affiliate member of the FDI has to be done in consultation with the current member association in that particular country.

Simonsen

So if the current association does not want to recognize the alternative organization...?

Discussion

Gonzales-Giralda

Not really, that is not the case. I mean there are countries where we have two associations, like Portugal, for instance. We have the association incorporating the new dentists being trained in that country. So we can have, of course, two associations from the same country.

But going back to overtreatment. If government policy is based on the fact that the more dentists there are in the market the lower the fees will be and that this will actually work in the public's favor — this is a false assumption. In the United States, for instance, in some states, as you know, they have introduced "denturism." Denturism has been lobbied in the Capitol just because it was going to provide lower fees to the population. That has not been the case at all. Once denturism has been legalized in that particular state the denturist will charge as much, if not more, than what dentists charge.

The more dentists you have in a country, of course, the more competition you introduce, and the more overtreatment as well. So governments should really listen to the advice, for instance, of the national dental associations when it comes to cutting down the number of dental schools, reducing the number of those that they have, reducing dental student intake, and so on. Because otherwise the government becomes mainly responsible for overtreatment.

Simonsen

Thank you very much. – George Zarb.

Zarb

I think you have to be very careful about addressing the issue of overtreatment. What do you mean by overtreatment? Because if you talk about overtreatment, then presumably there is such a thing as undertreatment and ideal treatment. I wish we would leave this discussion out.

Simonsen

Who was it who said this morning: a hungry dentist is something? Who was this?

Zarb

A hungry dentist is a dangerous dentist.

Simonsen

Yes – who said that ? Was it Ivar Mjör? I guess we can credit him since he is not here?

Zarb

Yes, it was Ivar [Mjör]. In a profession which is self-regulated and which personifies and manifests the highest in ethics, I think it is inappropriate to be talking about overtreatment. As my colleague said: you talk about ethical therapy or unethical therapy.

Simonsen

Don't you think we have to look at reality?

Zarb

If it is reality, there must be a definition for it. Would somebody like to define what overtreatment is?

Simonsen

Harald Löe?

Löe

I do not want to define overtreatment, but I would like to comment on something that has been called overtreatment in the United States. There is a tremendous interest among some practices in temporomandibular joint problems. And, of course, this is a very specific area of research at the moment with very little hard science going on. We have a hard time getting research activities in this area. And the clinical approach to management of temporomandibular joint problems is open to everyone, almost, and there is a lot of light cavalry, I would say, in this particular area.

That has been called overtreatment — when people do not get the right treatment or perhaps they may not have been in need of treatment. But diagnosis of TMJ problems has been more in the interests of the practitioner than to the benefit of the patient. There is no denying that this is going on at some level of activity.

I think this is typical in areas where there is a weak scientific basis for the subject. And I think that is why it is important to bring science along in all areas to clarify both the relationship of diagnosis to the pathogenesis, and of the diagnosis to the treatment.

So that is one area that is being accused of overtreatment.

Simonsen

I can't get Dr Zarb to say any more. I agree that overtreatment is hard to define but I believe that some public health systems have documented tremendous variations in the type and frequency of treatment in different dental offices with essentially the same type of patient pool. This would indicate that there are some whose criteria for the replacement of an amalgam, for example, is far more lenient than others. Some would say that those who replace an amalgam at the slightest sign of a marginal defect, or who restore teeth on the suspicion of incipient caries, all in the name of

doing what they believe to be the best for their patients, are guilty of overtreatment. It's too bad Ivar [Mjör] is not here to give us his wisdom on this issue.
Dr Braun.

Braun

I think we have got another very important factor. The factor of research was mentioned as a most important one. But a very similar important one is, of course, our closer cooperation with the dental industry and the dental trade. Because our coming together here in Berlin and this magnificent symposium should have been done, actually, by the FDI. But the FDI is not able to combine, perhaps, such a really important scientific meeting.

Simonsen

Dr Dugoni.

Dugoni

I would like to comment in the area because I think, for instance, Mr Haase's program is an example of industry and the dental profession working together to provide education. So often that's not done. Industry in my opinion is product oriented. They advertise with multimillions of dollars for products. If they'd used more dollars for health education, for dental education, to educate the public — in my opinion they would get an even bigger market share. They get a greater share of the marketplace as the profession gets busier and the public takes advantage of more care.

I believe that we have to get that message out to industry to do more with the profession. There is certainly a large segment of industry that does participate. For instance, in the United States, Procter and Gamble accepted the challenge of the American Dental Association to have a major program to educate the public on the importance of periodontal health. And I think that is a meaningful program to date. They probably put 5 to 6 million dollars into that program.

I think additional programs must be done whether it be continued education of a dentist, which Ray White talked about earlier, or the public. The public is demanding such sophisticated care in some instances that only segments of the profession are able to deliver. And I think that aspect is important: education of the profession. But equally important is education of the public. The dental trade needs to have a closer alliance with the profession. The profession has a concern, I think, about being seen to be in bed with industry. But in the 21st century there has to be a marriage between industry and the profession, in the best interests of the public.

Simonsen

Mr Haase would like to say something.

Haase

Please allow me to point out one thing. You know, Dr Dugoni, you mentioned that industry has to work closer together with your profession and I really want you to understand that I do not regard a publisher as "industry." Publishing companies should, in my opinion, be primarily regarded as communicators. We build bridges and we deliver information. And, please forgive me, we are really not an industry. Sometimes I wish I had a product that goes on and on and on.

Simonsen

Thank you. – Dr Mmembe.

Mmembe

I just wish to endorse very heartily what Dr Dugoni has said about the relationship between the profession and industry, by giving an example of what has happened in Zambia.

Zambia has been successful in dental health education purely through the assistance of the dental industry in the country. Particularly that of Colgate-Palmolive. They have continued to support our efforts. There is no way we would have been able to reach the people to the extent we have in the country without the assistance of the dental industry. And it is not only the people who are benefiting from this sort of assistance, but also the company itself. In one instance we went to a rural area and the children at that school decided to put on an entertainment show. They were busy singing songs of praise for Colgate-Palmolive which showed that the advertising campaign is also percolating through to segments of the population where they did not think it was reaching.

But they have also not only confined themselves to improving dentistry through education. They have also provided assistance to the government. This year they gave the government access to one million kwacha which in dollars does not amount to much, but in kwacha it certainly is a lot of money. And this was purely to try to help the government to improve the country.

This is, I believe, an important area for the profession to address itself. We really should promote the idea that we are working together towards achieving the goal of improved dentistry.

Simonsen

I am delighted to hear this discussion about industry and the beneficial effects of close cooperation between industry and governments and dental organizations. But, regrettably, I think I must bring our session to a close.

The words or the themes that remain with me after our discussions today are:

1. *Research:* the need for basic research as the foundation for future progress.

2. *Prevention:* the need for aggressive preventive efforts, particularly in the developing nations as they emerge into the 21st century.
3. *Working together:* industry and the profession combining their resources for the benefit of society. As Dr Dugoni put it so well, "A marriage between industry and the profession, in the best interests of the public."

Also, I think there has been general agreement that *different countries require different health care systems.* What is good, for example, for the United States may not be the answer in South Africa, Zambia, or the Soviet Union.

And I am left with an inner appeal, an inner feeling, that we all need to do whatever we can to help our brothers and sisters of the world in the less fortunate countries than we happen to be born in — help them to provide the kind of health and dental care that we are so fortunate to be a part of. Because it certainly is very clear from this meeting that there are millions and millions of people around the world who are not fortunate enough to get even the most basic medical or dental care — the kind of care that we take for granted.

This meeting came about from an idea that Mr Haase gave to me at a meeting in London. Those of you who know Mr Haase know that he is very good at planting seeds. We were sitting in a hotel in London and he said: "You know I want to have this meeting. I want to bring the people together from 25 or more countries of the world to celebrate the 40-year anniversary of the International Quintessence Publishing Group and the 20-year anniversary of *Quintessence International.*" So we walked around a little and pulled out your names. From that meeting, of about 2 years ago I think, we have come together and had a most productive and fruitful day together.

It has been a long day but a good day. You have all done a tremendous job, particularly those of you whose language is not English. I am in great admiration of all of your splendid presentations today. You did an excellent job.

Perhaps Mr Haase would like to say the last few words. Thank you all.

Haase

This is not another speech. But I really admire all of you for your discipline, for your preparation for this meeting. And I don't know how to thank you but to give you all my greatest respect for coming and for spending so much time giving us such as wonderful symposium. Thank you.

And I would like to thank Dr Simonsen for preparing everything in detail so well and for keeping all of us in good order over the past 12 hours, or maybe more, of this meeting.

This symposium has been a great example to the world of dentistry. We have shown that it can be done — that so many different kinds of people can discuss topics of mutual interest, although from very different backgrounds, for 12 hours together without losing discipline. My greatest respect to you all.

Thank you very much!